Personalized Nursing and Health Care

Personalized Nursing and Health Care

Editors

Riitta Suhonen
Minna Stolt
David Edvardsson

MDPI • Basel • Beijing • Wuhan • Barcelona • Belgrade • Manchester • Tokyo • Cluj • Tianjin

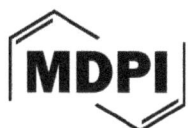

Editors

Riitta Suhonen
Department of Nursing Science
University of Turku
Turku
Finland

Minna Stolt
Department of Nursing Science
University of Turku
Turku
Finland

David Edvardsson
School of Nursing & Midwifery
La Trobe University
Melbourne
Australia

Editorial Office
MDPI
St. Alban-Anlage 66
4052 Basel, Switzerland

This is a reprint of articles from the Special Issue published online in the open access journal *Journal of Personalized Medicine* (ISSN 2075-4426) (available at: www.mdpi.com/journal/jpm/special_issues/personalized_nursing).

For citation purposes, cite each article independently as indicated on the article page online and as indicated below:

LastName, A.A.; LastName, B.B.; LastName, C.C. Article Title. *Journal Name* **Year**, *Volume Number*, Page Range.

ISBN 978-3-0365-7459-2 (Hbk)
ISBN 978-3-0365-7458-5 (PDF)

© 2023 by the authors. Articles in this book are Open Access and distributed under the Creative Commons Attribution (CC BY) license, which allows users to download, copy and build upon published articles, as long as the author and publisher are properly credited, which ensures maximum dissemination and a wider impact of our publications.

The book as a whole is distributed by MDPI under the terms and conditions of the Creative Commons license CC BY-NC-ND.

Contents

About the Editors ix

Riitta Suhonen, Minna Stolt and David Edvardsson
Personalized Nursing and Health Care: Advancing Positive Patient Outcomes in Complex and Multilevel Care Environments
Reprinted from: *J. Pers. Med.* **2022**, *12*, 1801, doi:10.3390/jpm12111801 1

Jenni Sipilä, Anne-Marie Mäkelä, Sasu Hyytiä and Minna Stolt
How to Measure Foot Self-Care? A Methodological Review of Instruments
Reprinted from: *J. Pers. Med.* **2023**, *13*, 434, doi:10.3390/jpm13030434 5

María Torres-Lacomba, Beatriz Navarro-Brazález, María José Yuste-Sánchez, Beatriz Sánchez-Sánchez, Virginia Prieto-Gómez and Fernando Vergara-Pérez
Women's Experiences with Compliance with Pelvic Floor Home Exercise Therapy and Lifestyle Changes for Pelvic Organ Prolapse Symptoms: A Qualitative Study
Reprinted from: *J. Pers. Med.* **2022**, *12*, 498, doi:10.3390/jpm12030498 23

Simon Kocbek, Primož Kocbek, Lucija Gosak, Nino Fijačko and Gregor Štiglic
Extracting New Temporal Features to Improve the Interpretability of Undiagnosed Type 2 Diabetes Mellitus Prediction Models
Reprinted from: *J. Pers. Med.* **2022**, *12*, 368, doi:10.3390/jpm12030368 39

Beatriz Navarro-Brazález, Fernando Vergara-Pérez, Virginia Prieto-Gómez, Beatriz Sánchez-Sánchez, María José Yuste-Sánchez and María Torres-Lacomba
What Influences Women to Adhere to Pelvic Floor Exercises after Physiotherapy Treatment? A Qualitative Study for Individualized Pelvic Health Care
Reprinted from: *J. Pers. Med.* **2021**, *11*, 1368, doi:10.3390/jpm11121368 49

Ana Ramos, César Fonseca, Lara Pinho, Manuel Lopes, Henrique Oliveira and Adriana Henriques
Functional Profile of Older Adults Hospitalized in Convalescence Units of the National Network of Integrated Continuous Care of Portugal: A Longitudinal Study
Reprinted from: *J. Pers. Med.* **2021**, *11*, 1350, doi:10.3390/jpm11121350 61

Tosin Popoola, Joan Skinner and Martin Woods
Exploring the Social Networks of Women Bereaved by Stillbirth: A Descriptive Qualitative Study
Reprinted from: *J. Pers. Med.* **2021**, *11*, 1056, doi:10.3390/jpm11111056 73

Fernanda Loureiro, Luís Sousa and Vanessa Antunes
Use of Digital Educational Technologies among Nursing Students and Teachers: An Exploratory Study
Reprinted from: *J. Pers. Med.* **2021**, *11*, 1010, doi:10.3390/jpm11101010 85

Marco Clari, Michela Luciani, Alessio Conti, Veronica Sciannameo, Paola Berchialla and Paola Di Giulio et al.
The Impact of the COVID-19 Pandemic on Nursing Care: A Cross-Sectional Survey-Based Study
Reprinted from: *J. Pers. Med.* **2021**, *11*, 945, doi:10.3390/jpm11100945 99

Elena Mejías-Gil, Elisa María Garrido-Ardila, Jesús Montanero-Fernández, María Jiménez-Palomares, Juan Rodríguez-Mansilla and María Victoria González López-Arza
Kinesio Taping vs. Auricular Acupressure for the Personalised Treatment of Primary Dysmenorrhoea: A Pilot Randomized Controlled Trial
Reprinted from: J. Pers. Med. **2021**, 11, 809, doi:10.3390/jpm11080809 111

Cheryl Lin, Rungting Tu, Brooke Bier and Pikuei Tu
Uncovering the Imprints of Chronic Disease on Patients' Lives and Self-Perceptions
Reprinted from: J. Pers. Med. **2021**, 11, 807, doi:10.3390/jpm11080807 123

Marlena van Munster, Johanne Stümpel, Franziska Thieken, David J. Pedrosa, Angelo Antonini and Diane Côté et al.
Moving towards Integrated and Personalized Care in Parkinson's Disease: A Framework Proposal for Training Parkinson Nurses
Reprinted from: J. Pers. Med. **2021**, 11, 623, doi:10.3390/jpm11070623 135

Birute Bartkeviciute, Vita Lesauskaite and Olga Riklikiene
Individualized Health Care for Older Diabetes Patients from the Perspective of Health Professionals and Service Consumers
Reprinted from: J. Pers. Med. **2021**, 11, 608, doi:10.3390/jpm11070608 151

Riitta Suhonen, Katja Lahtinen, Minna Stolt, Miko Pasanen and Terhi Lemetti
Validation of the Patient-Centred Care Competency Scale Instrument for Finnish Nurses
Reprinted from: J. Pers. Med. **2021**, 11, 583, doi:10.3390/jpm11060583 165

Júlio Belo Fernandes, Sónia Belo Fernandes, Ana Silva Almeida, Diana Alves Vareta and Carol A. Miller
Older Adults' Perceived Barriers to Participation in a Falls Prevention Strategy
Reprinted from: J. Pers. Med. **2021**, 11, 450, doi:10.3390/jpm11060450 177

Guido Edoardo D'Aniello, Davide Maria Cammisuli, Alice Cattaneo, Gian Mauro Manzoni, Enrico Molinari and Gianluca Castelnuovo
Effect of a Music Therapy Intervention Using Gerdner and Colleagues' Protocol for Caregivers and Elderly Patients with Dementia: A Single-Blind Randomized Controlled Study
Reprinted from: J. Pers. Med. **2021**, 11, 455, doi:10.3390/jpm11060455 187

Shirin Vellani, Veronique Boscart, Astrid Escrig-Pinol, Alexia Cumal, Alexandra Krassikova and Souraya Sidani et al.
Complexity of Nurse Practitioners' Role in Facilitating a Dignified Death for Long-Term Care Home Residents during the COVID-19 Pandemic
Reprinted from: J. Pers. Med. **2021**, 11, 433, doi:10.3390/jpm11050433 197

Shuyu Han, Yaolin Pei, Lina Wang, Yan Hu, Xiang Qi and Rui Zhao et al.
The Development of a Personalized Symptom Management Mobile Health Application for Persons Living with HIV in China
Reprinted from: J. Pers. Med. **2021**, 11, 346, doi:10.3390/jpm11050346 213

Ewa Kupcewicz, Elżbieta Grochans, Helena Kadučáková, Marzena Mikla, Aleksandra Bentkowska and Adam Kupcewicz et al.
Personalized Healthcare: The Importance of Patients' Rights in Clinical Practice from the Perspective of Nursing Students in Poland, Spain and Slovakia—A Cross-Sectional Study
Reprinted from: J. Pers. Med. **2021**, 11, 191, doi:10.3390/jpm11030191 225

David Ramiro-Cortijo, Maria de la Calle, Vanesa Benitez, Andrea Gila-Diaz, Bernardo Moreno-Jiménez and Silvia M. Arribas et al.
Maternal Psychological and Biological Factors Associated to Gestational Complications
Reprinted from: *J. Pers. Med.* **2021**, *11*, 183, doi:10.3390/jpm11030183 . . . . **239**

About the Editors

Riitta Suhonen

Ph.D., RN Riitta Suhonen is Professor in Nursing Science and has a speciality Gerontological Nursing Science since 2011. RS is the Director of the Doctoral Programme in Nursing Science (DPNurs). She is the fellow (FEANS) of the European Academy of Nursing Science (board and scientific committee member) and Member of the Academia Europaea. RS has a part-time position of Nursing Director in the Turku University Hospital and City of Turku, Welfare Services Division since 2016. RS has worked in the Department of Nursing Science since 2008 and formerly as a quality and development manager in health care district understanding of the healthcare systems, nurse leader and registered nurse. She has served as the former associate editor of the Nursing Open (Wiley) and Nursing Ethics (Sage).

Minna Stolt

My research, function and health, from foot to head, focuses on health from functional perspective. I am interested in evaluating patients' functional health, quality of care, and rehabilitation in different levels of health care; patients' own strategies to care for and promote their own functional health; and to evaluate the competence of health care professionals to provide care and rehabilitation. The basis for this research lies in foot healh research in different age groups and contexts. My research area belongs to research strategy in the Department of Nursing Science in the Clinical Quality research program.

My Ph.D. study (2013) focused on foot health in older people and I developed the Foot Health Assessment Instrument to be used in clinical nursing care. My post doctoral study concentrated on occupational health care, namely in foot health in nurses. My current research deals with functional health and rehabilitation in patients with long-term conditions, such as rheumatoid arthritis.

David Edvardsson

Professor Edvardsson is a recognized international authority in research across care sciences, health promotion and population health, and ageing and dementia. His ongoing scientific research is focused across five themes, health-promotion, care and support for older people; global and population health, ill-health, and burden of disease; developing positive health outcome measures and health-promoting interventions; person-centred care, health and quality of life; and health-promoting environments.

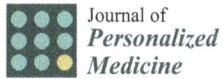

Editorial

Personalized Nursing and Health Care: Advancing Positive Patient Outcomes in Complex and Multilevel Care Environments

Riitta Suhonen [1,2,*], Minna Stolt [1] and David Edvardsson [3]

1. Department of Nursing Science, University of Turku, 20014 Turku, Finland
2. Welfare Services Division, Turku University Hospital, 20014 Turku, Finland
3. School of Nursing & Midwifery, La Trobe University, Melbourne, VIC 3086, Australia
* Correspondence: riisuh@utu.fi

This Special Issue of the *Journal of Personalised Medicine* invited manuscripts that further establish the current state of science relating to personalized nursing and health care. We welcomed manuscripts that highlight and further the knowledge base conceptually, instrumentally, observationally and experimentally, with sound theoretical and methodological underpinnings and implications for research, theory and clinical work in the disciplines of nursing, medicine, allied health and beyond. As there has been a rapid development in the academic literature over the last ten years in terms of papers relating to individualization, personalization, patient-, client-, consumer- and person-centredness, with work on conceptual, instrumental, observational and experimental levels, this theme seemed timely and relevant [1,2].

The individuality of care and services is essential for the realisation of healthcare quality, ethical obligations and the development of a deeper understanding of user perspectives necessary for health care, health policy development and increasing patient choice [3]. Healthcare systems in countries should be based on the comprehensive need assessment of individual clients [4,5] and patients to provide individualised, personalised or tailored care [6]. Personalized medical care should not only improve the patient's situation by providing the right diagnosis, prevention or treatment; it also needs to be tailored according to individual characteristics, situation, context, and environment to support people's health power, health careers and thus, their self-management and independent living [7,8]. This is highly important as health care systems have taken responsibility for care that also warrants the increasing responsibility of people's own self-management [9,10]. In order to support self-care, an individualised assessment of care needs is needed; furthermore, individual client's and patient's active participation in determining care and co-designing services is necessary [11]. Self-care is of vital importance for sustainable healthcare; however, it is not sufficiently emphasised. Knowing the clients and patients, assessing their individual needs and responding to these needs in an individualised manner has been found effective, and even cost-effective. Such initiative requires individualised or tailored interventions that are effective in care delivery. However, the complex multilevel interplay between care and service networks for patients, especially for older people, is rarely studied.

Individualised treatment and nursing care is an activity carried out by professionals and provides the perception of personalised care; it can act as an indicator of person-centeredness, requiring person-centred behaviour and other forms of competence [12,13]. Such care does not appear in and of itself, and health professionals need to support new-comers to in providing individualised or person-centred care for citizens [14]. Individualised care and patient-centeredness can be seen as a process or specific set of nursing or other care activities which produce positive patient outcomes [15]. However, there is a need to change the shift from system and professional-centred activities to patient-centeredness and orientation to build usable and effective care options for different groups

Citation: Suhonen, R.; Stolt, M.; Edvardsson, D. Personalized Nursing and Health Care: Advancing Positive Patient Outcomes in Complex and Multilevel Care Environments. *J. Pers. Med.* 2022, 12, 1801. https://doi.org/10.3390/jpm12111801

Received: 8 October 2022
Accepted: 17 October 2022
Published: 1 November 2022

Publisher's Note: MDPI stays neutral with regard to jurisdictional claims in published maps and institutional affiliations.

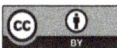

Copyright: © 2022 by the authors. Licensee MDPI, Basel, Switzerland. This article is an open access article distributed under the terms and conditions of the Creative Commons Attribution (CC BY) license (https://creativecommons.org/licenses/by/4.0/).

of people, including individualised environments that support self-management and independence [16,17]. However, health system reforms have not necessarily taken into account the processes from the client's point of view and there is also a lack of studies focusing on the care environment of older people. There is also a need to increase the multidisciplinarity of care assessment, planning, delivery and evaluation, where different professions and disciplines work with the person at the centre of care and treatment; there has never been a better time to do this than now due to developments in precision medicine, personalized treatment and care, digitalisation [18] and consumer/community participation. All these contemporary trends and support systems can facilitate increased agency on behalf of patients/persons in need of care and can facilitate the health literacy and agency needed to individualise care directed by the person with health needs [19]. However, some further developments are needed to improve the 'individual/person literacy' on behalf of health care professionals and how this information is collected, shared and implemented in care decisions [20]. Standards and structures can also restrict the sharing of agency, power, expertise and accountability of healthcare decisions and actions, particularly in the specialized healthcare space. However, as this Special issue demonstrates, there are rapid developments in the space of personalised medicine and care, which indicate a promising future ahead.

We hope to provide an interesting and comprehensive reading experience with this Special issue. We thank all the authors and editorial office professionals for their contributions to this Special Issue; we also thank the journal and publication platform for providing us with the opportunity to collect multi-disciplinary work covering various important approaches. This Special Issue highlights the scientific advancements in the field as well as meaningful results that can be used to advance healthcare systems.

Author Contributions: Conceptualization R.S., M.S. and D.E.; Writing—original draft preparation, R.S.; Writing—review and editing, M.S. and D.E. All authors have read and agreed to the published version of the manuscript.

Funding: This research received no external funding.

Institutional Review Board Statement: Not applicable.

Informed Consent Statement: Not applicable.

Data Availability Statement: Not applicable.

Conflicts of Interest: The authors declare no conflict of interest.

References

1. Byrne, A.L.; Baldwin, A.; Harvey, C. Whose centre is it anyway? Defining person-centred care in nursing: An integrative review. *PLoS ONE* **2020**, *15*, e0229923. [CrossRef] [PubMed]
2. Sillner, A.Y.; Madrigal, C.; Behrens, L. Person-Centered Gerontological Nursing: An Overview Across Care Settings. *J. Gerontol. Nurs.* **2021**, *47*, 7–12. [CrossRef] [PubMed]
3. Vellani, S.; Boscart, V.; Escrig-Pinol, A.; Cumal, A.; Krassikova, A.; Sidani, S.; Zheng, N.; Yeung, L.; McGilton, K.S. Complexity of Nurse Practitioners' Role in Facilitating a Dignified Death for Long-Term Care Home Residents during the COVID-19 Pandemic. *J. Pers. Med.* **2021**, *11*, 433. [CrossRef] [PubMed]
4. Han, S.; Pei, Y.; Wang, L.; Hu, Y.; Qi, X.; Zhao, R.; Zhang, L.; Sun, W.; Zhu, Z.; Wu, B. The Development of a Personalized Symptom Management Mobile Health Application for Persons Living with HIV in China. *J. Pers. Med.* **2021**, *11*, 346. [CrossRef] [PubMed]
5. Suhonen, R.; Lahtinen, K.; Stolt, M.; Pasanen, M.; Lemetti, T. Validation of the Patient-Centred Care Competency Scale Instrument for Finnish Nurses. *J. Pers. Med.* **2021**, *11*, 583. [CrossRef] [PubMed]
6. Lin, C.; Tu, R.; Bier, B.; Tu, P. Uncovering the Imprints of Chronic Disease on Patients' Lives and Self-Perceptions. *J. Pers. Med.* **2021**, *11*, 807. [CrossRef] [PubMed]
7. Bartkeviciute, B.; Lesauskaite, V.; Riklikiene, O. Individualized Health Care for Older Diabetes Patients from the Perspective of Health Professionals and Service Consumers. *J. Pers. Med.* **2021**, *11*, 608. [CrossRef] [PubMed]
8. Kocbek, S.; Kocbek, P.; Gosak, L.; Fijačko, N.; Štiglic, G. Extracting New Temporal Features to Improve the Interpretability of Undiagnosed Type 2 Diabetes Mellitus Prediction Models. *J. Pers. Med.* **2022**, *12*, 368. [CrossRef] [PubMed]

9. Navarro-Brazález, B.; Vergara-Pérez, F.; Prieto-Gómez, V.; Sánchez-Sánchez, B.; Yuste-Sánchez, M.J.; Torres-Lacomba, M. What Influences Women to Adhere to Pelvic Floor Exercises after Physiotherapy Treatment? A Qualitative Study for Individualized Pelvic Health Care. *J. Pers. Med.* **2021**, *11*, 1368. [CrossRef] [PubMed]
10. Popoola, T.; Skinner, J.; Woods, M. Exploring the Social Networks of Women Bereaved by Stillbirth: A Descriptive Qualitative Study. *J. Pers. Med.* **2021**, *11*, 1056. [CrossRef] [PubMed]
11. Fernandes, J.B.; Fernandes, S.B.; Almeida, A.S.; Vareta, D.A.; Miller, C.A. Older Adults' Perceived Barriers to Participation in a Falls Prevention Strategy. *J. Pers. Med.* **2021**, *11*, 450. [CrossRef] [PubMed]
12. van Munster, M.; Stümpel, J.; Thieken, F.; Pedrosa, D.J.; Antonini, A.; Côté, D.; Fabbri, M.; Ferreira, J.J.; Růžička, E.; Grimes, D.; et al. Moving towards Integrated and Personalized Care in Parkinson's Disease: A Framework Proposal for Training Parkinson Nurses. *J. Pers. Med.* **2021**, *11*, 623. [CrossRef] [PubMed]
13. Kupcewicz, E.; Grochans, E.; Kaduĉáková, H.; Mikla, M.; Bentkowska, A.; Kupcewicz, A.; Andruszkiewicz, A.; Jóźwik, M. Personalized Healthcare: The Importance of Patients' Rights in Clinical Practice from the Perspective of Nursing Students in Poland, Spain and Slovakia-A Cross-Sectional Study. *J. Pers. Med.* **2021**, *11*, 191. [CrossRef] [PubMed]
14. Clari, M.; Luciani, M.; Conti, A.; Sciannameo, V.; Berchialla, P.; Di Giulio, P.; Campagna, S.; Dimonte, V. The Impact of the COVID-19 Pandemic on Nursing Care: A Cross-Sectional Survey-Based Study. *J. Pers. Med.* **2021**, *11*, 945. [CrossRef] [PubMed]
15. Ramiro-Cortijo, D.; de la Calle, M.; Benitez, V.; Gila-Diaz, A.; Moreno-Jiménez, B.; Arribas, S.M.; Garrosa, E. Maternal Psychological and Biological Factors Associated to Gestational Complications. *J. Pers. Med.* **2021**, *11*, 183. [CrossRef] [PubMed]
16. D'Aniello, G.E.; Cammisuli, D.M.; Cattaneo, A.; Manzoni, G.M.; Molinari, E.; Castelnuovo, G. Effect of a Music Therapy Intervention Using Gerdner and Colleagues' Protocol for Caregivers and Elderly Patients with Dementia: A Single-Blind Randomized Controlled Study. *J. Pers. Med.* **2021**, *11*, 455. [CrossRef] [PubMed]
17. Mejías-Gil, E.; Garrido-Ardila, E.M.; Montanero-Fernández, J.; Jiménez-Palomares, M.; Rodríguez-Mansilla, J.; González López-Arza, M.V. Kinesio Taping vs. Auricular Acupressure for the Personalised Treatment of Primary Dysmenorrhoea: A Pilot Randomized Controlled Trial. *J. Pers. Med.* **2021**, *11*, 809. [CrossRef] [PubMed]
18. Loureiro, F.; Sousa, L.; Antunes, V. Use of Digital Educational Technologies among Nursing Students and Teachers: An Exploratory Study. *J. Pers. Med.* **2021**, *11*, 1010. [CrossRef] [PubMed]
19. Ramos, A.; Fonseca, C.; Pinho, L.; Lopes, M.; Oliveira, H.; Henriques, A. Functional Profile of Older Adults Hospitalized in Convalescence Units of the National Network of Integrated Continuous Care of Portugal: A Longitudinal Study. *J. Pers. Med.* **2021**, *11*, 1350. [CrossRef] [PubMed]
20. Torres-Lacomba, M.; Navarro-Brazález, B.; Yuste-Sánchez, M.J.; Sánchez-Sánchez, B.; Prieto-Gómez, V.; Vergara-Pérez, F. Women's Experiences with Compliance with Pelvic Floor Home Exercise Therapy and Lifestyle Changes for Pelvic Organ Prolapse Symptoms: A Qualitative Study. *J. Pers. Med.* **2022**, *12*, 498. [CrossRef] [PubMed]

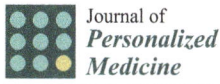

Review

How to Measure Foot Self-Care? A Methodological Review of Instruments

Jenni Sipilä [1], Anne-Marie Mäkelä [2], Sasu Hyytiä [3] and Minna Stolt [1,4,*]

1. Department of Nursing Science, University of Turku, 20520 Turku, Finland
2. Department of Nursing Science, Turku University Hospital, University of Turku, 20520 Turku, Finland
3. Pihlajalinna Pikku Huopalahti, 00300 Helsinki, Finland
4. Department of Nursing Science, University of Eastern, 70211 Kuopio, Finland
* Correspondence: minna.stolt@utu.fi; Tel.: +358-469237973

Abstract: Foot self-care is an important element of caring for and promoting foot health. However, little is known about the validity and reliability of existing foot self-care instruments. The purpose of this review is to describe and analyze the focus, content, and psychometric evidence of existing instruments for measuring foot self-care. A methodological review of three international scientific databases—Medline (PubMed), CINAHL (Ebsco), and Embase—was conducted in May 2022. The search produced 3520 hits, of which 53 studies were included in the final analysis based on a two-phase selection process. A total of 31 instruments were identified, of which six were observed to have been used more than once. Subsequently, the methodological quality of these six instruments was evaluated. It is noted that although a considerable variety of instruments are used in measuring foot self-care, only a small proportion are used consistently. In general, the psychometric testing instruments seem to primarily focus on analyzing content validity and homogeneity. In the future, comprehensive testing of instrument psychometrics could enhance the cumulative evidence of the methodological quality of these instruments. Furthermore, researchers and clinicians can use the information in this review to make informed choices when selecting an instrument for their purposes.

Keywords: foot; foot self-care; instrument; measurement; methodological review

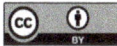

1. Introduction

Foot self-care is an important element of caring for and promoting foot health. Active and proper foot self-care help maintain foot health and prevent foot problems. Notably, foot problems are particularly prevalent in older people [1,2] and people with long-term health problems [3–6], such as diabetes mellitus and rheumatic conditions, thus emphasizing the urgent need for implementing preventive foot self-care. In this context, it is necessary to have valid instruments for evaluating patients' foot self-care. However, a systematic summary of existing foot self-care instruments is lacking in the literature.

Self-care, in general, has become a central component of health care and patients' own resources in terms of caring for, maintaining, and promoting their own health [7]. Foot self-care is a demanding daily task that entails maintaining fine motor skills, general mobility, and upper limb dexterity with sufficient muscle strength [8]. Although a universally agreed-upon definition of foot self-care is lacking, this review defines it as individuals' own activities directed at caring for their own feet, including skin and nail care, foot pain, and use of proper footwear [9]. Foot self-care is important in caring for different foot disorders, such as dry skin, flatfoot, hallux valgus, and metatarsalgia. To conduct foot self-care, it requires competence [10], including personal knowledge, skills, motivation, and physical ability. In this context, proper knowledge relates to evidence and good practice guidelines about foot self-care. Furthermore, skills refer to individuals' abilities to conduct activities, such as skin moisturisation or nail cutting, according to evidence-based guidelines and recommendations. In addition, motivation is also significant for regularly caring for one's feet.

Adherence to foot self-care among people/patients is diverse. Although foot self-care is considered important by patients, it is generally conducted unsystematically [8]. In fact, the importance of preventive foot self-care is often recognized when foot problems have already occurred [11]. Poor or improper foot self-care can, in turn, negatively affect one's foot health status. For example, the foot self-care activities of patients with diabetes who suffer from foot ulcers have been demonstrated to be improper [12,13]. Therefore, a systematic measurement of patients' foot self-care is required to identify potential gaps in their competence.

The evaluation of the validity and reliability of foot self-care instruments is a constant process, as they are used in various contexts and populations. Therefore, cumulative evidence is needed to prove the validity and reliability of a particular instrument. A single study can only provide evidence of the psychometrics in a certain sample and, therefore, cannot be regarded as the only source of evidence. This indicates that robust reporting of the instruments' development process and the results of their psychometric testing are needed to gather relevant evidence of their validity and reliability. Moreover, instruments used as self-reported outcome tools are useful only if there is evidence to support the interpretation of their obtained scores [14]. Therefore, accurate interpretations of reliability and validity considering different settings and samples can be made only when such kinds of necessary information are available. Furthermore, this information aids researchers in understanding the instrument development process, testing, and its results. From a clinical point of view, such information provides an opportunity to use instruments that have been consistently assessed as reliable.

The validity and reliability of foot- and ankle-related instruments have increasingly been under investigation. However, the target of most studies has been the assessment of foot and ankle symptoms and functions rather than foot self-care. For example, recent reviews have prominently focused on patient-reported outcome measures (PROMs) in foot and ankle orthopaedics to reveal variability and deficits in methodological quality and instrumentation [15,16] and highlighted many studies that have used non-validated instruments [17] with limited evidence of their psychometric properties [18]. Similarly, a substantial variability in the measurement properties of instruments assessing foot-related disabilities was identified in the studies focusing on patients with rheumatoid arthritis [19,20]. In contrast, foot- and ankle-related studies conducted on people with diabetes mellitus seemed to maintain a sufficient level of methodological rigour and used valid instruments to measure issues, such as diabetic neuropathy [21]. However, a review focusing on foot self-care instruments still seems to be lacking.

Previous reviews on the impact of foot care education on foot self-care have criticized the heterogeneity of the available assessment tools [22,23]. These instruments focused on measuring changes in knowledge levels, foot care behaviour, and foot health [23]. Moreover, they were developed for the purposes of a single study and measured the technical competence to carry out a certain skill or regularity of desired foot care behaviour rather narrowly [23]. Furthermore, the content areas that the instruments focus on and their validity remain unclear. Furthermore, the lack of validated outcome tools hampers the precision of the instruments' measurements and their ability to measure changes in behaviour, thus revealing flaws in their evaluation of the impact of foot care education.

Poorly conducted foot self-care can increase the risk of foot complications [24] and seriously decrease the level of foot health [25]. Thus, the proper evaluation of foot self-care requires valid and reliable instruments. To address this challenge, a methodological psychometric review of existing foot self-care instruments could promote and facilitate their use in clinical practice and research. Therefore, the purpose of this review is to describe and analyse the focus, content, and psychometric evidence of existing instruments that measure foot self-care. The ultimate goal is to gather and provide information regarding the accurate assessment of foot self-care and the measurement properties of individual instruments.

Therefore, the primary questions that this review seeks to answer are as follows:
(1) What is the focus and content of the instruments that measure foot self-care?
(2) What is the psychometric evidence for these foot self-care instruments?

2. Materials and Methods

2.1. Design

This study was conducted by applying a methodological review design. The reporting process was carried out in accordance with the Preferred Reporting Items for Systematic Reviews and Meta-Analyses (PRISMA) statement [26]. Moreover, a review protocol was planned, but not published, prior to conducting the review.

2.2. Eligibility Criteria

The identified studies were included in the sample for this investigation if they: (1) Were an empirical primary study with a focus on foot self-care; (2) Included an instrument that measures foot self-care (subjective or objective); (3) Provided evidence of psychometric properties of the foot self-care instrument; and (4) Written in English. The exclusion criteria for the studies included (1) Theoretical discussion papers or (2) The use of general self-care instruments.

2.3. Information Sources and Search Strategy

A methodological review was conducted across three international scientific databases (Medline (PubMed), CINAHL (Ebsco), and Embase) in May 2022. The search sentence was ((foot[Title/Abstract]) AND (self[Title/Abstract])) AND (care[Title/Abstract] OR caring[Title/Abstract] OR manage[Title/Abstract] OR management[Title/Abstract] OR efficacy[Title/Abstract]). This search was limited to the title and abstract levels and to studies written in English. Furthermore, no time limit was applied. Moreover, although the review protocol was planned a priori, it was neither published nor registered.

2.4. Selection Process

The process of selecting the relevant studies included screening the records and evaluating their eligibility against the inclusion and exclusion criteria (Figure 1). All duplicate records were excluded in the screening phase. Following this, the titles and abstracts of the studies were inspected by two independent researchers (A-MM, MS). After reaching a consensus, the full texts of the included studies were read and evaluated. After each step, the researchers discussed their selections to ultimately reach a consensus. In cases of disagreement, a third researcher was consulted.

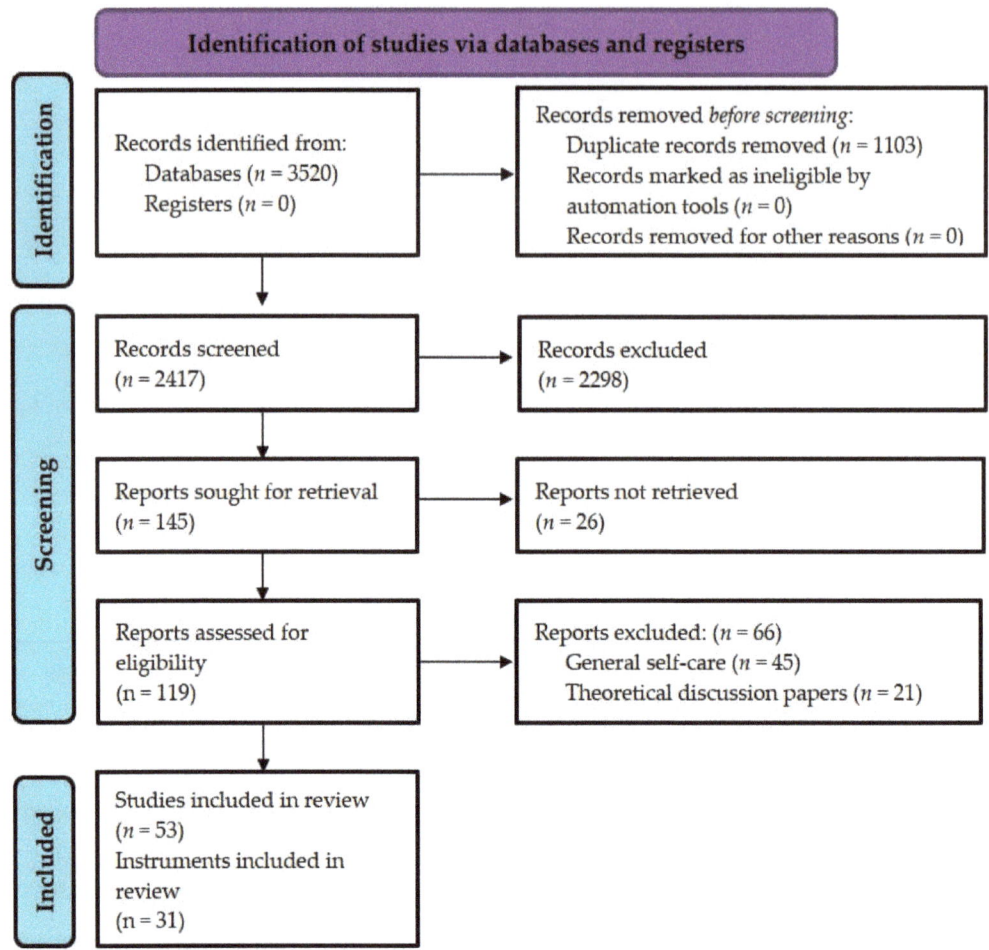

Figure 1. Flowchart of the study selection process.

2.5. Data Collection Process and Data Items

A spreadsheet was developed particularly for the purposes of this review. It included the following information: author, year of publication, country of origin, aim of the study, name of the instrument, measurement focus, number of items, response options, and a list of studies using the particular instrument. While retrieving the data, the study authors' original expressions for the instruments were used without inducing any additional interpretation.

2.6. Quality Appraisal

The Mixed Methods Appraisal Tool (MMAT, version 2018) [27] was used to evaluate the methodological quality of the selected studies. The MMAT consists of seven items: two general and five design-related items. The response to each item was registered in terms of a three-point scale (yes, no, and can't tell).

2.7. Synthesis of Results

The instruments used by patients to measure their performed activities related to foot self-care were first identified from the original articles. After identification, they were listed and classified into groups according to their names. Notably, some of these instruments were used in multiple studies, while the revised versions of some were also reported.

Subsequently, the articles were categorized into studies that (a) Reported original instrument development research; (b) Reported further validation of a certain instrument; and (c) Used instruments without considering any information regarding their validation or psychometric testing. Based on this categorization, instruments that were used in multiple studies were identified, and further analysis was conducted on them.

Descriptive information of each instrument on the item level was gathered to a separate table. Items were grouped based on their characteristics to show which foot self-care content areas were present in these instruments. To have an understanding of item coverage, the number of items describing a certain aspect of foot self-care was summed up.

The psychometric properties of each instrument were analyzed using the framework proposed by Zwakhalen and colleagues [28], which includes 10 items that cover the most crucial aspects of validity and reliability: (1) Known origin of the items; (2) Sufficient sample for testing (number of participants); (3) Analysis of, and justification for, content validity; (4) Level of criterion validity achieved using correlation; (5) Construct validity in relation to other appropriate knowledge tests; (6) Construct validity of differentiation; (7) Homogeneity; (8) Inter-rater reliability (confirmed through observation or noted in activity); (9) Intra-rater or test–retest reliability; and (10) Feasibility. Each item was scored as either 0, 1, or 2 by the two researchers according to the relevant scoring criteria [28]. To gather an overall level of psychometric evidence, the scores were summed up. On summing up the scores, the maximum score stood at 20, with a higher score representing a higher level of the analyzed psychometric property. Originally, these criteria were created to evaluate a pain assessment tool for people with memory disorders [28]. Although the psychometric properties assessed in the original study are universal, the assessment criteria of this study were modified to correspond to foot self-care content. Moreover, the criteria suggested by Zwakhalen and her colleagues [28] have been previously used to assess the psychometric properties of instruments [29]. Notably, this framework was developed based on the methodological literature as a quality judgement criterion for instruments in nursing and health research.

3. Results

3.1. Study Selection

The search produced a total of 3520 hits ($n = 1449$ for Medline and PubMed, $n = 466$ for CINAHL and $n = 1605$ for Embase). After removing duplicates, 2417 hits were included in the study selection phase. Subsequently, 119 studies were selected after screening the titles and abstracts of the studies. Following this, based on the full texts of the selected studies, 53 that met the eligibility criteria were included in the final analysis.

3.2. Study Characteristics

A total of 31 instruments used in 53 studies were identified for further analysis (Supplementary Table S1). These instruments were observed to predominantly measure self-reported foot self-care behaviours or activities. The number of items in the instruments ranged from 4 to 29, while a five-point response scale was primarily used to indicate the frequency of activities related to foot self-care. Out of these 31 instruments, 25 were used only once or were developed for the purpose of a single study. In addition, six instruments were unnamed. Therefore, the analysis of psychometric properties targeted the instruments ($n = 6$) that were used more than once.

3.3. Description of the Analysed Instruments

This section provides a detailed description of the six instruments that were employed in multiple studies considered in the sample selected for this investigation.

The Diabetes Foot Self-care Behavior Scale (DFSBS) [30] measures the frequency of foot self-care behaviour. It entails seven items: checking the bottom of the feet and between toes, washing between toes, drying between toes after washing, applying lotion, inspecting the insides of shoes, and breaking in new shoes. Furthermore, this scale has two parts. Part 1 assesses the number of days that a respondent performs a certain behaviour during a 1-week period using the five-point scale (0 days, 1–2 days, 3–4 days, 5–6 days, 7 days). Meanwhile, Part 2 evaluates the frequency at which a respondent performs a certain foot self-care behaviour (5-point scale from 1 = never to 5 = always). These ratings are summed up to arrive at a score, with higher scores indicating a better performance of foot self-care behaviour [30]. This section may be divided by subheadings. It should provide a concise and precise description of the experimental results, their interpretation, as well as the experimental conclusions that can be drawn.

The Summary of Diabetes Self-Care Activities (SDSCA) [31] is a self-report instrument dealing with diabetes self-management. It covers all the self-care areas related to diabetes: general diet, specific diet, exercise, blood-glucose testing, foot care, and smoking. Since specific parts of this instrument can be used separately, many studies investigated in this review were observed to implement the foot care section of the SDSCA, which consists of five items that help to identify the number of days in a week that a person has performed diabetes foot self-care activities: feet washing, feet soaking, drying between the toes after washing, foot checks, and footwear inspection. The response to each item is registered on a scale from 0 to 7, based on the number of days that the person performed the activity (the higher the mean, the better the care) [31].

The Nottingham Assessment of Functional Footcare (NAFF) [32] is a self-report instrument for assessing the foot care behaviour of people with diabetes. This tool accounts for a total of 29 items to measure the extent to which people comply with recommended foot care behaviours. Response options for this instrument are provided on a four-point scale ranging from "rarely" to "most of the time." The sum of the items' scores is then calculated, with a higher score indicating better foot self-care [32].

The Diabetic Foot Self-Care Questionnaire of the University of Malaga, Spain (DFSQ-UMA) [33] was formulated to evaluate foot self-care among patients with diabetes. It consists of 16 questions that are divided into three domains: personal self-care, podiatric care, and shoes and socks. Each item is scored on a five-point response scale (1 = very inadequate; 5 = very adequate), while some items explore the frequency of a determined self-care activity (1 = never; 5 = always) [33].

The Foot Self-Care Behaviour Questionnaire [34] measures the frequency of performing foot care behaviour based on 17 items divided into two subscales: preventive foot self-care (nine items) and potentially foot-damaging behaviour (eight items). Similarly, two different response scales are used: a six-point scale (i.e., twice a day, daily, every other day, twice a week, once a week, or never) and a four-point scale (i.e., always, most of the time, occasionally, or never). The responses are summed up, wherein a higher score indicates more preventive and potentially damaging behaviours.

The Foot Self-Care Observation Guide (FSCOG) [35] is an objective observation measurement for detecting foot self-exam components. It consists of 16 items divided into three categories: foot care (five items), foot check (three items), and foot safety (eight items). The responses are provided on a five-point scale (1 = never, 2 = occasionally, 3 = sometimes, 4 = frequently, and 5 = always), and then the responses are summarized (range 15–75) with a higher score indicating better foot self-care behaviour.

3.4. Methodological Quality of the Included Studies

The methodological quality of the selected studies, as assessed by the MMAT [27], was found to be acceptable (Supplementary Table S2). However, the main deficit observed in the descriptive quantitative studies was related to non-response bias. Furthermore, the blinding of the assessors was seldom achieved in the randomized controlled trials. For the non-randomized studies, the main shortcoming was recognized as accounting for the confounders of the analysis.

3.5. Focus and Content of the Instruments

The selected instruments were implemented for primarily measuring the frequency of foot self-care (DFSBS [30]; SDSCA [31]; DFSQ-UMA [33], foot self-care activities (DFSQ-UMA [33]) and compliance with recommended foot care (NAFF [32]).

At the item level (Table 1), the focus was predominantly on the selection of the type of footwear (n = 15), followed by questions related to socks (n = 8), footwear assessment (n = 7), foot inspection (n = 7), drying the feet after washing (n = 6), and skin care (n = 6). A few other items that were targeted for evaluation include walking barefoot (n = 4), skin moisturization (n = 4), foot washing (n = 3), nail cutting (n = 3), attitude towards foot self-care (n = 2), and foot soaking (n = 1).

Table 1. Content and number of items in the instruments measuring foot self-care.

Name of Instrument, Reference	Number of Items	Foot Inspection	Foot Wash	Foot Soaking	Drying the Feet	Skin Care	Skin Moisturization	Nail Cutting	Foot Warming	Footwear Assessment	Selection and Type of Footwear	Socks	Walking Barefoot	Attitude toward Foot Self-Care
Diabetes Foot Self-Care Behavior Scale (DFSBS) [30]	7	2	1		1	1				2				
Summary of Diabetes Self e Care Activities (SDSCA) [31]	4	1		1	1					1				
Nottingham Assessment of Functional Footcare (NAFF) [32]	29	1	1		2	3	2	1	4	2	7	4	2	
Diabetic foot self-care questionnaire of the University of Malaga, Spain (DFSQ-UMA) [33]	15	2			2	1		1	1		4	2		2
Foot Self-Care Behaviour (FSCB) questionnaire [34]	17	1	1		2	1	1	2	1	4	2	2		
The Foot Self-Care Observation Guide (FSCOG) [35]	16	3	1	1	3	1	1		2	1	3	1		
number of items/content		10	4	1	7	9	5	4	7	8	16	11	5	2

3.6. Psychometric Evidence of the Instruments

The evidence on the psychometric properties of the instruments varied (Table 2, Supplementary Table S3). First, it should be noted that all the assessed foot self-care instruments were developed based on comprehensive literature reviews. In addition, some authors (NAFF [32] and FSCOG [35]) incorporated foot care recommendations or guidelines to strengthen the theoretical basis of their instruments.

Table 2. Psychometric evidence of six instruments measuring foot self-care, analysed against the criteria proposed by Zwakhalen and colleagues [28].

Instrument	Origin of Items	Number of Participants	Content	Criterion	Validity Construct I: in Relation to Other Tests	Construct II: Differentiates	Homogeneity	Intra-Rater	Reliability Test-Retest	Feasibility	Total Score
Diabetes foot self-care behavior scale (DFSBS)											
Diabetes foot self-care behavior scale (DFSBS) [30]	2	2	2	2	2	2	2	0	0	2	16
Use of DFSBS in Iran [36]	2	2	2	0	0	0	2	0	0	0	8
Use of DFSCBS in Taiwan [37]	2	2	0	0	0	0	2	0	0	0	6
Use of DFSBS in State of Palestine [38]	2	2	2	0	0	0	2	0	2	0	10
Use of DFSBS in Malaysia [39]	2	2	2	0	0	0	0	0	0	0	6
Use of DFSBS in Turkey [40]	2	2	0	0	0	0	1	0	0	0	5
Use of DFSBS in Malaysia [41]	2	2	2	0	0	0	1	0	0	2	9
The Summary of Diabetes Self-Care Activities (SDSCA): foot care											
Use of SDSCA in United States [42]	2	2	0	0	0	0	0	0	0	0	4
Use of SDSCA in Tanzania [12]	2	2	0	0	0	0	0	0	0	0	4
Use of SDSCA in Brazil [43]	0	2	0	0	0	0	0	0	0	0	2
Use of SDSCA in Filippines [44]	2	2	0	0	0	0	0	0	0	0	4

Table 2. Cont.

Instrument	Origin of Items	Number of Participants	Validity				Reliability			Feasibility	Total Score
			Content	Criterion	Construct I: in Relation to Other Tests	Construct II: Differentiates	Homogeneity	Intra-Rater	Test-Retest		
Use of SDSCA in South Africa [45]	2	2	0	0	0	0	0	0	0	2	6
The Diabetes Self-Care Activities Questionnaire (DSQ) [46]	2	2	0	0	0	0	0	0	0	0	4
Nottingham Assessment of Functional Foot-Care questionnaire (NAFF)											
The Nottingham Assessment of Functional Footcare, original study [32]	2	2	0	0	0	2	1	0	2	2	11
The use of NAFF in United Kingdom [47]	2	2	0	0	0	2	1	0	2	0	9
The use of NAFF in United Kingdom [48]	2	2	0	0	0	0	0	0	0	0	4
The use of NAFF in United Kingdom [49]	2	2	2	0	0	0	2	0	0	0	8
Diabetic foot self-care questionnaire of the University of Malaga, Spain (DFSQ-UMA)											
Diabetic foot self-care questionnaire of the University of Malaga, Spain (DFSQ-UMA) [33]	2	2	2	2	2	2	2	0	2	2	18
The use of DFSQ-UMA in Spain [50]	2	2	0	0	0	0	0	0	0	0	4

Table 2. Cont.

Instrument	Origin of Items	Number of Participants	Validity				Reliability			Feasibility	Total Score
			Content	Criterion	Construct I: in Relation to Other Tests	Construct II: Differentiates	Homogeneity	Intra-Rater	Test-Retest		
Foot Self-Care Behaviour (FSCB) questionnaire											
The use of FSCB in Australia [51]	2	2	2	0	0	0	2	0	0	0	8
The use of FSCB in Australia [52]	2	2	0	0	0	0	0	0	0	0	4
The Foot Self-Care Observation Guide											
Original study [35]	2	2	1	0	0	0	1	0	2	2	10
Gökdeniz & Sahin 2020 [53]	2	2	0	0	0	0	2	0	0	0	6

The DFSBS [30] was originally tested comprehensively on a sample of 295 patients with diabetes. Evidence of its content validity, construct validity, differentiation, and internal consistency was also provided. In addition, its feasibility was tested using a pilot test [30]. Over time, the DFSBS has been translated into Arabic [38], Iranian [36], Malay [39,41], and Turkish [40] languages. Moreover, several studies that provide evidence of the instrument's construct validity and internal consistency [36,38–41] have been conducted. However, no evidence of its criterion or construct validity was provided, while its reliability testing focused only on homogeneity. Notably, its feasibility was evaluated by a few studies in pilot testing [30,38,39].

Limited reports could be acquired on the psychometric evidence for the SDSCA [31]. Only one study reported evaluating the feasibility of the instrument through a pilot study [45]. Meanwhile, it was noted that the NAFF [47] was tested for content validity and homogeneity [49].

The DFSQ–UMA [33] was found to be based on a comprehensive literature review followed by careful item operationalization. In addition, extensive testing of its psychometric properties was conducted. The original study thoroughly reported the instrument development process and provided evidence of its validity and reliability in a sample of patients with diabetes [33]. However, its intra-rater reliability was not tested.

The Foot Self-Care Behaviour Questionnaire [34] demonstrated both content validity and homogeneity. Furthermore, the Foot Self-Care Observation Guide [35] reported sufficient evidence of its content validity, internal consistency, test-retest reliability, and feasibility.

3.7. Synthesis of the Results

There are several instruments available for measuring foot self-care, all of which especially focus on foot self-care among people with diabetes. However, among the investigated studies, only six instruments were used more than once, thus providing scattered psychometric evidence. In addition, although the instruments were tested for validity and reliability, the testing process for the different instruments varied, with their predominant focus being on content validity and homogeneity.

4. Discussion

The current study identified six instruments that measure foot self-care, all of which focus primarily on patients with diabetes. Although each instrument had sufficient evidence supporting its usefulness in evaluating foot self-care, they focused mostly on content validity and homogeneity. This indicates the need for systematic and comprehensive psychometric testing of these instruments. In addition, a wealth of instruments used in single studies was found to have limited evidence of their development processes and psychometrics. Moreover, with the increasing volume of tools used for this purpose, duplication and variability were some of the challenges faced in choosing specific instruments among the available ones.

The selected instruments varied in terms of their complexity regarding the items and factors covered. A clear definition of the construct is necessary to search for the most accurate instrument in terms of a given context [54]. In this context, foot self-care is a complex construct that encompasses knowledge (to know what to do and how), skills (how to care for the feet in real life by implementing the correct procedures), and attitude (motivation for carrying out foot self-care). However, since there is currently no standardized definition of foot self-care, the selected instruments were free to measure different kinds of factors related to foot self-care. The main content of the instruments was related to foot inspection, the type of footwear, socks, and the warming of the feet. This is probably because these areas are theoretically relevant and fundamental when it comes to feet care for patients with diabetes. However, in the future, a concept analysis of foot self-care could be beneficial for improving the measurement focus of foot self-care instruments. The NAFF [32] was found to be the most comprehensive instrument covering a wide number of foot self-care activities. Moreover, the target population in the studies was predominantly patients with diabetes. Therefore, constructing an instrument for measuring basic foot self-care activities performed by the general population could be relevant for population-based health promotion programmes.

Although the construct of interest is generally clearly defined when searching for an appropriate instrument, one should be aware of whether development study and psychometric testing of the specific instrument on the target population were performed [54].

In the future, a strong emphasis should be placed on testing construct validity and reliability in terms of an instrument's intra-rater and test-retest (stability) reliability. A particularly significant need is to conduct further psychometric evaluation studies on existing instruments and adapt them accordingly, focusing especially on the psychometric properties that are rarely evaluated, such as reliability, measurement error, and responsiveness [14,16]. From a clinical perspective, more information on the clinical feasibility of the evaluated instruments is necessary. To address this issue, researchers could benefit from planning a detailed testing procedure for their instruments. Since all the elements of validity and reliability are impossible to test in a single study, collecting data from different settings and participants, such as patients under home care or those having long-term health conditions like rheumatoid arthritis, could help cumulate more evidence and, in turn, improve the methodological quality of the instruments. Moreover, researchers should not rely solely on internal consistency as an indicator of reliability [14].

Given the variety of instruments that are currently available, understanding the quality of evidence about an instrument for evaluating its measurement properties is essential to make an informed selection of the most appropriate tool and properly assess foot self-care in the population of interest. The consistent use of instruments that have been assessed as valid and reliable allows for the systematic and credible monitoring and comparison of measured results [16]. This highlights the need for a clear definition of foot self-care to help focus future research accordingly.

Authors should discuss the results and how they can be interpreted from the perspective of previous studies and of the working hypotheses. The findings and their implications should be discussed in the broadest context possible. Future research directions may also be highlighted.

Limitations

The results of this review need to be interpreted while also considering some limitations. First, although the literature search on the selected databases was comprehensive, adding more databases would have provided more hits. In addition, the systematic search conducted across the three databases provided several duplicates, indicating overlapping content. To ensure accurate and comprehensive search terms, pilot searches were conducted, and the search terms were modified and approved by the research team. One researcher (MS) conducted the search, while the study selection was handled by two independent researchers (A-MM, MS). No discrepancies that needed intervention by a third researcher evaluation were encountered. Moreover, data retrieval and analysis were conducted by two researchers (JS, MS) to ensure the transparency of the analysis.

This review was limited to studies published in English. As a result, studies published in other languages that deal with the development of good-quality instruments or the measurement properties of the selected studies were omitted. Therefore, further research can focus on studies conducted in other languages. Moreover, the selected framework developed by Zwakhalen and colleagues [28] represents a general structure for evaluating the psychometric qualities of health measurement scales.

5. Conclusions

Although many instruments were identified as potentially suitable for evaluating foot self-care, deficits in demonstrating adequate measurement properties were recognized across all the domains of reliability and validity. Particularly, the evidence of the instruments' sensitivity to detecting changes in foot self-care is required before they are used as outcome instruments, such as for interventions.

The number of items evaluated in the selected studies ranged from 4 to 29. This supports the need for a concise instrument to minimize patient burden, maximize patient engagement, and ensure the collection of meaningful data [16].

A considerable variety of instruments are used to measure foot self-care, with a small proportion being used consistently. Moreover, substantial variability exists in their level of methodological rigour. Foot self-care instruments are important indicators of patients' competence in promoting and maintaining their foot health. With precise, well-targeted, and sensitive instruments, health care professionals may be able to monitor the progress of their patients' foot self-care and evaluate the impact of educational foot health interventions [14]. In addition, in terms of their clinical utility, foot self-care instruments are important for enhancing patients' engagement, outcome evaluation, and the evaluation of their motivation for carrying out foot health care. Future research should focus on testing the psychometric properties of the instruments as it could provide the benefit of incorporating tests from modern test theory, such as Rasch analysis. Most importantly, researchers and clinicians can take recourse to the information provided in this review to make informed choices when selecting an instrument for their purposes.

Supplementary Materials: The following supporting information can be downloaded at: https://www.mdpi.com/article/10.3390/jpm13030434/s1, Table S1: Descriptive information about the instruments included in the review. Table S2: Methodological quality of included studies (n = 53) using MMAT tool. Table S3: Detailed analysis of psychometric evidence of six instruments measuring foot self-care, analysed against the criteria proposed by Zwakhalen and colleagues [28,30–53,55–84].

Author Contributions: Conceptualization, M.S. and A.-M.M.; methodology, J.S., A.-M.M., S.H. and M.S.; formal analysis, J.S. and M.S.; resources, M.S.; writing—original draft preparation, J.S., A.-M.M., S.H. and M.S..; writing—review and editing, M.S. and S.H.; supervision, M.S.; project administration, M.S.; funding acquisition, M.S. All authors have read and agreed to the published version of the manuscript.

Funding: This research was funded by Turku University Hospital, grant number 13240.

Institutional Review Board Statement: Not applicable.

Data Availability Statement: The data presented in this study are available on request from the corresponding author.

Conflicts of Interest: The authors declare no conflict of interest.

References

1. Muchna, A.; Najafi, B.B.; Wendel, C.S.; Schwenk, M.; Armstrong, D.G.; Mohler, J. Foot problems in older adults associations with incident falls, frailty syndrome, and sensor-derived gait, balance, and physical activity measures. *J. Am. Podiatr. Med. Assoc.* **2018**, *108*, 126–139. [CrossRef] [PubMed]
2. Kunkel, D.; Mamode, L.; Burnett, M.; Pickering, R.; Bader, D.; Donovan-Hall, M.; Cole, M.; Ashburn, A.; Bowen, C. Footwear characteristics and foot problems in community dwelling people with stroke: A cross-sectional observational study. *Disabil. Rehabil.* **2022**, 1–8. [CrossRef] [PubMed]
3. Wilson, O.; Hewlett, S.; Woodburn, J.; Pollock, J.; Kirwan, J. Prevalence, impact and care of foot problems in people with rheumatoid arthritis: Results from a United Kingdom based cross-sectional survey. *J. Foot Ankle Res.* **2017**, *10*, 46. [CrossRef] [PubMed]
4. Simonsen, M.B.; Hørslev-Petersen, K.; Cöster, M.C.; Jensen, C.; Bremander, A. Foot and ankle problems in patients with rheumatoid arthritis in 2019: Still an important issue. *ACR Open Rheumatol.* **2021**, *3*, 396–402. [CrossRef] [PubMed]
5. Tang, U.H.; Zügner, R.; Lisovskaja, V.; Karlsson, J.; Hagberg, K.; Tranberg, R. Foot deformities, function in the lower extremities, and plantar pressure in patients with diabetes at high risk to develop foot ulcers. *Diabet. Foot Ankle* **2015**, *6*, 27593. [CrossRef] [PubMed]
6. Bundó, M.; Vlacho, B.; Llussà, J.; Puig-Treserra, R.; Mata-Cases, M.; Cos, X.; Jude, E.B.; Franch-Nadal, J.; Mauricio, D. Prevalence and risk factors of diabetic foot disease among the people with type 2 diabetes using real-world practice data from Catalonia during 2018. *Front. Endocrinol.* **2022**, *13*, 1024904. [CrossRef]

7. WHO Regional Office for South-East Asia. Self Care for Health. Available online: https://apps.who.int/iris/handle/10665/205887 (accessed on 20 January 2022).
8. Miikkola, M.; Lantta, T.; Suhonen, R.; Stolt, M. Challenges of foot self-care in older people: A qualitative focus-group study. *J. Foot Ankle Res.* **2019**, *12*, 5. [CrossRef]
9. Omote, S.; Watanabe, A.; Hiramatsu, T.; Saito, E.; Yokogawa, M.; Okamoto, R.; Sakakibara, C.; Ichimori, A.; Kyota, K.; Tsukasaki, K. A foot-care program to facilitate self-care by the elderly: A non-randomized intervention study. *BMC Res. Notes* **2017**, *10*, 586. [CrossRef]
10. Cowan, D.T.; Norman, I.; Coopamah, V.P. Competence in nursing practice: A controversial concept—A focused review of literature. *Nurse Educ. Today* **2005**, *25*, 355–362. [CrossRef]
11. Matricciani, L.; Jones, S. Who cares about foot care? Barriers and enablers of foot self-care practices among non-institutionalized older adults diagnosed with diabetes: An integrative review. *Diabetes Educ.* **2015**, *41*, 106–117. [CrossRef]
12. Chiwanga, F.S.; Njelekela, M.A. Diabetic foot: Prevalence, knowledge, and foot self-care practices among diabetic patients in Dar es Salaam, Tanzania—A cross-sectional study. *J. Foot Ankle Res.* **2015**, *8*, 20. [CrossRef] [PubMed]
13. Hirpha, N.; Tatiparthi, R.; Mulugeta, T. Diabetic foot self-care practices among adult diabetic patients: A descriptive cross-sectional study. *Diabetes Metab. Syndr. Obes.* **2020**, *13*, 4779–4786. [CrossRef] [PubMed]
14. Martin, R.L.; Irrgang, J.J. A survey of self-reported outcome instruments for the foot and ankle. *J. Orthop. Sports Phys. Ther.* **2007**, *37*, 72–84. [CrossRef] [PubMed]
15. Sierevelt, I.N.; Zwiers, R.; Schats, W.; Haverkamp, D.; Terwee, C.B.; Nolte, P.A.; Kerkhoffs, G. Measurement properties of the most commonly used Foot- and Ankle-Specific Questionnaires: The FFI, FAOS and FAAM. A systematic review. *Knee Surg. Sports Traumatol. Arthrosc.* **2018**, *26*, 2059–2073. [CrossRef]
16. Lakey, E.; Hunt, K.J. Patient-reported outcomes in foot and ankle orthopedics. *Foot Ankle Orthop.* **2019**, *4*, 2473011419852930. [CrossRef]
17. Hijji, F.Y.; Schneider, A.D.; Pyper, M.; Laughlin, R.T. The popularity of outcome measures used in the foot and ankle literature. *Foot Ankle Spec.* **2020**, *13*, 58–68. [CrossRef]
18. Jia, Y.; Huang, H.; Gagnier, J.J. A systematic review of measurement properties of patient-reported outcome measures for use in patients with foot or ankle diseases. *Qual. Life Res.* **2017**, *26*, 1969–2010. [CrossRef]
19. Van der Leeden, M.; Steultjens, M.P.; Terwee, C.B.; Rosenbaum, D.; Turner, D.; Woodburn, J.; Dekker, J. A systematic review of instruments measuring foot function, foot pain, and foot-related disability in patients with rheumatoid arthritis. *Arthritis Rheumatol.* **2008**, *59*, 1257–1269. [CrossRef]
20. Ortega-Avila, A.B.; Ramos-Petersen, L.; Cervera-Garvi, P.; Nester, C.J.; Morales-Asencio, J.M.; Gijon-Nogueron, G. Systematic review of the psychometric properties of patient-reported outcome measures for rheumatoid arthritis in the foot and ankle. *Clin. Rehabil.* **2019**, *33*, 1788–1799. [CrossRef]
21. Fernández-Torres, R.; Ruiz-Muñoz, M.; Pérez-Panero, A.J.; García-Romero, J.; Gónzalez-Sánchez, M. Instruments of choice for assessment and monitoring diabetic foot: A systematic review. *J. Clin. Med.* **2020**, *9*, 602. [CrossRef]
22. Goodall, R.J.; Ellauzi, J.; Tan, M.; Onida, S.; Davies, A.H.; Shalhoub, J. A systematic review of the impact of foot care education on self efficacy and self care in patients with diabetes. *Eur. J. Vasc. Endovasc. Surg.* **2020**, *60*, 282–292. [CrossRef] [PubMed]
23. Paton, J.; Abey, S.; Hendy, P.; Williams, J.; Collings, R.; Callaghan, L. Behaviour change approaches for individuals with diabetes to improve foot self-management: A scoping review. *J. Foot Ankle Res.* **2021**, *14*, 1. [CrossRef] [PubMed]
24. Srinath, K.M.; Basavegowda, M.; Tharuni, N.S. Diabetic self care practices in rural Mysuru, Southern Karnataka, India—A need for Diabetes Self Management Educational (DSME) program. *Diabetes Metab. Syndr.* **2017**, *11*, S181–S186. [CrossRef] [PubMed]
25. Bonner, T.; Foster, M.; Spears-Lanoix, E. Type 2 Diabetes related foot care knowledge and foot self-care practice interventions in the United States: A systematic review of the literature. *Diabet. Foot Ankle* **2016**, *7*, 29758. [CrossRef]
26. Page, M.J.; McKenzie, J.E.; Bossuyt, P.M.; Boutron, I.; Hoffmann, T.C.; Mulrow, C.D.; Shamseer, L.; Tetzlaff, J.M.; Akl, E.A.; Brennan, S.E.; et al. The PRISMA 2020 statement: An updated guideline for reporting systematic reviews. *BMJ* **2021**, *372*, n71. [CrossRef]
27. Hong, Q.N.; Pluye, P.; Fabregues, S.; Bartlett, G.; Boardman, F.; Cargo, M.; Dagenais, P.; Gagnon, M.-P.; Griffiths, F.; Nicolau, B.; et al. *Mixed Methods Appraisal Tool (MMAT), Version 2018*; Registration of Copyright (#1148552); Canadian Intellectual Property Office: Gatineau, QC, Canada, 2018.
28. Zwakhalen, S.M.; Hamers, J.P.; Abu-Saad, H.H.; Berger, M.P. Pain in elderly people with severe dementia: A systematic review of behavioural pain assessment tools. *BMC Geriatr.* **2006**, *6*, 15. [CrossRef]
29. Kielo, E.; Suhonen, R.; Ylönen, M.; Viljamaa, J.; Wahlroos, N.; Stolt, M. A systematic and psychometric review of tests measuring nurses' wound care knowledge. *Int. Wound J.* **2020**, *17*, 1209–1224. [CrossRef]
30. Chin, Y.F.; Huang, T.T. Development and validation of a diabetes foot self-care behavior scale. *J. Nurs. Res.* **2013**, *21*, 19–25. [CrossRef]
31. Toobert, D.J.; Hampson, S.E.; Glasgow, R.E. The summary of diabetes self-care activities measure: Results from 7 studies and a revised scale. *Diabetes Care* **2000**, *23*, 943–950. [CrossRef]
32. Lincoln, N.B.; Jeffcoate, W.J.; Ince, P.; Smith, M.; Radford, K.A. Validation of a new measure of protective footcare behaviour: The Nottingham Assessment of Functional Footcare (NAFF). *Pract. Diabetes* **2007**, *24*, 207–211. [CrossRef]

33. Navarro-Flores, E.; Morales-Asencio, J.M.; Cervera-Marín, J.A.; Labajos-Manzanares, M.T.; Gijon-Nogueron, G. Development, validation and psychometric analysis of the diabetic foot self-care questionnaire of the University of Malaga, Spain (DFSQ-UMA). *J. Tissue Viability* **2015**, *24*, 24–34. [CrossRef]
34. Vileikyte, L.; Gonzalez, J.S.; Leventhal, H.; Peyrot, M.F.; Rubin, R.R.; Garrow, A.; Ulbrecht, J.S.; Cavanagh, P.R.; Boulton, A.J. Patient Interpretation of Neuropathy (PIN) questionnaire: An instrument for assessment of cognitive and emotional factors associated with foot self-care. *Diabetes Care* **2006**, *29*, 2617–2624. [CrossRef] [PubMed]
35. Borges, W.J.; Ostwald, S.K. Improving foot self-care behaviors with Pies Sanos. *West. J. Nurs. Res.* **2008**, *30*, 325–349. [CrossRef] [PubMed]
36. Bahador, R.S.; Afrazandeh, S.S.; Ghanbarzehi, N.; Ebrahimi, M. The impact of three-month training programme on foot care and self-efficacy of patients with diabetic foot ulcers. *J. Clin. Diagn. Res.* **2017**, *11*, IC01–IC04. [CrossRef] [PubMed]
37. Chin, Y.F.; Liang, J.; Wang, W.S.; Hsu, B.R.; Huang, T.T. The role of foot self-care behavior on developing foot ulcers in diabetic patients with peripheral neuropathy: A prospective study. *Int. J. Nurs. Stud.* **2014**, *51*, 1568–1574. [CrossRef]
38. Salameh, B.S.; Abdallah, J.; Naerat, E.O. Case-control study of risk factors and self-care behaviors of foot ulceration in diabetic patients attending primary healthcare services in Palestine. *J. Diabetes Res.* **2020**, *2020*, 7624267. [CrossRef]
39. Ahmad Sharoni, S.K.; Mohd Razi, M.N.; Abdul Rashid, N.F.; Mahmood, Y.E. Self-efficacy of foot care behaviour of elderly patients with diabetes. *Malays. Fam. Physician* **2017**, *12*, 2–8.
40. Şahin, S.; Cingil, D. Evaluation of the relationship among foot wound risk, foot self-care behaviors, and illness acceptance in patients with type 2 diabetes mellitus. *Prim. Care Diabetes* **2020**, *14*, 469–475. [CrossRef]
41. Ahmad Sharoni, S.; Abdul Rahman, H.; Minhat, H.S.; Shariff Ghazali, S.; Azman Ong, M.H. A self-efficacy education programme on foot self-care behaviour among older patients with diabetes in a public long-term care institution, Malaysia: A quasi-experimental pilot study. *BMJ Open* **2017**, *7*, e014393. [CrossRef]
42. Bell, R.A.; Arcury, T.A.; Snively, B.M.; Smith, S.L.; Stafford, J.M.; Dohanish, R.; Quandt, S.A. Diabetes foot self-care practices in a rural triethnic population. *Diabetes Educ.* **2005**, *31*, 75–83. [CrossRef]
43. Rezende Neta, D.S.; da Silva, A.R.; da Silva, G.R. Adherence to foot self-care in diabetes mellitus patients. *Rev. Bras. Enferm.* **2015**, *68*, 103–116. [PubMed]
44. Jordan, D.N.; Jordan, J.L. Foot self-care practices among Filipino American women with Type 2 Diabetes mellitus. *Diabetes Ther.* **2011**, *2*, 1–8. [CrossRef] [PubMed]
45. Dikeukwu, R.A.; Omole, O.B. Awareness and practices of foot self-care in patients with diabetes at Dr Yusuf Dadoo District Hospital, Johannesburg. *J. Clin. Endocrinol. Metab.* **2013**, *18*, 112–118. [CrossRef]
46. Batista, I.B.; Pascoal, L.M.; Gontijo, P.; Brito, P.; Sousa, M.A.; Santos Neto, M.; Sousa, M.S. Association between knowledge and adherence to foot self-care practices performed by diabetics. *Rev. Bras. Enferm.* **2020**, *73*, e20190430. [CrossRef] [PubMed]
47. Senussi, M.; Lincoln, N.; Jeffcoate, W. Psychometric properties of the Nottingham Assessment of Functional Footcare (NAFF). *Int. J. Ther. Rehabil.* **2011**, *18*, 330–334. [CrossRef]
48. Wendling, S.; Beadle, V. The relationship between self-efficacy and diabetic foot self-care. *J. Clin. Transl. Endocrinol.* **2015**, *2*, 37–41. [CrossRef] [PubMed]
49. Abdelhamid, F.M.; Taha, N.M.; Mohamed, E.H.; El-Khashab, M.N. Effect of self-management support program on improving diabetic foot care behaviors. *Int. J. Pharm. Sci. Rev. Res.* **2018**, *7*, 67–76.
50. González-de la Torre, H.; Quintana-Lorenzo, M.L.; Lorenzo-Navarro, A.; Suárez-Sánchez, J.J.; Berenguer-Pérez, M.; Verdú-Soriano, J. Diabetic foot self-care and concordance of 3 diabetic foot risk stratification systems in a basic health area of Gran Canaria. *Enferm. Clin.* **2020**, *30*, 72–81. [CrossRef]
51. Nguyen, T.; Edwards, H.; Do, T.; Finlayson, K. Effectiveness of a theory-based foot care education program (3STEPFUN) in improving foot self-care behaviours and foot risk factors for ulceration in people with type 2 diabetes. *Diabetes Res. Clin. Pract.* **2019**, *152*, 29–38. [CrossRef]
52. Perrin, B.M.; Swerissen, H.; Payne, C. The association between foot-care self efficacy beliefs and actual foot-care behaviour in people with peripheral neuropathy: A cross-sectional study. *J. Foot Ankle Res.* **2009**, *2*, 3. [CrossRef]
53. Gökdeniz, D.; Akgün Şahin, Z. Evaluation of knowledge levels about diabetes foot care and self-care activities in diabetic individuals. *Int. J. Low. Extrem. Wounds* **2022**, *21*, 65–74. [CrossRef] [PubMed]
54. Terwee, C.B.; Prinsen, C.; Chiarotto, A.; Westerman, M.J.; Patrick, D.L.; Alonso, J.; Bouter, L.M.; de Vet, H.; Mokkink, L.B. COSMIN methodology for evaluating the content validity of patient-reported outcome measures: A Delphi study. *Qual. Life Res.* **2018**, *27*, 1159–1170. [CrossRef] [PubMed]
55. Li, R.; Yuan, L.; Guo, X.-H.; Lou, Q.-Q.; Zhao, F.; Shen, L.; Zhang, M.-X.; Sun, Z.-L. The current status of foot self-care knowledge, behaviours, and analysis of influencing factors in patients with type 2 diabetes mellitus in China. *Int. J. Nurs. Sci.* **2014**, *1*, 266–271. [CrossRef]
56. Al Sayah, F.; Soprovich, A.; Qiu, W.; Edwards, A.L.; Johnson, J.A. Diabetic foot disease, Self-care and clinical monitoring in adults with Type 2 Diabetes: The Alberta's Caring for Diabetes (ABCD) cohort study. *Can. J. Diabetes* **2015**, *39*, S120–S126. [CrossRef] [PubMed]
57. Magbanua, E.; Lim-Alba, R. Knowledge and practice of diabetic foot care in patients with diabetes at Chinese General Hospital and Medical Center. *J. ASEAN Fed. Endocr. Soc.* **2017**, *32*, 123–131. [CrossRef]

58. Kurup, R.; Ansari, A.A.; Singh, J.; Raja, A.V. Wound care knowledge, attitudes and practice among people with and without diabetes presenting with foot ulcers in Guyana. *Diabet. Foot* **2019**, *22*, 24–31.
59. Perrin, B.M.; Swerissen, H.; Payne, C.B.; Skinner, T.C. Cognitive representations of peripheral neuropathy and self-reported foot-care behaviour of people at high risk of diabetes-related foot complications. *Diabet. Med.* **2014**, *31*, 102–106. [CrossRef]
60. Bohorquez Robles, R.; Compeán Ortiz, L.G.; González Quirarte, N.H.; Berry, D.C.; Aguilera Pérez, P.; Piñones Martínez, S. Knowledge and Practices of Diabetes Foot Care and Risk of Developing Foot Ulcers in México May Have Implications for Patients of Méxican Heritage Living in the US. *Diabetes Educ.* **2017**, *43*, 297–303. [CrossRef]
61. Sari, Y.; Upoyo, A.S.; Isworo, A.; Taufik, A.; Sumeru, A.; Anandari, D.; Sutrisna, E. Foot self-care behavior and its predictors in diabetic patients in Indonesia. *BMC Res. Notes* **2020**, *13*, 38. [CrossRef]
62. Schmidt, S.; Mayer, H.; Panfil, E.M. Diabetes foot self-care practices in the German population. *J. Clin. Nurs.* **2008**, *17*, 2920–2926. [CrossRef]
63. Ahmad Sharoni, S.K.; Abdul Rahman, H.; Minhat, H.S.; Shariff-Ghazali, S.; Azman Ong, M.H. The effects of self-efficacy enhancing program on foot self-care behaviour of older adults with diabetes: A randomised controlled trial in elderly care facility, Peninsular Malaysia. *PLoS ONE* **2018**, *13*, e0192417. [CrossRef] [PubMed]
64. Stolt, M.; Suhonen, R.; Puukka, P.; Viitanen, M.; Voutilainen, P.; Leino-Kilpi, H. Foot health and self-care activities of older people in home care. *J. Clin. Nurs.* **2012**, *21*, 3082–3095. [CrossRef]
65. Świątoniowska, N.; Chabowski, M.; Jankowska-Polańska, B. Quality of foot care among patients with diabetes: A study using a Polish version of the diabetes foot disease and foot care questionnaire. *J. Foot Ankle Surg.* **2020**, *59*, 231–238. [CrossRef] [PubMed]
66. Thomas, S.M.; Nitin, I.G.; Reddy, M.U.K.; Devi, S.H. A prospective study: Knowledge assessment and patient care of diabetic foot ulcer patients in tertiary care hospital. *Int. J. Pharm. Pharm. Sci.* **2017**, *9*, 104–110. [CrossRef]
67. Vatankhah, N.; Khamseh, M.E.; Noudeh, Y.J.; Aghili, R.; Baradaran, H.R.; Haeri, N.S. The effectiveness of foot care education on people with Type 2 Diabetes in Tehran, Iran. *Prim. Care Diabetes* **2009**, *3*, 73–77. [CrossRef] [PubMed]
68. Kruger, S.; Guthrie, D. Foot care: Knowledge retention and self-care practices. *Diabetes Educ.* **1992**, *18*, 487–490. [CrossRef] [PubMed]
69. Lael-Monfared, E.; Tehrani, H.; Moghaddam, Z.E.; Ferns, G.A.; Tatari, M.; Jafari, A. Health literacy, knowledge and self-care behaviors to take care of diabetic foot in low-income individuals: Application of extended parallel process model. *Diabetes Metab. Syndr.* **2019**, *13*, 1535–1541. [CrossRef]
70. Corbett, C.F. A randomized pilot study of improving foot care in home health patients with diabetes. *Diabetes Educ.* **2003**, *29*, 273–282. [CrossRef]
71. Fan, L.; Sidani, S.; Cooper-Brathwaite, A.; Metcalfe, K. Improving foot self-care knowledge, self-efficacy, and behaviors in patients with Type 2 Diabetes at low risk for foot ulceration: A pilot study. *Clin. Nurs. Res.* **2014**, *23*, 627–643. [CrossRef]
72. Li, J.; Gu, L.; Guo, Y. An educational intervention on foot self-care behaviour among diabetic retinopathy patients with visual disability and their primary caregivers. *J. Clin. Nurs.* **2019**, *28*, 2506–2516. [CrossRef]
73. Liang, R.; Dai, X.; Zuojie, L.; Zhou, A.; Meijuan, C. Two-year foot care program for minority patients with Type 2 Diabetes Mellitus of Zhuang Tribe in Guangxi, China. *Can. J. Diabetes* **2012**, *36*, 15–18. [CrossRef]
74. Makiling, M.; Smart, H. Patient-centered health education intervention to empower preventive diabetic foot self-care. *Adv. Skin Wound Care* **2020**, *33*, 360–365. [CrossRef] [PubMed]
75. Olson, J.M.; Hogan, M.T.; Pogach, L.M.; Rajan, M.; Raugi, G.J.; Reiber, G.E. Foot care education and self management behaviors in diverse veterans with diabetes. *Patient Prefer. Adherence* **2009**, *3*, 45–50. [CrossRef] [PubMed]
76. Sable-Morita, S.; Arai, Y.; Takanashi, S.; Aimoto, K.; Okura, M.; Tanikawa, T.; Maeda, K.; Tokuda, H.; Arai, H. Development and Testing of the Foot Care Scale for Older Japanese Diabetic Patients. *Int. J. Low. Extrem. Wounds* **2021**, 15347346211045033. [CrossRef] [PubMed]
77. Hanley, G.; Chiou, P.Y.; Liu, C.Y.; Chen, H.M.; Pfeiffer, S. Foot care knowledge, attitudes and practices among patients with diabetic foot and amputation in St. Kitts and Nevis. *Int. Wound J.* **2020**, *17*, 1142–1152. [CrossRef] [PubMed]
78. Ghasemi, Z.; Yousefi, H.; Torabikhah, M. The Effect of Peer Support on Foot Care in Patients with Type 2 Diabetes. *Iran. J. Nurs. Midwifery Res.* **2021**, *26*, 303–309.
79. Rossaneis, M.A.; Haddad, M.; Mathias, T.A.; Marcon, S.S. Differences in foot self-care and lifestyle between men and women with diabetes mellitus. *Rev. Lat. Am. Enfermagem.* **2016**, *24*, e2761. [CrossRef]
80. Bonner, T.; Guidry, J.; Jackson, Z. Association between foot care knowledge and practices among African Americans with Type 2 diabetes: An exploratory pilot study. *J. Natl. Med. Assoc.* **2019**, *111*, 256–261. [CrossRef]
81. Madarshahian, F.; Hassanabadi, M.; Koshniat Nikoo, M. Cognitive status and foot self care practice in overweight diabetics, engaged in different levels of physical activity. *J. Diabetes Metab. Disord.* **2014**, *13*, 31. [CrossRef]
82. Tuha, A.; Getie Faris, A.; Andualem, A.; Ahmed Mohammed, S. Knowledge and practice on diabetic foot self-care and associated factors among diabetic patients at Dessie Referral Hospital, Northeast Ethiopia: Mixed Method. *Diabetes Metab. Syndr. Obes.* **2021**, *14*, 1203–1214. [CrossRef]

83. Qasim, M.; Rashid, M.U.; Islam, H.; Amjad, D.; Ehsan, S.B. Knowledge, attitude, and practice of diabetic patients regarding foot care: Experience from a single tertiary care outpatient clinic. *Foot* **2021**, *49*, 101843. [CrossRef] [PubMed]
84. Ong, J.J.; Azmil, S.S.; Kang, C.S.; Lim, S.F.; Ooi, G.C.; Patel, A.; Mawardi, M. Foot care knowledge and self-care practices among diabetic patients in Penang: A primary care study. *Med. J. Malays.* **2022**, *77*, 224–231.

Disclaimer/Publisher's Note: The statements, opinions and data contained in all publications are solely those of the individual author(s) and contributor(s) and not of MDPI and/or the editor(s). MDPI and/or the editor(s) disclaim responsibility for any injury to people or property resulting from any ideas, methods, instructions or products referred to in the content.

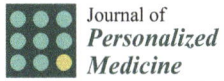

Article

Women's Experiences with Compliance with Pelvic Floor Home Exercise Therapy and Lifestyle Changes for Pelvic Organ Prolapse Symptoms: A Qualitative Study

María Torres-Lacomba, Beatriz Navarro-Brazález *, María José Yuste-Sánchez, Beatriz Sánchez-Sánchez, Virginia Prieto-Gómez and Fernando Vergara-Pérez

Physiotherapy in Women's Health (FPSM) Research Group, Physiotherapy Department, Faculty of Medicine and Health Sciences, University of Alcalá, 28805 Madrid, Spain; maria.torres@uah.es (M.T.-L.); marijo.yuste@uah.es (M.J.Y.-S.); beatriz.sanchez@uah.es (B.S.-S.); v.prieto@uah.es (V.P.-G.); fernando.vergara@uah.es (F.V.-P.)
* Correspondence: b.navarro@uah.es

Abstract: In this study, we aimed to investigate women's experiences with compliance with prescribed pelvic floor muscle exercises (PFMEs) and lifestyle changes 6–12 months after completing an individual pelvic floor physiotherapy program. This study was targeted to understanding factors affecting adherence to PFMEs and lifestyle changes to deal with pelvic organ prolapse (POP) symptoms. We designed this research as a descriptive qualitative study. We conducted this study from December 2016 to September 2017 in Madrid, Spain. Twenty-six women with symptomatic POP selected using a purposive sampling method participated in six focus groups and three one-to-one semi-structured interviews. Three authors coded and inductively analyzed transcript contents with iterative theme development. A thematic analysis revealed three main themes: (1) symptoms change; (2) PFMEs and lifestyle changes performance; and (3) a health practitioner–patient relationship. Women identified as adherent reported improvement in physical symptoms and emotional and general state as a result of the new knowledge achieved. Fear also promoted compliance with performing PFMEs and adopting lifestyle changes. Likewise, PFMEs preference and routine, integration of PFMEs and lifestyle changes into activities of daily living, support guides, therapeutic alliance, individual supervision, follow-up, and feedback were also identified as adherence facilitators. One of the biggest barriers that we identified was responsibility. Compliance with prescribed PFMEs and lifestyle changes can be improved with effective individual, women-centered, and supervised physiotherapy programs reducing symptoms, including exercises aligned with women's preferences that are easy to integrate in daily living, promoting knowledge and awareness of their condition, providing written or electronic guidelines, with routine follow-up visits offering both positive feedback and clear and consistent messages, and enhancing therapeutic alliance.

Keywords: pelvic organ prolapse; pelvic floor muscle exercises; lifestyle changes; therapeutic adherence; women's experience

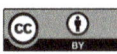

1. Introduction

Pelvic organ prolapse (POP) is a common condition affecting mostly postmenopausal women, with a peak age prevalence at 60–69 years [1,2]. The symptoms significantly impair women's daily activities and quality of life [1,3]. POP involves the descent of one or more perineal organs (uterus, bladder, and/or rectum) from the normal anatomic position into the vagina [4]. Widespread symptoms include feeling vaginal building or pressure in the pelvis, discomfort in the perineum, low back and pelvic pain, which are commonly associated with other urinary, bowel, and sexual symptoms, such as urinary incontinence, fecal incontinence, constipation, and sexual dysfunction that may or may not be related to POP [4–7]. Moreover, women with POP have reduced pelvic floor muscle (PFM) strength and greater PFM dysfunction, with more severe POP and urinary symptoms [8], and there are weaker PFM involuntary contractions during increases in intra-abdominal pressure such as coughing in women with POP stage I and II than in women without POP [9].

POP can be managed by surgery, conservative management (lifestyle advice, PFM training, and vaginal pessaries), or a combination of these [1,7,10,11]. Conservative treatments are often recommended if the POP is mild or surgery is not indicated. Additionally, surgical treatments are commonly associated with increased risk of postoperative complications and POP recurrence [11–13]. According to the latest meta-analysis, pelvic floor muscle exercises (PFMEs) can effectively improve POP symptoms and stage compared to controls [14]. Voluntary PFM contraction may improve support of the pelvic organs as well as their support in the normal anatomic position by contracting PFM before and during any increase in abdominal pressure such as abdominal straining, cough, etc. [14]. PFMEs are more strongly recommended, but their symptom reduction success rates decrease in the medium and long term as adherence to the program deteriorates [15,16]. Although adherence to PFMEs in the short and medium term has been investigated in women with urinary incontinence, women with POP likely also adhere less to PFME programs over time.

To the best of our knowledge, only one study explored adherence to a PFME program in five women with POP in New Zealand with a single data collection method: a one-to-one interview with a single researcher [17].

Thus, in this study, we aimed to investigate the experience with compliance with PFM home exercises and lifestyle changes in a group of women with POP who completed an 8 week supervised pelvic floor physiotherapy program combining PFM physiotherapy, PFM home exercises, and therapeutic education (which included lifestyle changes) in order to understand the factors that can facilitate or inhibit women's compliance with PFM home exercises and lifestyle changes for improving adherence and person-centered care.

2. Materials and Methods

2.1. Study Design

We conducted this qualitative research between December 2016 and September 2017 at the Research Unit of the Physiotherapy in Women's Health Research Group of the University of Alcalá (Madrid, Spain). We selected a descriptive qualitative design [18], and we conducted the study using focus groups and one-to-one interviews [19]. We used focus groups rather than individual interviews mainly because (a) sensitive and personal disclosures are more likely in a focus-group setting, (b) respondents are more likely to be candid when other similar people are present, (c) there is less individual pressure than in an in-depth interview, and (d) the moderator can more easily reintroduce a topic not sufficiently covered than in a one-to-one interview [20]. The study protocol was approved by the Ethics Committee for Clinical Research of the Príncipe de Asturias Hospital (OE10/2010) in Alcalá de Henares, Madrid, Spain. The study reporting followed the Standards for Reporting Qualitative Research (SRQR) guidelines [21], as well as the COREQ checklist [22]. We followed the ethical principles of the Declaration of Helsinki. All participants provided informed written consent.

2.2. Participants

Selected using a purposive sampling method [23], we considered 26 women diagnosed by their gynecologist, according to the POP-Quantification Scheme [4], with symptomatic POP, recruited from the Hospital Príncipe de Asturias (Madrid, Spain), and referred to a specialized women's health unit to receive an individual woman-centeredness program of pelvic floor physiotherapy to manage symptoms of POP for inclusion in the study. Women over 70 years of age, who gave birth within the six months prior to referral, with stage IV POP, with previous surgery for POP, with psychiatric disease, and who were not able to understand Spanish were excluded. Women who completed the physiotherapy program between 6 and 12 months prior to the start of the study were invited to participate.

The pelvic floor physiotherapy program consisted of 16 individual sessions over 8 weeks (two weekly sessions) with a women's health physiotherapist. The intervention included PFMEs with manual guidance and biofeedback progressing according to the PERFECT scheme from supine to standing and toward functional activities. Women also performed the PFMEs at home, prescribed one to three times per day during the eight-week intervention period. The program also included therapeutic education consisting of instruction with printed and audiovisual materials about the pelvic floor, pelvic floor dysfunctions, the identification of possible precipitating factors, weight loss, constipation, heavy lifting, coughing, high-impact exercise, knack, etc., together with individual strategies for implementing these measures [24]. Upon completion of the physiotherapy program, women were encouraged to continue PFMEs at home (once per day, at least three days per week) and to continue to comply with lifestyle changes.

2.3. Data Collection

Women who completed the pelvic floor physiotherapy program 6–12 months ago with an interest in participation were approached by the research team (M.J.Y.-S.) to determine their availability and convey arrangements with the researcher (M.T.-L.) for both conversational-style focus groups and one-to-one interviews. The six focus groups lasted 60 to 70 min each and involved 4, 3, 5, 4, 4, and 3 women, respectively. The three one-to-one interviews lasted 40 to 50 min each. All the focus groups and one-to one interviews were conducted by a facilitator (a physiotherapist experienced in focus groups and one-to one interviewing, M.T.-L.) in private, closed rooms at the Research Unit of the Physiotherapy in Women's Health Research Group of the University of Alcalá (Madrid, Spain) using a semi-structured approach. In addition, during the focus groups, the facilitator was supported by a qualified pelvic floor physiotherapist (B.N.-B.) who acted as an observer, taking hand-written field notes on nonverbal communications, other observations, etc. We generated the interview questions in the semi-structured guide (Appendix A) with regard to the literature on PFMEs adherence [17,25]. The questions were discussed by the study team: four qualified physiotherapists, two experienced in qualitative research (F.V.-P. and B.S.-S.) and the other two in women's health (B.N.-B. and M.T.-L.); an experienced gynecologist; and a midwife. All interviews were digitally audio-recorded and later transcribed verbatim by two researchers (B.N.-B. and V.P.-G.), with all women's names anonymized in the transcripts. We assigned different codes according to the type of interview (focus group or one-to-one interview) and to the women's intervention order.

2.4. Data Analysis

The analysis was conducted by three members of the research team (B.N.-B., F.V.-P., and M.T.-L.). A triangulation process (investigator and data collection) was conducted [26] to ensure rigor in research. We repeatedly read each transcript. Next, in an iterative and consensus process between three researchers, initial codes were generated and described, codes were grouped into higher-order categories, and then the categories were arranged under potential themes. We performed the transcription coding using ATLAS.ti version 6.1 software (Scientific Software Development GMBH, Berlin, Germany).

When the data being collected were repetitive and no new issues were emerging, we considered that data saturation was achieved, so we ceased collecting data [27]. This arose after six focus group interviews and three one-to-one interviews.

3. Results

Twenty-six women with symptomatic POP who completed a pelvic floor physiotherapy program 6–12 months ago participated in six focus groups and three one-to one interviews. Two women were Latin American, and the remaining were Caucasian. All women spoke and understood Spanish. The women's demographics and POP status are shown in Table 1.

Table 1. Women's demographics and prolapse status.

Parameter	Value
Age (years), X(SD)	57(9)
BMI (kg/m^2), X(SD)	25.1(4.7)
Menopause, n (%)	26 (92.8%)
Type of prolapse, n (%)	
Cystocele	20 (71.4%)
Hysterocele	12 (42.8%)
Rectocele	5 (5.3%)
Stage of prolapse, n (%)	
1	0 (0%)
2	21 (75%)
3	7 (25%)
4	0 (0%)
Other PFD	
Urinary incontinence	20 (76.9%)
SUI	11 (55%)
UUI	4 (2%)
MUI	12 (60%)
Anal incontinence	13 (46.4%)
Flat	12 (92.3%)
Flat & FI	1 (7.7%)
Time between physiotherapy program and interview (months), X (SD)	10.1 (1.4)
Pre-Post physiotherapy program changes	
P-QoL score (points), X (SD)	22.3 (5.6) *
PFDI-20 score (points), X (SD)	−28.4 (−19.3) **
PFM strength (cmH$_2$O), X (SD)	9.78 (2.48) ***

BMI: Body mass index; PFD: Pelvic floor dysfunction; SUI: stress urinary incontinence; UUI: urgency urinary incontinence; MUI: mixed urinary incontinence; FI: Fecal incontinence; P-QoL: Prolapse Quality of Life Questionnaire (* an improvement of 14.5 points is considered clinically relevant [28]); PFDI-20: Pelvic Floor Distress Inventory Short Form (** an improvement of 13.5 points is considered clinically relevant [29]); *** an improvement of 9 cmH$_2$O is considered clinically relevant [30]; PFM: Pelvic floor muscles; X (SD): Mean (Standard Deviation).

Women's experiences (facilitators and barriers) in complying with home PFMEs and lifestyle changes were identified in three themes: (1) symptom changes; (2) performance of PFMEs and lifestyle changes; (3) the health practitioner–patient relationship (Figure 1).

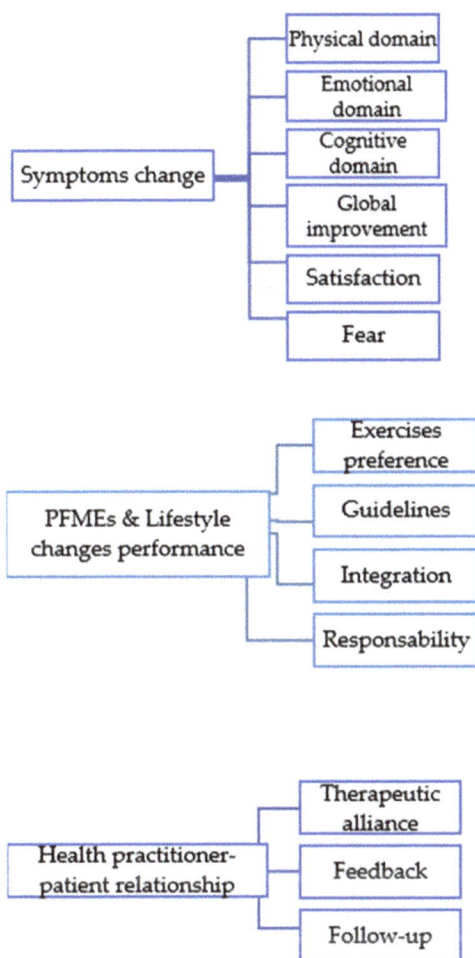

Figure 1. Summary of themes and codes. PFMEs: pelvic floor muscle exercises.

3.1. Theme 1: Symptom Changes

We identified improvement in physical symptoms as one of the main factors motivating compliance with home PFMEs and lifestyle changes, such as voluntary PFM contractions before and during activities that increase abdominal pressure such as weight bearing, coughing, etc. Women reported that having less of a bulging sensation in the vagina or a reduction in the episodes of urine leakage encouraged them to continue with the exercises.

> I am happy . . . I no longer leak urine . . . because before I had frequent leaks. It's what bothered and I disliked it the most . . . Now, yes, I feel calm because the exercises that have taught me . . . I'm fine. (FG3-POP-P5)

> At the moment I continue to do them [PFMEs and lifestyle changes], mainly contractions before weightbearing and coughing [knack], they have been very good for me, they have been very good for me, I feel much better because before, it seemed that I was walking with a ball there [she points to her vagina] all day, but now I don't feel anything [an expression of relief spread across her face]. Sometimes when I get constipated, I feel it a bit [the bulge

> into the vagina], although the position I learned to defecate is better for me, and of course, it is not the same as before coming here to do the exercises and learn those positions to urine, defecate, or contract before coughing, and those things that we learned here...at least I have felt that. (FG2-POP-P4)

We also found that the fear of worsening symptoms, or feeling the symptoms that they learned to control again, or of surgery as a reminder or trigger to resume the PFMEs and lifestyle changes were facilitating factors.

> As soon as I neglect myself and do the exercises less, or I have an allergy episode that I sneeze many times and I notice heaviness there [pelvis and vagina] or I start again with small leaks [urine leaks], I begin to do the exercise again, to contract [PFM] before sneezing, coughing, etc. Right away I think, I don't want to go back to be like before ... (FG3-POP-P5)

> I am afraid, afraid that everything will crumble and that is why I force myself to do it [PFMEs and lifestyle changes], because I am afraid. (FG6-POP-P2)

> Let's see, my neighbor has been operated and she has not been well. I think about the operation. So, the fear, right? I fear the operation, I know women who have put that surgical mesh on. Very bad. And after three months they have put it back on again, and... I don't want to go through that. (FG6-POP-P2)

> I'm afraid that it will fall more, that everything will collapse, and then that will stay dry, and I will get injured and have problems, that is, I am afraid that it will get worse. (Int-POP-P3)

This ability to control their symptoms produced an increase in confidence, security, and satisfaction.

> I was lost, emotionally lost, and everything has improved for me, because I did not know who to turn to and then I already met you one day. Well, my physical condition improved ... physically and mentally, I feel more secure. (FG2-POP-P3)

> I do it [PFMEs and lifestyle changes] to feel better, so that it doesn't get worse [POP] and improve my quality of life. (Int-POP-P3)

> You feel satisfied, you know that you can retain it [POP and urine leaks], that you can control it, and that you feel freer. (FG4-POP-P3)

> ... for me it has been a great benefit. I'm very happy" (Int-POP-P1)

They also reported perceiving a global improvement, an improvement in their sexual activity, and even in their quality of life.

> I have learned to control my muscles .... And to also facilitate many things in my body, to know how to control it as well. Sexually it also favors me, that is, it also stimulates many things. And to know my entire body. (FG1-POP-P1)

Women also associated these positive changes with their newly acquired knowledge and shared it with other women. New knowledge about the anatomy and physiology of the pelvic floor, pelvic floor dysfunctions, risk factors, management, how to correctly perform the PFMEs, etc., seemed give them a sense of control, facilitating adherence. The valuable knowledge gained was key to understanding the importance of incorporating PFMEs and lifestyle changes into their routines and living activities to improve their symptoms and thus prevent both POP and other pelvic floor dysfunctions from progressing.

> ... everything I have learned here has been surprising for me, and a satisfaction, I had no idea about so many things! Now, I know how important it is for me [PFMEs and lifestyle changes] and I even share it [new knowledge] with my daughters, my friends ... (Int-POP-P2)

> Knowing what you can do to improve, why you have to do it, understanding it, is fundamental ... Yes, yes, I already contract instinctively, especially when coughing and

sneezing, before gaining weight too, I control the stimulating drinks, I no hold myself for so long to go to the bathroom to urine, I defecate in a more adequate posture that helps me not to push . . . (FG3-POP-P3)

And I think that this pelvic floor program should be done for every woman from now on. To adolescents, that they learn everything that we have learned from now on... so that they learn from young, from before getting pregnant to take care of their pelvic floor and that what happens to us does not happen to them. (FG1-POP-P4)

3.2. Theme 2: Performance of PFMEs and Lifestyle Changes

In the theme of performing PFMEs and lifestyle changes, the experience of each woman with PFMEs was included. Women taught to perform the PFMEs felt they were performing them better and that, therefore, they had control (self-efficacy). In addition, the association of PFMEs with some everyday gestures (e.g., voluntary PFM contractions (Knack) before and during activities that increase abdominal pressure such as weight bearing, coughing, etc.,) act as a reminder to perform PFMEs. Therefore, these activities supported compliance.

But always the same, the one to maintain . . . I like and am good at. Although, I do PFMEs less than before, really, but everything I learned [lifestyle changes] I have fully integrated, and I no longer have to think about it, I just do it. (FG1-POP-P4)

I, for example, the one on "the ladder", well, the one on "the ladder" and the one "going down and up fast". I like them and I feel it very well. Also, the one to contract [Knack] before laughing or coughing, I like it a lot because it prevents me from leaks. (FG4-POP-P2)

Stand up, especially when I carry weight and sneeze or cough, I feel how it [knack] holds it [POP] inside [into the vagina]. (FG6-POP-P1)

That is the one I do best, of course . . . "the holding" and the knack, drinking, bathroom, etc. [lifestyle changes], that are totally integrated into my life. (Int-POP-P2)

Most of the women stated that integrating PFMEs and lifestyle changes into their daily life, the possibility of performing PFMEs in any place, and a PFME regular routine (routine of place, routine of time of day) made it easier to continue these changes. Most women claimed to be much more consistent with lifestyle changes, which they considered fully incorporated into their routines.

...what is easier to do, I see that I can do it [PFMEs] at any time. When I am standing, I am sitting, I am even washing the dishes, I am with the children, because I hold my baby in my arms, and of course, that forces me, because I know that I am going to force myself and that I am going to do it [Knack] at the same time....I take advantage of those moments. (FG3-POP-P5)

I take advantage of it the most, with the iron, you are standing up, you relax a little and come on, let's do it [PFMEs]. I really like that. (Int-POP-P2)

Yes, I am also . . . At work doing it [PFMEs] at all times . . . or waiting for the bus. (Int-POP-P3)

. . . well on Monday, Wednesday and Friday I do these [PFMEs], and on Tuesday and Thursday these others [PFMEs]. Always when I go to bed. (FG6-POP-P3)

I have incorporated them [PFMEs] into my gym routine, I do them three times a week that I go to the gym. And I also contract [Knack] when she taught me B. [Pelvic floor program Physiotherapist] during Pilates exercises. (FG4-POP-P4)

I always do them [PFMEs] after I shower in the morning, it is already routine and I always do them, just like contracting [Knack] before heavy load, I have already automated it. (Int-POP-P1)

However, several women reported a lack of criteria regarding the time of day of exercises, repetitions, and progression that made it difficult to perform PFMEs.

> And then when I suddenly remember and say to myself: come on, I'm going to do them at noon, even if it's on a carpet. I will always win something . . . . And then at night when I go to bed I say: Uffff! And again I have to do this . . . .. how many do I have to do, how I continue . . . ? (FG2-POP-P2)

> And especially when I look bad, I see that I need it and then I do them a few days, oh my God! Why have I stopped it? Pum pum . . . (FG4-POP-P3)

In addition, individualized ad hoc guides (written, spoken, or apps) providing reminders regarding PFME types, repetitions, progression, and lifestyle changes were described as support material that acted as a reminder facilitating adherence to PFMEs and lifestyle changes.

> What B. [pelvic floor program Physiotherapist] put in the notebook is what I exactly do, and so I don't forget. (FG3-POP-P1)

> I do what B. [pelvic floor program Physiotherapist] taught me, I have it here written down on a paper [written information], and very well. (Int-POP-P1)

> . . . I always have a small piece of paper, if I have a doubt...for example: I don't remember the progression of an exercise, so I look at the paper that I have on the bedside table, and I check the paper. (FG2-POP-P1)

> Well, I preferred to record it on my mobile phone, and that is how I always carry it with me, and if I don't remember something, I listen to it quickly, I do it on the subway when I go to work, and it suits me very well. (Int-POP-P3)

> The apps she [pelvic floor program Physiotherapist] taught me to do the exercises is fantastic, I carry it on my mobile and I do them with the app. I like it. (FG3-POP-P2)

Finally, the feeling of responsibility and the need to take care of themselves as they take care of others emerged from the sessions, mostly related as a barrier to integrating PFMEs in their daily living. Their roles as caregivers in the family negatively influenced their adherence to PFMEs, since they take care of the family first, and they do not pay enough attention to their self-care.

> It is our responsibility, the disease [POP], but we are not consistent, and we also think before of others, children, family. (FG5-POP-P4)

> We are not in the habit of spending time with ourselves. Because it is a bad habit and a bad practice of ourselves. So, we always make the mistake thinking "it doesn't matter". The last one, us. And we are not interested in ourselves. (FG5-POP-P3)

> Well, let's say that our will fails us, the truth is a bit for me that I think I had to be more responsible, and I haven't done them [PFMEs]. (Int-POP-P1)

> And we don't worry about ourselves. Always. And even if we don't have anything to do, we don't think about ourselves. (Int-POP-P3)

3.3. Theme 3: Healthcare Practitioner–Patient Relationship

The individualized pelvic floor physiotherapy program including follow-up sessions was identified as essential for performing PFMEs and for compliance with lifestyle changes.

> It is not the same as going to the gynecologist, and they tell you: look, do these exercises that will help you. And then, of course, you say: okay, I do them, but of course, you don't know if you do it well or do it poorly and of course, here they teach you how to do it. Also, how to urinate or defecate, which before you did not do as well as you should, and other things you do not know. So, it's different. (FG3-POP-P3)

> . . . and B. [pelvic floor program physiotherapist] has been giving me tricks, strategies, helping me to integrate them [PFMEs and lifestyle changes] into my life, to look for the moments . . . (FG4-POP-P3)

While we are here, we do it, we go, at least I do. And I know how to do it and if I do it well is because B. [pelvic floor program physiotherapist] tell me. And then we continue with the reviews. (Int-POP-P2)

I thank B. [pelvic floor program physiotherapist] who helped me to improve, because maybe if I did not come here ... well, uh ... when I also come here for follow-up, I remember to do it, it reinforces me. (Int-POP-P3)

In addition, the positive feedback of physiotherapists and other health professionals (mainly gynecologists) involved in the therapeutic approach also influenced adherence to PFMEs and lifestyle changes.

The gynecologist is happy, because he says: we have seen that many people have progressed, and we have seen that I have improved, and POP has been stabilized. (FG3-POP-P3)

And it also motivates me that the gynecologist has told me to continue exercising, that I am better and to continue. (FG5-POP-P1)

The physiotherapists of the program were identified as having a better approach to care than doctors and nurses. The women responded that the aspect of the physiotherapy program that they most valued was their patient, loving, listening, and helpful attitude, reflecting a person-centered attitude (therapeutic alliance).

... .and B. [pelvic floor program physiotherapist] has already taught me with love and patience, and we are learning, because I never knew, and in my country ... Well, I am not from here, but now, thank God, with the exercises that B. has taught me, I can. I am very happy and grateful. (FG2-POP-P4)

And here [pelvic floor program], I have felt very good, they [pelvic floor program physiotherapists] have treated me very well, with a lot of patience, they have listened to me, they have helped me, and I have learned a lot and I have improved. (FG6-POP-P2)

... for the learning we have had, that you can already carry it out to practice it in your daily life with a program that has been made for each of us, and well, if we do not come to the program, we would not have learned all this [PFMEs and lifestyle changes], me at least. You read four things, you know two or three, you know them in your own way, you don't know if it is well-done as well .... Well, for me it was the best, finding you [pelvic floor program physiotherapists]. (Int-POP-P3)

4. Discussion

In this study, we explored women's experiences with compliance with home PFMEs and lifestyles changes for POP symptoms and their facilitators and barriers. Our findings showed that most women, over time, do not perform PFMEs regularly (weekly); however, they comply with lifestyle changes. As shown in prior studies, decline in PFME compliance over time is normal [25,31]. Several researchers have investigated the factors that influence adherence to PFMEs, mainly in women with urinary incontinence, although none specifically addressed adherence to lifestyle changes [15,16,32–35]. Regarding POP, a single qualitative study analyzed adherence to PFME, but it also did not consider adherence to lifestyle changes [17]. So, to the best of our knowledge, this is the first study including factors affecting adherence to lifestyle changes (i.e., strategies for bladder control; contributing factors; knack application to manage everyday pelvic floor challenges; daily PFMEs for at least 15 days after a period of allergy, cold, weight bearing, etc.; performing PFMEs at the end of the sports activities involving weightbearing or impact, in addition to knack; etc.) [24,36–38].

Regarding the methodology, we used a descriptive design in order to understand and determine the experience of women who completed a supervised and individualized pelvic floor physiotherapy program including training for the long-term maintenance of PFMEs and lifestyle changes. This approach allowed us to explore women's experiences with adherence to PFMEs and lifestyle changes for POP from the their perspective and to understand the meanings that the women attach to their behavior [18]. In contrast to the phenomenological study by Hyland et al. [17], a key strength of our descriptive study is the data collection triangulation, combining one-to-one individual interviews and focus groups. The use of investigator triangulation further strengthened this study, resulting in a valid and comprehensive understanding of these phenomena [39].

Our approach produced three themes explaining the factors modifying adherence to PFMEs and lifestyle changes: (1) symptom changes; (2) performing PFMEs and lifestyle changes; and (3) the health practitioner–patient relationship.

4.1. Symptom Changes

Changes in symptoms were identified as an important factor modifying adherence. We found that both the improvement in and symptom relapse in those women who stopped performing the PFMEs or relaxed their changes in lifestyle, mainly knack, were powerful triggers of therapeutic adherence. Previous research in women with incontinence reported that women with more frequent urine leaks before and after PFMEs plus an education physiotherapy program were more adherent to PFMEs one year after physiotherapy than women with less frequent urine leaks [15]. Similarly, Abhyankarome et al. reported that women with POP ask for help based on the symptoms experienced. They explored women's experiences with seeking diagnosis and treatment for POP. They interviewed 22 women receiving POP care through U.K. NHS urogynecology services regarding experiences with seeking diagnosis and treatment for POP and their needs and priorities [40]. Lack of awareness of POP symptoms [40,41] due to mild symptoms resulted in women seeking less help and making less of a sustained effort to perform PFMEs, similar to women with urinary incontinence [15,34,42,43]. However, when women are aware of POP symptoms, when they feel their fear of symptoms worsening, and they feel fear of the condition progressing to the extent that surgery is the only achievable option [40], that is when PFME compliance increases. A wish to avoid surgery as long as possible is a motivator for seeking help and for performing PFMEs [40].

These symptoms can affect women's self-esteem, body image, and quality of life [40] and can have social, psychological, and sexual impacts. The more the symptoms progress, the more they affect quality of life, social well-being, and sexual health [44–46]. Ghetti et al. found, in their qualitative study describing the emotional burden experienced by forty-four women seeking treatment for POP, that women's psychological well-being is intimately related with their POP symptoms [47]. Salovey et al. reported that physical health and emotional states influence one another. Positive emotional states, such as the satisfaction expressed by the women in this study, and their empowerment regarding the control of their symptoms may promote healthy perceptions, beliefs, and physical well-being [48]. Women also linked satisfaction and sense of control to embodied knowledge. Women stated that gaps in their pelvic health knowledge have been addressed. Pintos-Díaz et al., in a qualitative study exploring the reasons Spanish women with urinary incontinence sought help, stated that women' have complaints about the overall lack of information. They also found that the knowledge of many women about pelvic floor and pelvic floor dysfunctions was based on beliefs or myths [43]. Pelvic health education is effective in dealing with myths, false beliefs, and misinformation about the pelvic floor and pelvic floor dysfunction [43]. Moreover, all women reported using their new knowledge, mainly lifestyle changes, and PFMEs. They even shared this information with others. Adherence was linked with knowledge. The more knowledgeable and insightful the women were about their pelvic floor and pelvic health, and the more they experienced an effect on their symptoms, the more they adhered to PFMEs [49]. These findings agree with those of other studies conducted in women with urinary incontinence [15,50,51].

This theme did not emerge the study by Hyland et al. [17]. This could be due to the clinical characteristics of the women in each study. Although women were homogeneous regarding the stage of POP (II and III) and they could also have been homogeneous in relation to the POP symptoms, whether the five women interviewed by Hyland et al. suffered from other pelvic floor dysfunctions is unknown. In our study, women also reported urinary incontinence (76.9%) and anal incontinence (46.4%) symptoms. POP often co-exists with other pelvic floor dysfunctions, mainly those involving urinary incontinence [5,12,52].

4.2. Performing PFMEs and Lifestyle Changes

Compliance with PFMEs and lifestyle changes was associated with regular routines and their integration into their daily lives, PFME movability, and PFME preference regarding control and self-efficacy. Most women performed the PFMEs, which allowed them to have more control and a greater sense of performing PFMEs effectively, which could be related to self-efficacy with a PFME-specific task. A woman's belief in her own ability to perform PFMEs seems to influence adherence to PFME as well as to predict the intention to adhere to PFMEs [15,36,53,54]. These findings agree with those of prior studies in women with urinary incontinence [34] as well as with the findings reported by Hyland et al. in women with POP symptoms [17].

Women also valued the individualized ad hoc guidelines because they explained PFME types, repetitions, progression, and some lifestyle changes. This support material acted as a reminder that facilitated adherence to PFMEs and lifestyle changes. Several studies have evaluated strategies to improve adherence to PFMEs [15,55–57] in women with urinary incontinence. Some researchers tested the efficacy of electronic reminders or exercise diaries, finding that these are effective in increasing adherence to PFMEs in an unsupervised approach [55–57]. As barriers to seeking treatment, Abhyankarome et al. reported that women with POP expressed forgetting to perform the exercises after some time. To recall the exercises, some of them used telephone apps or alarms as reminders and some paired the exercises with daily activities [40].

Women identified the largest barrier to PFME adherence as the feeling of responsibility and the need to take care of others. In the current study, not only did women prioritize others over themselves, but they also expressed their poor commitment to their own healthcare. This may be due to the role of women in society as family planners and caregivers [58,59], probably because of their feeling of moral and affective obligation [60,61]. Despite the social changes over the last decades and the increased involvement of men in caring for the family, women continue to be the main caregivers, at least in Spanish society [62]. These findings agree with those of Alewijse [15] and Hyland [17].

In studies on PFME adherence, adherence is associated with performing PFMEs, seldom with bladder training or with the functional use of pelvic floor muscles in activities of daily living. In our study, women stated that they were more compliant with the functional use of pelvic floor muscles in their day-to-day activities (i.e., knack) than with PFMEs. Moreover, the functional use of the pelvic floor muscles acts as a reminder to perform PFMEs, and therefore supports compliance. This is probably because knack is an effective tool in reducing urine loss, as well as a valid tool for reducing bladder neck movement, which can also minimize POP symptoms [63,64]. To the best of our knowledge, this is the first study exploring adherence to lifestyle changes (including functional use of the pelvic floor muscles) in women with POP symptoms.

4.3. Health Practitioner–Patient Relationship

Women in our study highlighted the importance of their relationship with healthcare professionals, mainly with the gynecologist and with physiotherapists. This could because these women underwent a previous pelvic floor physiotherapy program, and in this eight-week program, the physiotherapists had more opportunities to explain the program and have discussions with the women. The most valued aspect, as in Abhyankarome et al., was the physiotherapists' person-centered attitude. This issue has not emerged in other studies on adherence to PFMEs. This could be because those studies were less supervised or the interventions were unsupervised. The therapeutic relationship or therapeutic alliance seems to improve adherence, satisfaction, and quality of life [65].

This therapeutic alliance may have also been reinforced by the follow-ups and the univocal positive feedback from all of the health professionals involved in the diagnosis and treatment of the women in the study. The follow-up and feedback were described as a demand from women with symptoms of POP, expressing "a strong need for longer-term monitoring and periodic follow-up of prolapse symptoms following the appropriate training in PFME" [sic] [40]. These follow-ups and univocal positive feedback may have simultaneously reinforced self-efficacy [35].

Our findings of the experiences with long-term PFME adherence confirm those reported in the literature on women with urinary incontinence [15,16,25,32–34] and with POP symptoms [17]. Our findings also provide new evidence of the experiences of women with POP symptoms and adherence to lifestyle changes.

4.4. Limitations

The qualitative approach employed in this study also has some limitations. By nature, this approach prevents the generalization of the findings to further ethnically diverse groups. Although the purpose of qualitative research is not to generalize, our results can be extended mainly to Spanish-culture Caucasian women (although two Latin American women also participated) who have previously attended an individualized and supervised woman-centered pelvic floor physiotherapy program in an urban and outpatient academic and research women's health physiotherapy unit. Therefore, our findings cannot be extended to women with POP symptoms who have not visited a women's health clinic or specialist.

Although the interviewer (facilitator, M.T.-L.) was an independent researcher to the pelvic floor physiotherapy program that all women previously completed, the observer (B.N.-B.) in the focus groups interviews was one of the pelvic floor physiotherapy program physiotherapists. Therefore, women may also have said what they thought the physiotherapist would have wanted to hear. Nevertheless, the fact that the women and one of the researchers had a relationship may have contributed to a safe, confidential, and conducive environment for women to talk about their intimate stories.

5. Conclusions

To conclude, long-term compliance with prescribed PFMEs and lifestyle changes can improve with effective, individual, women-centered, and supervised pelvic floor physiotherapy programs, thereby reducing symptoms. The program should include exercises agreeing with women's preferences that are easy to integrate into their activities of daily living, promoting knowledge and awareness of their condition, providing written or electronic guidelines adapted to the specific needs of women, with routine follow-up visits offering both positive feedback and clear and consistent messages from all of the healthcare professionals involved, and enhancing the therapeutic alliance.

An increased understanding of the facilitators of and barriers to performing PFMEs and lifestyle changes may help providers better understand women's needs and provide individualized care.

Author Contributions: Conceptualization, M.T.-L. and F.V.-P.; methodology, M.T.-L., F.V.-P. and B.N.-B.; software, V.P.-G.; validation, M.J.Y.-S., V.P-G. and B.S.-S..; formal analysis, M.T.-L., F.V.-P. and B.N.-B.; investigation, M.T.-L., F.V.-P. and B.N.-B.; resources, M.T.-L.; writing—original draft preparation, M.T.-L.; writing—review and editing, M.T.-L., F.V.-P. and B.N.-B.; visualization, B.S.-S.; supervision, M.T.-L.; project administration, M.J.Y.-S.; funding acquisition, M.T.-L. All authors have read and agreed to the published version of the manuscript.

Funding: This research is part of a study funded by the Health Institute Carlos III (Protocol PI10/01756) of the Spanish Health Ministry.

Institutional Review Board Statement: The study was conducted according to the guidelines of the Declaration of Helsinki and approved by the Ethics Committee of at the Hospital Príncipe de Asturias (protocol number: OE10/2010) in Alcalá de Henares (Madrid), Spain, and with the 1964 Helsinki declaration and its later amendments or comparable ethical standards.

Informed Consent Statement: Informed consent was obtained from all the subjects involved in the study.

Data Availability Statement: Data are held securely by the research team and may be available upon reasonable request and with relevant approvals in place.

Conflicts of Interest: The authors declare no conflict of interest.

Appendix A

Interview Guide

What do you think the pelvic floor muscle exercises are for? What do you think are its effects?
What do you think the lifestyle changes are for? What do you think are its effects?
Can you tell me about the kind of things you do when you do pelvic floor muscle exercises?
Where are you?
What time of day?
What exercises do you practice the most? Why?
What exercises do you practice the least? Why?
What do you think makes it easier to do the exercises?
What do you think makes it difficult to do the exercises?
Tell me about how your exercises fit into a typical day
Tell me about how your exercises fit into a typical week
How do you go about fitting these exercises in?
Can you tell me about your lifestyle changes? What have you adopted?
Where are you?
What time of day?
What do you think makes it easier lifestyle changes?
What do you think makes it difficult lifestyle changes?
Tell me about how your lifestyle changes into a typical day
Tell me about how your lifestyle changes into a typical week
How do you go about fitting these lifestyle changes in?
What things get in the way of you doing your exercises? And making your lifestyle changes?
How do you cope with these "barriers"?
What have you found useful to keep you going with exercising?
What have you found useful to keep you going with lifestyle changes?

References

1. Bugge, C.; Adams, E.J.; Gopinath, D.; Stewart, F.; Dembinsky, M.; Sobiesuo, P.; Kearney, R. Pessaries (mechanical devices) for managing pelvic organ prolapse in women. *Cochrane Database Syst. Rev.* **2020**, *11*, Cd004010. [PubMed]
2. de Albuquerque Coelho, S.C.; de Castro, E.B.; Juliato, C.R. Female pelvic organ prolapse using pessaries: Systematic review. *Int. Urogynecology J.* **2016**, *27*, 1797–1803. [CrossRef] [PubMed]
3. Pakbaz, M.; Persson, M.; Löfgren, M.; Mogren, I. 'A hidden disorder until the pieces fall into place'—A qualitative study of vaginal prolapse. *BMC Women's Health* **2010**, *10*, 18. [CrossRef] [PubMed]
4. Bo, K.; Frawley, H.C.; Haylen, B.T.; Abramov, Y.; Almeida, F.G.; Berghmans, B.; Bortolini, M.; Dumoulin, C.; Gomes, M.; McClurg, D.; et al. An International Urogynecological Association (IUGA)/International Continence Society (ICS) joint report on the terminology for the conservative and nonpharmacological management of female pelvic floor dysfunction. *Neurourol. Urodyn.* **2017**, *36*, 221–244. [CrossRef] [PubMed]
5. Hunskaar, S.; Burgio, K.L.; Clark, A.; Lapitan, M.C.; Nelson, R.; Sillen, U. Epidemiology of Urinary (UI) and Faecal (FI) Incontinence and Pelvic Organ Prolapse (POP). In *Incontinence*, 3rd ed.; Abrams, P., Cardozo, L., Khoury, S., Wein, A., Eds.; International Continence Society: Bristol, UK, 2005; pp. 255–312.
6. Barber, M.D.; Neubauer, N.L.; Klein-Olarte, V. Can we screen for pelvic organ prolapse without a physical examination in epidemiologic studies? *Am. J. Obstet. Gynecol.* **2006**, *195*, 942–948. [CrossRef]
7. Hagen, S.; Stark, D. Conservative prevention and management of pelvic organ prolapse in women. *Cochrane Database Syst. Rev.* **2011**, *12*, CD003882. [CrossRef] [PubMed]

8. Borello-France, D.F.; Handa, V.L.; Brown, M.B.; Goode, P.; Kreder, K.; Scheufele, L.L.; Weber, A.M. Pelvic-floor muscle function in women with pelvic organ prolapse. *Phys. Ther.* **2007**, *87*, 399–407. [CrossRef] [PubMed]
9. Slieker-ten Hove, M.; Pool-Goudzwaard, A.; Eijkemans, M.; Steegers-Theunissen, R.; Burger, C.; Vierhout, M. Pelvic floor muscle function in a general population of women with and without pelvic organ prolapse. *Int. Urogynecology J.* **2010**, *21*, 311–319. [CrossRef] [PubMed]
10. Hagen, S.; Glazener, C.; McClurg, D.; Macarthur, C.; Elders, A.; Herbison, P.; Wilson, D.; Toozs-Hobson, P.; Hemming, C.; Hay-Smith, J.; et al. Pelvic floor muscle training for secondary prevention of pelvic organ prolapse (PREVPROL): A multicentre randomised controlled trial. *Lancet (Lond. Engl.)* **2017**, *389*, 393–402. [CrossRef]
11. Maher, C.; Feiner, B.; Baessler, K.; Christmann-Schmid, C.; Haya, N.; Brown, J. Surgery for women with anterior compartment prolapse. *Cochrane Database Syst. Rev.* **2016**, *11*, CD004014. [CrossRef]
12. Friedman, T.; Eslick, G.D.; Dietz, H.P. Risk factors for prolapse recurrence: Systematic review and meta-analysis. *Int. Urogynecology J.* **2018**, *29*, 13–21. [CrossRef] [PubMed]
13. Mangir, N.; Roman, S.; Chapple, C.R.; MacNeil, S. Complications related to use of mesh implants in surgical treatment of stress urinary incontinence and pelvic organ prolapse: Infection or inflammation? *World J. Urol.* **2020**, *38*, 73–80. [CrossRef] [PubMed]
14. Li, C.; Gong, Y.; Wang, B. The efficacy of pelvic floor muscle training for pelvic organ prolapse: A systematic review and meta-analysis. *Int. Urogynecology J.* **2016**, *27*, 981–992. [CrossRef] [PubMed]
15. Alewijnse, D.; Metsemakers, J.F.; Mesters, I.E.; van den Borne, B. Effectiveness of pelvic floor muscle exercise therapy supplemented with a health education program to promote long-term adherence among women with urinary incontinence. *Neurourol. Urodyn.* **2003**, *22*, 284–295. [CrossRef] [PubMed]
16. Bø, K.; Kvarstein, B.; Nygaard, I. Lower urinary tract symptoms and pelvic floor muscle exercise adherence after 15 years. *Obstet. Gynecol.* **2005**, *105 Pt 1*, 999–1005. [CrossRef]
17. Hyland, G.; Hay-Smith, J.; Treharne, G. Women's experiences of doing long-term pelvic floor muscle exercises for the treatment of pelvic organ prolapse symptoms. *Int. Urogynecology J.* **2014**, *25*, 265–271. [CrossRef]
18. Sandelowski, M. Whatever happened to qualitative description? *Res. Nurs. Health* **2000**, *23*, 334–340. [CrossRef]
19. Lambert, S.D.; Loiselle, C.G. Combining individual interviews and focus groups to enhance data richness. *J. Adv. Nurs.* **2008**, *62*, 228–237. [CrossRef]
20. Guest, G.; Namey, E.; Taylor, J.; Eley, N.; McKenna, K. Comparing focus groups and individual interviews: Findings from a randomized study. *Int. J. Soc. Res. Methodol.* **2017**, *20*, 693–708. [CrossRef]
21. O'Brien, B.C.; Harris, I.B.; Beckman, T.J.; Reed, D.A.; Cook, D.A. Standards for reporting qualitative research: A synthesis of recommendations. *Acad. Med. J. Assoc. Am. Med. Coll.* **2014**, *89*, 1245–1251. [CrossRef]
22. Tong, A.; Sainsbury, P.; Craig, J. Consolidated criteria for reporting qualitative research (COREQ): A 32-item checklist for interviews and focus groups. *Int. J. Qual. Health Care J. Int. Soc. Qual. Health Care* **2007**, *19*, 349–357. [CrossRef] [PubMed]
23. Gill, S.L. Qualitative Sampling Methods. *J. Hum. Lact. Off. J. Int. Lact. Consult. Assoc.* **2020**, *36*, 579–581. [CrossRef] [PubMed]
24. Sánchez-Sánchez, B.; Arranz-Martín, B.; Navarro-Brazález, B.; Vergara-Pérez, F.; Bailón-Cerezo, J.; Torres-Lacomba, M. How Do We Assess Patient Skills in a Competence-Based Program? Assessment of Patient Competences Using the Spanish Version of the Prolapse and Incontinence Knowledge Questionnaire and Real Practical Cases in Women with Pelvic Floor Disorders. *Int. J. Environ. Res. Public Health* **2021**, *18*, 2377. [CrossRef] [PubMed]
25. Bø, K. Adherence to pelvic floor muscle exercise and long-term effect on stress urinary incontinence. A five-year follow-up study. *Scand. J. Med. Sci. Sports* **1995**, *5*, 36–39. [CrossRef] [PubMed]
26. Carter, N.; Bryant-Lukosius, D.; DiCenso, A.; Blythe, J.; Neville, A.J. The use of triangulation in qualitative research. *Oncol. Nurs. Forum* **2014**, *41*, 545–547. [CrossRef] [PubMed]
27. Gibbs, L.; Kealy, M.; Willis, K.; Green, J.; Welch, N.; Daly, J. What have sampling and data collection got to do with good qualitative research? *Aust. N. Z. J. Public Health* **2007**, *31*, 540–544. [CrossRef] [PubMed]
28. Farthmann, J.; Mengel, M.; Henne, B.; Grebe, M.; Watermann, D.; Kaufhold, J.; Stehle, M.; Fuenfgeld, C. Improvement of pelvic floor-related quality of life and sexual function after vaginal mesh implantation for cystocele: Primary endpoint of a prospective multicentre trial. *Arch. Gynecol. Obstet.* **2016**, *294*, 115–121. [CrossRef] [PubMed]
29. Wiegersma, M.; Panman, C.M.; Berger, M.Y.; De Vet, H.C.; Kollen, B.J.; Dekker, J.H. Minimal important change in the pelvic floor distress inventory-20 among women opting for conservative prolapse treatment. *Am. J. Obstet. Gynecol.* **2017**, *216*, e391–e397. [CrossRef] [PubMed]
30. Navarro-Brazález, B.; Prieto-Gómez, V.; Prieto-Merino, D.; Sánchez-Sánchez, B.; McLean, L.; Torres-Lacomba, M. Effectiveness of Hypopressive Exercises in Women with Pelvic Floor Dysfunction: A Randomised Controlled Trial. *J. Clin. Med.* **2020**, *9*, 1149. [CrossRef] [PubMed]
31. Alewijnse, D.; Mesters, I.; Metsemakers, J.; van den Borne, B. Predictors of long-term adherence to pelvic floor muscle exercise therapy among women with urinary incontinence. *Health Educ. Res.* **2003**, *18*, 511–524. [CrossRef] [PubMed]
32. Borello-France, D.; Burgio, K.L.; Goode, P.S.; Markland, A.D.; Kenton, K.; Balasubramanyam, A.; Stoddard, A.M. Adherence to behavioral interventions for urge incontinence when combined with drug therapy: Adherence rates, barriers, and predictors. *Phys. Ther.* **2010**, *90*, 1493–1505. [CrossRef] [PubMed]

33. Borello-France, D.; Burgio, K.L.; Goode, P.S.; Ye, W.; Weidner, A.C.; Lukacz, E.S.; Jelovsek, J.E.; Bradley, C.S.; Schaffer, J.; Hsu, Y.; et al. Adherence to behavioral interventions for stress incontinence: Rates, barriers, and predictors. *Phys. Ther.* **2013**, *93*, 757–773. [CrossRef] [PubMed]
34. Hay-Smith, E.J.C.; Ryan, K.; Dean, S. The silent, private exercise: Experiences of pelvic floor muscle training in a sample of women with stress urinary incontinence. *Physiotherapy* **2007**, *93*, 53–61. [CrossRef]
35. Milne, J.L.; Moore, K.N. Factors impacting self-care for urinary incontinence. *Urol. Nurs.* **2006**, *26*, 41–51.
36. Alewijnse, D.; Mesters, I.E.; Metsemakers, J.F.; van den Borne, B.H. Program development for promoting adherence during and after exercise therapy for urinary incontinence. *Patient Educ. Couns.* **2002**, *48*, 147–160. [CrossRef]
37. Fitz, F.F.; Gimenez, M.M.; de Azevedo Ferreira, L.; Matias, M.M.P.; Bortolini, M.A.T.; Castro, R.A. Effects of voluntary pre-contraction of the pelvic floor muscles (the Knack) on female stress urinary incontinence-a study protocol for a RCT. *Trials* **2021**, *22*, 484. [CrossRef]
38. Imamura, M.; Williams, K.; Wells, M.; McGrother, C. Lifestyle interventions for the treatment of urinary incontinence in adults. *Cochrane Database Syst. Rev.* **2015**, *12*, Cd003505. [CrossRef]
39. Barusch, A.S.; Gringeri, C.E.; George, M. Rigor in Qualitative Social Work Research: A Review of Strategies Used in Published Articles. *Soc. Work. Res.* **2011**, *35*, 11–19. [CrossRef]
40. Abhyankar, P.; Uny, I.; Semple, K.; Wane, S.; Hagen, S.; Wilkinson, J.; Guerrero, K.; Tincello, D.; Duncan, E.; Calveley, E.; et al. Women's experiences of receiving care for pelvic organ prolapse: A qualitative study. *BMC Women's Health* **2019**, *19*, 45. [CrossRef]
41. Rada, M.P.; Jones, S.; Falconi, G.; Milhem Haddad, J.; Betschart, C.; Pergialiotis, V.; Doumouchtsis, S.K. A systematic review and meta-synthesis of qualitative studies on pelvic organ prolapse for the development of core outcome sets. *Neurourol. Urodyn.* **2020**, *39*, 880–889. [CrossRef]
42. Burns, P.A.; Pranikoff, K.; Nochajski, T.H.; Hadley, E.C.; Levy, K.J.; Ory, M.G. A comparison of effectiveness of biofeedback and pelvic muscle exercise treatment of stress incontinence in older community-dwelling women. *J. Gerontol.* **1993**, *48*, M167–M174. [PubMed]
43. Pintos-Díaz, M.Z.; Alonso-Blanco, C.; Parás-Bravo, P.; Fernández-de-Las-Peñas, C.; Paz-Zulueta, M.; Fradejas-Sastre, V.; Palacios-Ceña, D. Living with Urinary Incontinence: Potential Risks of Women's Health? A Qualitative Study on the Perspectives of Female Patients Seeking Care for the First Time in a Specialized Center. *Int. J. Environ. Res. Public Health* **2019**, *16*, 3781. [CrossRef] [PubMed]
44. Jelovsek, J.E.; Barber, M.D. Women seeking treatment for advanced pelvic organ prolapse have decreased body image and quality of life. *Am. J. Obstet. Gynecol.* **2006**, *194*, 1455–1461. [CrossRef] [PubMed]
45. Lowder, J.L.; Ghetti, C.; Nikolajski, C.; Oliphant, S.S.; Zyczynski, H.M. Body image perceptions in women with pelvic organ prolapse: A qualitative study. *Am. J. Obstet. Gynecol.* **2011**, *204*, 441.e441–445. [CrossRef] [PubMed]
46. Mattsson, N.K.; Karjalainen, P.K.; Tolppanen, A.M.; Heikkinen, A.M.; Sintonen, H.; Härkki, P.; Nieminen, K.; Jalkanen, J. Pelvic organ prolapse surgery and quality of life-a nationwide cohort study. *Am. J. Obstet. Gynecol.* **2020**, *222*, 588.e510–588.e581. [CrossRef] [PubMed]
47. Ghetti, C.; Skoczylas, L.C.; Oliphant, S.S.; Nikolajski, C.; Lowder, J.L. The Emotional Burden of Pelvic Organ Prolapse in Women Seeking Treatment: A Qualitative Study. *Female Pelvic Med. Reconstr. Surg.* **2015**, *21*, 332–338. [CrossRef] [PubMed]
48. Salovey, P.; Rothman, A.J.; Detweiler, J.B.; Steward, W.T. Emotional states and physical health. *Am. Psychol.* **2000**, *55*, 110–121. [CrossRef]
49. Hay-Smith, J.; Dean, S.; Burgio, K.; McClurg, D.; Frawley, H.; Dumoulin, C. Pelvic-floor-muscle-training adherence "modifiers": A review of primary qualitative studies-2011 ICS State-of-the-Science Seminar research paper III of IV. *Neurourol. Urodyn.* **2015**, *34*, 622–631. [CrossRef] [PubMed]
50. Frawley, H.C.; McClurg, D.; Mahfooza, A.; Hay-Smith, J.; Dumoulin, C. Health professionals' and patients' perspectives on pelvic floor muscle training adherence-2011 ICS State-of-the-Science Seminar research paper IV of IV. *Neurourol. Urodyn.* **2015**, *34*, 632–639. [CrossRef] [PubMed]
51. Fernandes, A.; Palacios-Ceña, D.; Hay-Smith, J.; Pena, C.C.; Sidou, M.F.; de Alencar, A.L.; Ferreira, C.H.J. Women report sustained benefits from attending group-based education about pelvic floor muscles: A longitudinal qualitative study. *J. Physiother.* **2021**, *67*, 210–216. [CrossRef]
52. Rortveit, G.; Subak, L.L.; Thom, D.H.; Creasman, J.M.; Vittinghoff, E.; Van Den Eeden, S.K.; Brown, J.S. Urinary incontinence, fecal incontinence and pelvic organ prolapse in a population-based, racially diverse cohort: Prevalence and risk factors. *Female Pelvic Med. Reconstr. Surg.* **2010**, *16*, 278–283. [CrossRef] [PubMed]
53. Picha, K.J.; Howell, D.M. A model to increase rehabilitation adherence to home exercise programmes in patients with varying levels of self-efficacy. *Musculoskelet. Care* **2018**, *16*, 233–237. [CrossRef] [PubMed]
54. Chen, S.Y.; Tzeng, Y.L. Path analysis for adherence to pelvic floor muscle exercise among women with urinary incontinence. *J. Nurs. Res. JNR* **2009**, *17*, 83–92. [CrossRef] [PubMed]
55. Sugaya, K.; Owan, T.; Hatano, T.; Nishijima, S.; Miyazato, M.; Mukouyama, H.; Shiroma, K.; Soejima, K.; Masaki, Z.; Ogawa, Y. Device to promote pelvic floor muscle training for stress incontinence. *Int. J. Urol. Off. J. Jpn. Urol. Assoc.* **2003**, *10*, 416–422. [CrossRef] [PubMed]

56. Sampselle, C.M.; Messer, K.L.; Seng, J.S.; Raghunathan, T.E.; Hines, S.H.; Diokno, A.C. Learning outcomes of a group behavioral modification program to prevent urinary incontinence. *Int. Urogynecology J. Pelvic Floor Dysfunct.* **2005**, *16*, 441–446. [CrossRef] [PubMed]
57. Sacomori, C.; Berghmans, B.; Mesters, I.; de Bie, R.; Cardoso, F.L. Strategies to enhance self-efficacy and adherence to home-based pelvic floor muscle exercises did not improve adherence in women with urinary incontinence: A randomised trial. *J. Physiother.* **2015**, *61*, 190–198. [CrossRef] [PubMed]
58. Guberman, N.; Maheu, P.; Maillé, C. Women as family caregivers: Why do they care? *Gerontologist* **1992**, *32*, 607–617. [CrossRef] [PubMed]
59. Halper, L.R.; Cowgill, C.M.; Rios, K. Gender bias in caregiving professions: The role of perceived warmth. *J. Appl. Soc. Psychol.* **2019**, *49*, 549–562. [CrossRef]
60. Calasanti, T.; King, N. Taking 'Women's Work' 'Like a Man': Husbands' Experiences of Care Work. *Gerontologist* **2007**, *47*, 516–527. [CrossRef]
61. Helgeson, V.S.; Fritz, H.L. A theory of unmitigated communion. *Personal. Soc. Psychol. Rev. Off. J. Soc. Personal. Soc. Psychol. Inc* **1998**, *2*, 173–183. [CrossRef]
62. Pérez-Fuentes, M.d.C.; Herrera-Peco, I.; Jurado, M.d.M.M.; Oropesa, N.F.; Gázquez Linares, J.J. Predictors of Threat from COVID-19: A Cross-Sectional Study in the Spanish Population. *J. Clin. Med.* **2021**, *10*, 692. [CrossRef] [PubMed]
63. Miller, J.M.; Perucchini, D.; Carchidi, L.T.; DeLancey, J.O.; Ashton-Miller, J. Pelvic floor muscle contraction during a cough and decreased vesical neck mobility. *Obstet. Gynecol.* **2001**, *97*, 255–260. [PubMed]
64. Miller, J.M.; Sampselle, C.; Ashton-Miller, J.; Hong, G.R.; DeLancey, J.O. Clarification and confirmation of the Knack maneuver: The effect of volitional pelvic floor muscle contraction to preempt expected stress incontinence. *Int. Urogynecology J. Pelvic Floor Dysfunct.* **2008**, *19*, 773–782. [CrossRef] [PubMed]
65. Babatunde, F.; MacDermid, J.; MacIntyre, N. Characteristics of therapeutic alliance in musculoskeletal physiotherapy and occupational therapy practice: A scoping review of the literature. *BMC Health Serv. Res.* **2017**, *17*, 375.

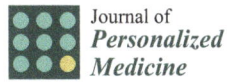

Article

Extracting New Temporal Features to Improve the Interpretability of Undiagnosed Type 2 Diabetes Mellitus Prediction Models

Simon Kocbek [1,*], Primož Kocbek [2], Lucija Gosak [2], Nino Fijačko [2] and Gregor Štiglic [1,2,3]

[1] Institute of Informatics, Faculty of Electrical Engineering and Computer Science, University of Maribor, 2000 Maribor, Slovenia; gregor.stiglic@um.si
[2] Faculty of Health Sciences, University of Maribor, 2000 Maribor, Slovenia; primoz.kocbek@um.si (P.K.); lucija.gosak2@um.si (L.G.); nino.fijacko@um.si (N.F.)
[3] Usher Institute, University of Edinburgh, Edinburgh EH8 9YL, UK
* Correspondence: simon.kocbek1@um.si

Citation: Kocbek, S.; Kocbek, P.; Gosak, L.; Fijačko, N.; Štiglic, G. Extracting New Temporal Features to Improve the Interpretability of Undiagnosed Type 2 Diabetes Mellitus Prediction Models. *J. Pers. Med.* **2022**, *12*, 368. https://doi.org/10.3390/jpm12030368

Academic Editors: Riitta Suhonen, Minna Stolt and David Edvardsson

Received: 6 December 2021
Accepted: 25 February 2022
Published: 28 February 2022

Publisher's Note: MDPI stays neutral with regard to jurisdictional claims in published maps and institutional affiliations.

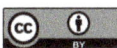

Copyright: © 2022 by the authors. Licensee MDPI, Basel, Switzerland. This article is an open access article distributed under the terms and conditions of the Creative Commons Attribution (CC BY) license (https://creativecommons.org/licenses/by/4.0/).

Abstract: Type 2 diabetes mellitus (T2DM) often results in high morbidity and mortality. In addition, T2DM presents a substantial financial burden for individuals and their families, health systems, and societies. According to studies and reports, globally, the incidence and prevalence of T2DM are increasing rapidly. Several models have been built to predict T2DM onset in the future or detect undiagnosed T2DM in patients. Additional to the performance of such models, their interpretability is crucial for health experts, especially in personalized clinical prediction models. Data collected over 42 months from health check-up examinations and prescribed drugs data repositories of four primary healthcare providers were used in this study. We propose a framework consisting of LogicRegression based feature extraction and Least Absolute Shrinkage and Selection operator based prediction modeling for undiagnosed T2DM prediction. Performance of the models was measured using Area under the ROC curve (AUC) with corresponding confidence intervals. Results show that using LogicRegression based feature extraction resulted in simpler models, which are easier for healthcare experts to interpret, especially in cases with many binary features. Models developed using the proposed framework resulted in an AUC of 0.818 (95% Confidence Interval (CI): 0.812–0.823) that was comparable to more complex models (i.e., models with a larger number of features), where all features were included in prediction model development with the AUC of 0.816 (95% CI: 0.810–0.822). However, the difference in the number of used features was significant. This study proposes a framework for building interpretable models in healthcare that can contribute to higher trust in prediction models from healthcare experts.

Keywords: diabetes mellitus type 2; prediction model; LogicRegression; interpretability

1. Introduction

Morbidity and mortality are often results of Type 2 diabetes mellitus (T2DM). In addition, T2DM presents a substantial financial drain for individuals and families, health systems, and societies. Globally, the incidence and prevalence of T2DM are increasing rapidly [1]. In 2017, it was estimated that 425 million people had any diabetes (approx. 5.5% of the worldwide population), of which 90% had T2DM. According to projection estimations, the prevalence is going to increase substantially in the coming years; by 2045, for example, a 48% increase of prevalence from the above numbers is expected, or in absolute numbers, an estimated 629 million people (approx. 6.6% of the worldwide population) are expected to be suffering from any diabetes [2]. T2DM can also lead to a substantially increased risk of macrovascular and microvascular disease, especially in inadequate glycemic control [3]. Impaired fasting glucose typically leads to slow progression of T2DM and, more importantly, its symptoms may remain undetected for many years.

Electronic Health Records (EHR) enable researchers to perform predictive modeling by providing a large amount of data [4] and many links have been found between patient health, the environment, and clinical decisions [5]. Nowadays, data mining techniques are applied to various fields of science, including healthcare and medicine [6]. Usually, techniques such as pattern recognition, disease prediction, and classification are used. Although multiple methods are available to build prediction models, prediction accuracy and data validity are often not realistic for model application in practice. Models usually perform well in specific datasets used to build the prediction models but are frequently not adapted sufficiently well when used on other datasets [7].

There is growing interest in clinical prediction, but models' interpretation is rarely based on end-user needs [8], and there is a lack of model interpretability techniques [9]. Interpretability of results based on predictive models is crucial in critical areas such as healthcare and is essential for adopting models. People often do not understand predictive models and therefore do not trust them [10]. LogicRegression can be used to improve the interpretability of predictive models.

LogicRegression is an adaptive classification and regression procedure which searches for Boolean (logic) combinations of binary variables that best explain the variability in the outcome [11,12]. LogicRegression looks for logical combinations of binary features. We can explain the variability of the outcome feature and thus reveal the features and interactions related to the response and whether they have predictive capabilities [11].

The purpose of this paper is to use LogicRegression to make final models less complex (i.e., with less features) and the features that appear in the interpretation of predictive models much more understandable. This is also important for health professionals, as they do not have the necessary knowledge to apply prediction models or interpret the results obtained. This is also important from the patient's point of view and the provision of personalized healthcare. Simple interpretation will make it easier for the patient to understand the operation of the predictive model and outcome. The paper presents an example of using extracted features using Logic Regression to improve the personalized interpretability of the prediction models to the end-users.

2. Materials and Methods

2.1. Data

EHR data consisted of health check-ups and prescribed drugs data from four Slovenian primary healthcare providers for a period of approximately 3.5 years from 12 December 2014 to 27 July 2018. Data for 21,138 medical records and 114 potential useful features were exported from the healthcare information systems after the on-site anonymization process. Our first step was the removal of features with more than 20% of missing data (73 potential features remain). Since our focus when building prediction models was on the fasting plasma glucose level (FPGL) measurement (mmol/L) and results of Finnish Diabetes Risk Score (FINDRISC) features, which included Age, Gender, BMI, Waist circumference, Active_30_min, Medication, High_BS, Grocer, and Diab_fam we selected cases with all those values present (4086 such cases remained). We next removed (a) cases with more than 50% of the features were not available (4067 cases left), (b) removed all duplicate entries (in cases of multiple patient visits only the most recent visit was included) (3535 cases left), (c) cases not having a previous diabetes diagnosis (3176 cases left) and entries where: (d) FPGL was not reported giving us a total of 3120 records of patient visits were left for development of a prediction model to estimate the risk of undiagnosed T2DM. Data included demographics, questionnaire answers for lifestyle choices, physiological measurements, and prescribed medications for two time periods.

Binary features were created for prescribed drugs and questionnaire responses, which resulted in nine numeric and 161 binary features where specific drug related feature was coded as positive in cases where a patient was prescribed with the specific drug during the last 4 months prior to the visit. The target feature was binary, where positive cases were defined as having FPGL higher than 6.1 mmol/L consisting of 24.71% (n = 771) of patient visits.

We imputed the remaining missing values using the MissForest based approach [7], which on average meant features with 12.25% missing values as we initially already removed features with 20% or more missing values. MissForest is used to impute missing values particularly in the case of mixed-type data. It can be used to impute continuous and/or categorical data including complex interactions and nonlinear relations. The summary information of the basic predictive and target features can be seen in Table 1. Please see Table A1 for list of all features used in the experiments.

Table 1. Summary table basic predictive and target features for healthcare centers.

Original Feature Name	Description	FPGL $\leq$ 6.1 mmol/L [75.29% [n = 2349]]	FPGL > 6.1 mmol/L [24.71% [n = 771]]
Age [mean (standard deviation – SD)]	Age in years	56.07 (SD = 13.2)	61.77 (SD = 10.98)
Gender_M [%(n)]	Percentage of males	37.16 (n = 873)	54.47 (n = 420)
BMI [mean (SD)]	Body mass index	28.89 (SD = 5.39)	32.16 (SD = 13.21)
WC [mean (SD)]	Waist circumference in cm	96.25 (SD = 13.89)	103.48 (SD = 13.8)
Active_30_min (Q2) [%(n)]	Active at least 30 minutes a day?	64.88 (n = 1524)	52.27 (n = 403)
Medication (Q3) [%(n)]	Blood pressure medication?	40.19 (n = 944)	60.18 (n = 464)
High_BS [%(n)] (Q4)	Ever measured high blood sugar?	7.32 (n = 172)	47.47 (n = 366)
Grocer [%(n)] (Q18)	Eat vegetable/fruit daily?	90.59 (n = 2128)	78.99 (n = 609)
Diab_fam [%(n)] (Q6)	Diabetes in family?	69.65 (n = 1636)	61.74 (n = 476)
FPGL [mean (SD)]	Fasting plasma glucose level	5.26 (SD = 0.44)	6.74 (SD = 0.8)

2.2. Experimental Setup

The data were split into 80% to derive five extracted features using Logic Regression [13] and 20% to build and evaluate the final prediction models.

Finally, we created three datasets with the following features: all numeric and binary (170), all numeric and logic (14), and all numeric, binary, and logic features (175). On each dataset, we built a predictive model separately using the same training data.

The Least Absolute Shrinkage and Selection Operator (LASSO) [13] was used to build prediction models. We repeated each 10-fold cross-validation ten times to estimate the variance in Area under the ROC curve (AUC) that was used as our classification performance metric.

3. Results

We split the results in this section into two parts. First, we present selected logic attributes extracted from the dataset for the undiagnosed T2DM prediction use case. Next, we present the performance evaluation of the model.

3.1. Feature Extraction Using LogicRegression Approach

To demonstrate the practical example of using LogicRegression based extraction of new features to improve interpretability of the prediction models, we provide the results of the first cross-validation run.

The selected use case resulted in five logic features (Table 2) extracted from the complete set of features.

In Table 3, we list all features that were selected in at least 50% of runs in our experiments with LASSO on the dataset with numeric and logic features, while Table 4 lists features for the dataset with numeric, binary and logic features. Frequency (freq) shows in how many experiment runs each feature appeared in the final set of features.

Table 2. Extracted logic features with corresponding LogicRegression rules and descriptions.

Feature	Rule	Description
L1	(ATC_J01EE01 or (not Q41))	Prescribed sulfadiazine and trimethoprim, or never measured high blood sugar.
L2	Q51	Seldom eat fruit and vegetable.
L3	((ATC_M01AE02 and ATC_J01CE10) or (not SE))	Prescribed naproxen and benzathine phenoxymethylpenicillin or not socially endangered.
L4	Q494	Daily consumption of alcohol in the last 12 months.
L5	(MSE or ATC_D01AE15)	Medium socially endangered or prescribed antifungals for dermatological use.

Table 3. Selected features with the Least Absolute Shrinkage and Selection Operator (LASSO) on the dataset with numeric and logic features.

Feature	Freq	Description
−Gender	100	Gender
+Blood_pressure	100	Blood pressure
+Heart_beat	100	Heart_beat
+Age	100	Age
+BMI	100	Body mass index
+WC	100	Waist circumference
−L1	100	Logic feature 1
−L2	100	Logic feature 2
−L3	100	Logic feature 3
−Body_height	99	Body height
+Body_weight	83	Body weight

Table 4. Selected features with LASSO on the dataset with binary, numeric, and logic features.

Feature	Freq	Description
−L3	100	Logic feature 3
−L4	100	Logic feature 4
+L5	100	Logic feature 5
+Blood_pressure	100	Blood pressure
+WC	100	Waist circumference in cm
+Heart_beat	100	Heart_beat
+Age	100	Age in years
+Q45	100	Ever measured high blood sugar? Yes
−Gender	100	Gender
+Q32	93	Using drug(s) for lowering blood pressure
+Body_weight	87	Body weight
−Non_smoker	87	Non-smoker
+L2	79	Logic attribute 2
−Q321	78	Most often used oil is vegetable oil
−Non_drinker	77	No alcohol consumption
−Q583	75	Handle stress with hardship
+Q62	74	Parent, brother, or sister have diabetes
+BMI	69	Body Mass Index
−Q161	63	2 meals per day on average
−Q301	51	No habit of using salt at the table

It can be observed that L1, L2, and L3 were used by prediction models derived from the data in all folds of all evaluation runs. Thus, confirming a high contribution of extracted logic features.

In the case of results from a much wider set of features (Table 4), we can see a higher variance in selection by the final prediction models. Four (L2, L3, L4, L5) logic features can be found among the varaibles that were selected in at least 50% of evaluation runs.

3.2. Performance Evaluation

In Figure 1, we summarize AUC and a selected number of features for all three datasets: no_logic (numeric and binary features), all_logic (numeric, binary, and logic features), and num_logic (numeric and logic features).

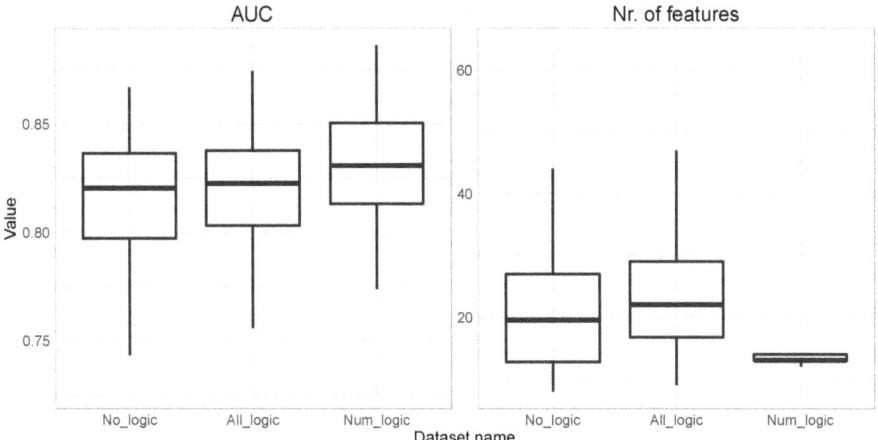

Figure 1. Selected features with the Least Absolute Shrinkage and Selection Operator (LASSO) on the dataset with numeric and logic features.

We can observe a slowly increasing average AUC from 0.816 (Standard Deviation (SD)) = 0.03) in no_logic to 0.819 (SD = 0.03) in all_logic and finally 0.829 (SD = 0.03) in the num_logic dataset. When looking at the number of selected feature averages and its variation, we can observe that it slowly increases from 21.7 (SD = 11.18) in no_logic to 23.7 (SD = 10.09) in all_logic but it then almost halves to 13.35 (SD = 0.63) in the num_logic dataset. The SD is steadily increasing in the first two cases, but then it decreases sharply to below 1 (SD = 0.63), which means that out of the 100 repetitions in 92 cases 13 or 14 features were selected in the num_logic dataset. This indicates a very stable final prediction models when comparing num_logic based solutions to no_logic or all_logic.

4. Discussion and Conclusions

In this paper, we compared three dimensionality reduction approaches to improve the interpretability of undiagnosed T2DM prediction models (Please note that the calibration of a prediction models was not the scope of this paper and presents a limitation). A simple LASSO regression approach is compared to two variants where a pre-selection of predictive features is conducted on the training set using LogicRegression to consequently simplify a final set of features obtained by the LASSO regression. We kept all original features with added logic features in the first variant, while in the second variant, we kept only numeric and logic features.

Results showed that logic features resulted in simpler models with lower number of features, which are potentially easier to interpret by healthcare experts. This is especially important in the field of personalized medicine. Measured AUC was similar to more complex models, where all features were included. It should be noted that although our method resulted in a lower number of features, some of the logic features may not be straightforward to interpret (e.g., the feature L3 in this paper). To address this issue, we plan to include an interactive system in our future work, where the user would specify the maximum number of original features included in generated logic features in cases where the final model would include many complex logic features. As a result of the current work, in cases when some of the final features are hard to interpret, we recommend that the user uses LogicRegression settings to adjust the complexity of final logic features for achieving satisfactory results.

When healthcare professionals and patients know which features are important in obtaining the outcome of a prediction model and how they can be combined, it helps to understand and increase the level of trust in the decision-making systems [10]. With greater interpretability of the model, we better understand and interpret the forecast for end-users and improve the support in decision-making for health professionals based on data [14]. More complex models such as deep neural networks [15] allow high accuracy but are difficult to explain. Simple models (e.g., decision trees) are less accurate but allow for more straightforward explanations [16]. Therefore, sophisticated machine learning models usually offer better performance than traditional simple models but are difficult for health professionals to understand. However, in many cases simple models also provide good classification performance, which is not significantly different from more complex models [17]. Our results confirm this hypothesis. Comprehensible models are known for their contribution to higher trust in prediction models from the end-users in healthcare.

Interpretability techniques are often categorized according to the time period used to develop the machine learning model [14]. Pre-model approaches are independent of the model and may be employed prior to making a choice on which model to use. Our approach presented in this study belongs in this group of interpretability approaches along with techniques such as Principal Component Analysis (PCA), t-Distributed Stochastic Neighbor Embedding (t-SNE), and some clustering techniques. While Molnar [18] classifies PCA, t-SNE, and clustering methods as interpretable methods, it is worth noting that the interpretability of attributes transformed using PCA, embeddings, or clusters cannot provide comprehensible medical interpretation, but can be used to visualize the results and highlight patterns of interest from an interpretability standpoint. The proposed approach is much more interpretable, despite the possible complex combinations of features that might occur as a result of LogicRegression.

During the experiments, we also observed the unstable behavior of logic regression, where different logic features were selected with each run of the cross-validation. Although this did not influence the average number of selected features it resulted in instability of the interpretability of the model. Another limitation are the combinations of the features used in extracted features. For example, the first extracted feature (L1) suggested that checking whether a person did not experience elevated blood sugar in the past should be accompanied by checking for sulfadiazine and trimethoprim use in the last 4 months – this extracted feature works as a protective factor as seen from Table 3. We see this as a disadvantage of logic regression since different conclusions can be made based on selected features. This could be resolved to some extent by using exhaustive search methods to extract logic features resulting in extremely long running times, presenting another drawback, especially in cases where personalized models would be built. To personalize the solution even further, it would be worth exploring the prediction model development for each specific patient at the time of the examination using the subset of the data where patients similar to the examined patient would be assigned a higher weight in comparison to other patients (boosting principle).

Although our work is the field of healthcare, we believe that our results can also be applied in other emerging fields of applied prediction modeling where interpretability of results is important such as security [19] or ecology [20]. In future work, we will explore effectiveness of our methods in the broader field of security, specifically, to help us understand how misinformation (e.g., intentionally misleading information) is being spread.

Author Contributions: Conceptualization, S.K., P.K. and G.Š.; methodology, S.K., P.K. and G.Š.; software, S.K., P.K. and G.Š.; validation, S.K., P.K. and G.Š.; formal analysis, S.K. and P.K.; investigation, S.K., P.K., L.G. and G.Š.; resources, P.K. and G.Š.; data curation, S.K. and P.K.; writing—original draft preparation, S.K., P.K., L.G. and G.Š.; writing—review and editing, S.K., P.K., L.G., N.F. and G.Š.; visualization, P.K.; supervision, G.Š.; project administration, G.Š.; funding acquisition, G.Š. All authors have read and agreed to the published version of the manuscript.

Funding: This research was funded by Slovenian Research Agency (grants number ARRS N2-0101 and ARRS P2-0057) and the European Union's Horizon 2020 Research and Innovation Program under the Cybersecurity CONCORDIA project (GA No. 830927).

Institutional Review Board Statement: Not applicable.

Informed Consent Statement: Not applicable.

Data Availability Statement: Restrictions apply to the availability of these data. Data was obtained from Nova vizija d.d. and are available from the authors with the permission of Nova vizija d.d.

Conflicts of Interest: The authors declare no conflict of interest.

Appendix A

Table A1. List of original features with description and their possible values. Please note that Nominal features were processed in such a way that for each possible value a new feature was generated. For example, the feature Q43 resulted in three features for each possible value (new features were named Q431, Q432 and Q433). Drug features are marked with the Anatomical Therapeutic Chemical (ATC) classification. The final set contained 170 features.

Name	Description	Value
Age	Age of the patient	Numeric
Gender	Gender of the patient	Male, Female
BMI	Body Mass Index of the patient	Numeric
Blood_pressure	Blood pressure of the patient	Numeric
WC	Waist circumference of the patient	Numeric
Heart_beat	Heart beat of the patient	Numeric
Body_weight	Body weight of the patient	Numeric
Body_height	Body height of the patient	Numeric
Smoking_status	Smoking status of the patient	Non-smoker, Smoker, Ex-smoker, Passive smoker
Eating_habits	Assessment of eating habits	Adequate, Satisfactory, Inadequate
Drinking_status	Drinking status	Abstinent, Less risky drinking, Risky, Harmful, Addictive
SDH	Social determinants of health	Not threatened, Medium threatened, Threatened
PAS	Physical activity status	Sufficient, Borderline, Insufficient
Stress	Level of stress	Not threatened, Threatened
RD	Risk of depression	No significant risk of depression, Risk of depression
Q18	How often do you usually eat vegetables?	Never Points, 4-6 times a week, 1x a day, More than 1x a day
Q16	How many meals do you eat on average per day?	2 or less, 3 to 5, 6 or more
Q2	Are you physically active for at least 30 min/day?	Yes, No

Table A1. *Cont.*

Name	Description	Value
Q3	Do you take medication to lower your blood pressure?	Yes, No
Q30	Do you have a habit of salting dishes at the table?	Yes, No
Q32	On average, which type of fat do you use most in food preparation or as a spread?	Vegetable oils, Cream, Butter, Lard, Hard margarines, Soft margarines, High-fat spreads, Low-fat spreads, Chocolate spread, Peanut butter, Pate, Cream Spread, Mayonnaise
Q4	Have you ever had your blood sugar measured?	Yes, No
Q43	How many times in a typical week do you engage in vigorous physical activity for at least 25 minutes each time to the point where you are breathing and sweating?	0 or 1 times per week, 2 times per week, 3 or more times per week
Q44	How many times in a typical week do you engage in moderate physical activity for at least 30 minutes each time, to the extent that you breathe a little faster and warm up?	0 or 1 times per week, 2 to 4 times per week, 5 or more times per week
Q47	How often have you drunk drinks containing alcohol in the last 12 months?	Never, Once a month or less, 2 to 4 times a month, 2 to 3 times a week, 4 or more times a week
Q48	In the last 12 months, how many measures of a drink containing alcohol did you usually have when you were drinking?	Zero to 1 measure, 2 measures, 3 or 4 measures, 5 or 6 measures, 7 or more
Q49	In the last 12 months, how often have you had 6 or more sips on one occasion for men and 4 or more sips on one occasion for women?	Never, Less than once a month, 1 to 3 times a month, 1 to 3 times a week, Daily or almost daily
Q51	In the last 12 months, how often have you needed an alcoholic drink in the morning to recover from excessive drinking the day before?	Never, Less than once a month, 1 to 3 times a month, 1 to 3 times a week, Daily or almost daily
Q57	How often do you feel tense, stressed or under a lot of pressure?	Never, Rarely, Occasionally, Often, Every day
Q58	How do you manage the tensions, stresses and pressures you experience in your life?	Easily, Able to, Able to with more efforts, Very difficult, Can't
Q59	How often in the past 2 weeks have you felt little interest and satisfaction in the things you do?	Not at all, A few days, More than half the days, Almost every day
Q6	Does family have diabetes?	No, Outer family, Inner family
Q60	How often have you felt depressed, depressed, despairing in the past 2 weeks?	Not at all, A few days, More than half the days, Almost every day

Table A1. *Cont.*

Name	Description	Value
Q69	Please indicate the last school you attended.	Primary school incomplete, Primary school, 2 or 3-year vocational school, 4-year secondary school or gymnasium, Graduate, Postgraduate
Q70	What is your current employment status?	Employed, Self-employed, Unemployed, Student, Retired, Disabled pensioner, Permanently disabled, Housewife
Q71	How do you get through the month based in income?	Good, Occasional problems, I have problems
ATC_A02BC01	Omeprazole	Binary (0,1)
ATC_A02BC02	Pantoprazole	Binary (0,1)
ATC_A11CC05	Colecalciferol	Binary (0,1)
ATC_B01AC06	Acetylsalicylic acid	Binary (0,1)
ATC_C03BA11	Indapamide	Binary (0,1)
ATC_C07AB07	Bisoprolol	Binary (0,1)
ATC_C09AA04	Perindopril	Binary (0,1)
ATC_D01AC01	Clotrimazole	Binary (0,1)
ATC_D01AE15	Terbinafine	Binary (0,1)
ATC_D07AC13	Mometasone	Binary (0,1)
ATC_G04BD09	Trospium	Binary (0,1)
ATC_J01CA04	Amoxicillin	Binary (0,1)
ATC_J01CE10	Benzathine phenoxymethylpenicillin	Binary (0,1)
ATC_J01CR02	Amoxicillin and beta-lactamase inhibitor	Binary (0,1)
ATC_J01EE01	Sulfadiazine /trimethoprim	Binary (0,1)
ATC_J01FA10	Azithromycin	Binary (0,1)
ATC_M01AB05	Diclofenac	Binary (0,1)
ATC_M01AE01	Ibuprofen	Binary (0,1)
ATC_M01AE02	Naproxen	Binary (0,1)
ATC_N02AJ13	Tramadol and paracetamol	Binary (0,1)
ATC_N02BB02	Metamizole sodium	Binary (0,1)
ATC_N02BE01	Paracetamol	Binary (0,1)
ATC_N05BA08	Bromazepam	Binary (0,1)
ATC_N05BA12	Alprazolam	Binary (0,1)
ATC_N05CF02	Zolpidem	Binary (0,1)
ATC_R01AD09	Mometasone	Binary (0,1)
ATC_R03AC02	Salbutamol	Binary (0,1)
ATC_R03AL01	Fenoterol and ipratropium bromide	Binary (0,1)
ATC_R06AE07	Cetirizine	Binary (0,1)
ATC_R06AX13	Loratadine	Binary (0,1)
ATC_S01AA12	Tobramycin	Binary (0,1)

References

1. Einarson, T.R.; Acs, A.; Ludwig, C.; Panton, U.H. Prevalence of cardiovascular disease in type 2 diabetes: A systematic literature review of scientific evidence from across the world in 2007–2017. *Cardiovasc. Diabetol.* **2018**, *17*, 83. [CrossRef]
2. International Diabetes Federation. *IDF Diabetes Atlas 2021*, 10th ed.; IDF: Brussels, Belgium, 2021.
3. Mohammedi, K.; Woodward, M.; Marre, M.; Colagiuri, S.; Cooper, M.; Harrap, S.; Mancia, G.; Poulter, N.; Williams, B.; Zoungas, S.; et al. Comparative effects of microvascular and macrovascular disease on the risk of major outcomes in patients with type 2 diabetes. *Cardiovasc. Diabetol.* **2017**, *16*, 95. [CrossRef]
4. Steele, A.J.; Denaxas, S.C.; Shah, A.D.; Hemingway, H.; Luscombe, N.M. Machine learning models in electronic health records can outperform conventional survival models for predicting patient mortality in coronary artery disease. *PLoS ONE* **2018**, *13*, e0202344. [CrossRef] [PubMed]
5. La Cava, W.; Bauer, C.; Moore, J.H.; Pendergrass, S.A. Interpretation of machine learning predictions for patient outcomes in electronic health records. *AMIA Annu. Symp. Proc.* **2019**, *2019*, 572–581.
6. Birjandi, S.M.; Khasteh, S.H. A survey on data mining techniques used in medicine. *J. Diabetes Metab. Disord.* **2021**, *20*, 2055–2071. [CrossRef]
7. Stekhoven, D.J.; Bühlmann, P. Missforest—Non-parametric missing value imputation for mixed-type data. *Bioinformatics* **2012**, *28*, 112–118. [CrossRef]
8. Barda, A.J.; Horvat, C.M.; Hochheiser, H. A qualitative research framework for the design of user-centered displays of explanations for machine learning model predictions in healthcare. *BMC Med. Inform. Decis. Mak.* **2020**, *20*, 257. [CrossRef]
9. Elshawi, R.; Al-Mallah, M.H.; Sakr, S. On the interpretability of machine learning-based model for predicting hypertension. *BMC Med. Inform. Decis. Mak.* **2019**, *19*, 146. [CrossRef] [PubMed]
10. Lakkaraju, H.; Bach, S.H.; Leskovec, J. Interpretable decision sets: A joint framework for description and prediction. In Proceedings of the 22nd ACM SIGKDD International Conference on Knowledge Discovery and Data Mining, San Francisco, CA, USA, 13–17 August 2016; pp. 1675–1684.
11. Schwender, H.; Ruczinski, I. Logic regression and its extensions. *Adv. Genet.* **2010**, *72*, 25–45. [PubMed]
12. Ruczinski, I.; Kooperberg, C.; LeBlanc, M. Logic regression. *J. Comput. Graph. Stat.* **2003**, *12*, 475–511. [CrossRef]
13. Friedman, J.; Hastie, T.; Tibshirani, R. Regularization paths for generalized linear models via coordinate descent. *J. Stat. Softw.* **2010**, *33*. [CrossRef]
14. Stiglic, G.; Kocbek, P.; Fijacko, N.; Zitnik, M.; Verbert, K.; Cilar, L. Interpretability of machine learning-based prediction models in healthcare. *Wiley Interdiscip. Rev. Data Min. Knowl. Discov.* **2020**, *10*, e1379. [CrossRef]
15. Emmert-Streib, F.; Yang, Z.; Feng, H.; Tripathi, S.; Dehmer, M. An introductory review of deep learning for prediction models with big data. *Front. Artif. Intell.* **2020**, *3*, 4. [CrossRef] [PubMed]
16. Lim, T.S.; Loh, W.Y.; Shih, Y.S. A comparison of prediction accuracy, complexity, and training time of thirty-three old and new classification algorithms. *Mach. Learn.* **2000**, *40*, 203–228. [CrossRef]
17. Stiglic, G.; Kocbek, S.; Pernek, I.; Kokol, P. Comprehensive decision tree models in bioinformatics. *PLoS ONE* **2012**, *7*, e33812. [CrossRef]
18. Molnar, C. *Interpretable Machine Learning*; Lulu.com: Research Triangle, NC, USA, 2020.
19. Brigugilio, W.R. Machine Learning Interpretability in Malware Detection. Ph.D. Dissertation, University of Windsor, Windsor, ON, Canada, 2020.
20. Lucas, T.C. A translucent box: Interpretable machine learning in ecology. *Ecol. Monogr.* **2020**, *90*, e01422. [CrossRef]

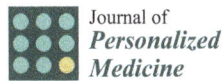

Article

What Influences Women to Adhere to Pelvic Floor Exercises after Physiotherapy Treatment? A Qualitative Study for Individualized Pelvic Health Care

Beatriz Navarro-Brazález, Fernando Vergara-Pérez, Virginia Prieto-Gómez *, Beatriz Sánchez-Sánchez, María José Yuste-Sánchez and María Torres-Lacomba

Physiotherapy in Women's Health (FPSM) Research Group, Physiotherapy Department, Faculty of Medicine and Health Sciences, University of Alcalá, 28871 Alcalá de Henares, Spain; b.navarro@uah.es (B.N.-B.); fernando.vergara@uah.es (F.V.-P.); beatriz.sanchez@uah.es (B.S.-S.); marijo.yuste@uah.es (M.J.Y.-S.); maria.torres@uah.es (M.T.-L.)
* Correspondence: v.prieto@uah.es; Tel.: +34-91-885-4828

Abstract: Conservative treatment of pelvic floor dysfunction (PFD) includes therapeutic exercise for pelvic floor muscle (PFM) training or other complementary exercise modalities, such as hypopressive exercises. However, the long-term effectiveness of the conservative treatment depends on a patient's adherence to the exercises and the integration of professional health advice into their daily life. The objective of this study was to establish the adherence experience of women with diagnosed PFD in home-based exercises after an intensive face-to-face physiotherapy treatment. A qualitative study from an interpretive paradigm was developed. Semi-structured individual and group interviews were performed 6 months after finishing individual physiotherapy treatment. The interviews were recorded, fully transcribed and analyzed thematically by creating categories. Thirty-one women were interviewed. The women reported that their adherence to home PFM exercises depended on the exercise program itself, its efficacy, their personal experiences with the exercises, intrinsic factors such as self-awareness or beliefs, and extrinsic factors, such as professional or instrumental feedback. Thus, therapeutic adherence could be more likely with effective physiotherapy programs that include mutually agreed home exercises and simple movements women can build into their daily lives. Improving awareness and knowledge of the pelvic region and the importance of PFM treatment as well as consideration for potential worsening of PFD will also encourage women to adhere to the exercises.

Keywords: pelvic floor muscle exercises; pelvic floor dysfunction; qualitative research; therapeutic exercise; therapeutic adherence; women's health physiotherapy

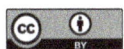

1. Introduction

The pelvic floor muscles (PFM) play an important role in the preservation of urinary and anal continence, in pelvic organ support and in sexual function, among others [1]. The weakness and loss of PFM properties are associated with the development and maintenance of pelvic floor dysfunctions (PFD) [2,3]. Prevalence studies estimate that PFD affect up to 40% of women [4], including symptoms of urinary incontinence (UI), pelvic organ prolapse (POP), and anal incontinence (AI), which are the most frequent PFD. The first line of treatment for mild PFD is focused on specific PFM exercises [5,6], which can involve a therapeutic education program [7] to provide knowledge and self-management strategies to women. In addition, global exercise modalities, such as hypopressive exercises, have recently begun to be included in PFD treatment [8–10], to train the PFM in coordination with posture and adjacent muscles. However, the long-term effectiveness of conservative treatment does not seem to depend exclusively on the exercise method. Patient adherence to a prescribed exercise program and to health professional advice seems to be one of the determining variables to ensure the success of the treatment in the short and long term [11].

The determining factors of therapeutic adherence to PFM exercises have been analyzed and classified based on patient personal parameters or factors dependent on physiotherapeutic performance. Motivation, perceived self-efficacy and benefit expectations are identified as personal facilitating factors, while misconceptions, false beliefs or low body awareness are presented as personal adherence barriers. Regarding physiotherapy treatment, a structured program and close supervision are positive adherence factors, and a high number of sessions and abstract concepts are associated with poor adherence [12–14].

Hay-Smith et al. [15] inquired about the experiences of women in performing PFM exercises at home and observed that a high degree of self-efficacy was needed, which could be improved with individualized educational programs. Recent qualitative studies in women with PFD point to the patient's demand for [16] and the perceived usefulness [17] of a structured educational program on the functions and dysfunctions of the pelvic floor, on risk factors and on coping strategies. However, further studies to understand and delve into the patient's experiences are required to develop more long-term effective and patient-centered programs [18,19].

In a previously published randomized clinical trial [8], women who experienced stress or mixed urinary incontinence, anal incontinence, or mild pelvic organ prolapse received physiotherapy treatment. Participants were randomly allocated to either PFM training and an educational strategy (PFMT group), or to hypopressive exercises and an educational strategy (HE group), or to PFM training plus hypopressive exercises and an educational strategy (PFMT+HE group). The three programs were conducted individually and face-to-face by the same physiotherapist specialized in women's health. The physiotherapy treatment lasted 8 weeks, with two visits of 45 min each week. Moreover, women were advised to carry out 15 min of daily home exercises based on the specifications of the physiotherapist depending on the intervention group. Despite the difference between the study exercises, the three groups showed similar adherence data, not being able to understand or deepen the reasons for continuing or abandoning the home guidelines.

Therefore, the aim of the present study was to establish the experience of women to adhere to home exercises recommended by their physiotherapist after completing an intensive face-to-face treatment, which included PFM exercises and/or hypopressive exercises and an individually tailored educational program.

2. Materials and Methods

2.1. Research Team and Reflexibility

From October 2014 to June 2016, semi-structured individual interviews and focus groups were conducted. The personal interviews were carried out by the physiotherapist who performed the 2 months of individual treatments. This assumed that the participants knew the physiotherapist, and a prior relationship of trust could have been established. The physiotherapist (B.N.-B.) was a woman with more than 5 years of professional experience in women's health and with previous experience in qualitative interviews. The focus groups were led by another woman physiotherapist (B.S.-S.), a university professor, who also specialized in women's health and was experienced in qualitative research interviews. She was not connected with the study in order to achieve the appearance of a new perspective [20], and the participants did not know her. All the interviews began with the presentation of the objective of the study, the guarantee of the confidentiality of the contributions and the request for permission to record the audio of the interviews.

2.2. Study Design

A qualitative descriptive study was developed from an interpretative paradigm design to present the women's perspectives on the phenomenon of adherence [21] to the pelvic floor exercise program after a randomized clinical trial [8]. The Clinical Research Committee of the Principe de Asturias Hospital (OE20/2013) approved the study, which was registered at ClinicalTrials.gov (NCT02259712). The consolidated criteria for reporting qualitative research (COREQ) were followed for reporting [22].

2.3. Participant Selection and Setting

Purposive sampling was used to select women from the three intervention groups. Women who were included in the randomized clinical trial and were in the follow-up period after the physiotherapy treatment were invited to participate in the qualitative study. The inclusion criteria were to have completed the 2 months of physiotherapy treatment in any of the three study groups, for a period of between 3 and 6 months to have elapsed after its completion, to have availability to attend the interview, speak Spanish fluently and to freely agree to participate. Since no statistically significant differences were found in the adherence of the three study groups, the qualitative study was proposed and aimed at all participants, regardless of the assigned treatment group. The capture of the individual interviews was carried out in person during the physiotherapy reviews, inviting participants to carry out the interview at a time that best suited them. Group interviews were scheduled, and the participants were contacted by phone to give them a face-to-face appointment.

A total of 20 individual semi-structured face-to-face interviews were completed: nine interviews of women allocated to the PFMT group, six interviews of women in the HE group, and five interviews of participants who were in the PFMT+HE group. Furthermore, three group interviews were conducted, one for each intervention group with the participation of three to five women in each group. Three participants rejected the interview due to time incompatibility. The appointments were developed in a private room at the FPSM-RG laboratory at the University of Alcalá (Madrid, Spain). During the interviews, only the participants and the interviewer were present.

Since the age of the participants [23], the PFD symptoms, or the improvement found with the physiotherapy treatment could influence the results of the interviews [14], a descriptive analysis of the sample was carried out. This description only provides a descriptive character of the participant and not a criterion for interpretive analysis. To verify normal distribution of the data, the Kolmogorov–Smirnov statistical test was used. The normal quantitative variables were described with means and standard deviations. The categorical variables were described with absolute frequencies and percentages. For this statistical analysis, the IMB SPSS Statistics version 20 software was used.

The mean age of the participants was 49.74 (10.78) years, with a BMI of 26.01 (4.88) kg/m^2, 16 (51.6%) of them had experienced menopause, and in relation to the history of pregnancy and childbirth had an average of 2 (1) vaginal deliveries. Annual household income indicated that the study population belonged to the middle class; 35.5% of the women had a university education, 51.6% had a basic education, and one participant indicated that she had never attended school. All the participants suffered from some PFD, since it was an inclusion criterion, presenting UI in 87.1%, IA in 48.4%, and POP in 51.6% of the women. Comparison of PFM strength and quality of life survey results before and after the physiotherapy treatment indicated improvements in all participants. Table 1 shows the characteristics of the sample in more detail.

Table 1. Demographic and clinical data of the participating women.

Clinical Characteristics	$n = 31$
Age years, (SD)	49.74 (10.78)
BMI kg/m^2, (SD)	26.01 (4.88)
Menopause, n (%)	16 (51.6%)
Parity, (SD)	2 (1)
Education	
Never went to school n (%)	1 (3.2%)
Primary school n (%)	7 (22.6%)
Secondary school n (%)	9 (29%)
Vocational Education and Training/ Certificate of Higher Education n (%)	3 (9.7%)
University degree n (%)	11 (35.5%)

Table 1. *Cont.*

Clinical Characteristics	n = 31	
Annual income		
<12,000 €	8 (25.8%)	
12,000–24,000 €	9 (29%)	
24,000–36,000 €	11 (35.5%)	
36,000–48,000 €	2 (6.5%)	
>48,000 €	1 (3.2%)	
Pelvic floor dysfunction	31 (100%)	
UI, n (%)	27 (87.1%)	
AI, n (%)	15 (48.4%)	
POP, n (%)	16 (51.6%)	
Modified Oxford scale	Pre-treatment	Post-treatment
0 n (%)	1 (3.2%)	0
1 n (%)	3 (9.7%)	1 (3.2%)
2 n (%)	4 (12.9%)	1 (3.2%)
3 n (%)	15 (48.4%)	3 (9.7%)
4 n (%)	8 (25.8%)	7 (22.6%)
5 n (%)	0	19 (61.3%)
Manometry cmH2O, (SD)	20.23 (14.71)	30.04 (16.94)
PFDI-20 total, (SD)	76.44 (43.11)	49.23 (43.8)
PFIQ-7 total, (SD)	23.81 (52.37)	9.52 (23.81)

n: Number; SD: Standard deviation; BMI: Body mass index; UI: Urinary incontinence; AI: Anal incontinence; POP: Pelvic organ prolapse; PFDI-20: Pelvic Floor Distress Inventory Short Form; PFIQ-7: Pelvic Floor Impact Questionnaire Short Form.

2.4. Data Collection

Prior to the start of the interviews, a group of three physiotherapists, specializing in women's health (M.T.-L. and M.Y.-S.) and qualitative research (F.V.-P.), and a gynecologist developed referral questions (Table 2). After the guide questions were prepared, they were presented to the interviewers to consider if they needed any changes. A pilot test was carried out with a participant. This interview was excluded because it was not recorded and was only conducted to ensure the understandability and relevance of the questions.

Table 2. Guide questions for the individual and focal group interviews.

Number	Question
1	What do you think is the effect of the exercises? What do you think they are good for?
2	At what time of the day do you practice them?
3	What exercises do you practice the most? Why?
4	What exercises do you practice the least? Why?
5	What do you think makes it easier to practice the exercises?
6	What do you think makes it difficult to practice the exercises?
7	What responsibility do you think you have to improve your symptoms?
8	Are the exercises worth doing?
9	Was attending the pelvic floor physiotherapy program worth it?
10	Have you included exercises at some point in your daily life? When?
11	Do you associate the exercises with any situation with a preventive objective?

All the interviews included in this study were audio recorded with participant permission. No field notes were taken, the interviews were conducted only once, and the interview transcriptions were not returned to participants.

The mean duration was 24 min for individual interviews and 65 min for focal group interviews. Data saturation was considered when the information collected was consistent with the previous interviews. This fact was shared and discussed with the physiotherapists who participated in transcribing the interviews.

2.5. Data Analysis

Five physiotherapist members of the FPSM-RG (B.N.-B., F.V.-P, V.P.-G., M.T.-L. and B.S.-S.) manually transcribed the recorded interviews. Different codes were established as part of the intervention group allocation, to sort the interview (individual or in group) and the participant intervention order, with the purpose of securing the women's anonymity. Researchers' triangulation process was performed, where three physiotherapist members analyzed the resultant texts (B.N.-B., F.V.P and M.T.-L.). In an iterative consensus process, the researchers conducted an open and axial coding since a previous theoretical framework was not used, as well as related codes and categories. The transcription encoding was performed using the ATLAS.ti version 6.1 software (Scientific Software Development GMBH, Berlin, Germany). The interviews and the categorization of the themes were carried out in Spanish. Quotes and categories were later translated into English.

3. Results

Five themes emerged from the literal transcription analyses: the exercise program, the program efficacy, personal experiences with exercises, intrinsic factors, and extrinsic factors (Table 3).

Table 3. Main themes and codes extracted from participants' interviews.

Themes	Code	Positive	Negative
Exercise program	How to access	- The privilege to be attended to. - This program was free, and in private health care would have a high cost.	- No derivation for other health professionals. - Low public awareness of program existence. - Not all women can benefit from this program.
	Access time	- Started when it could be adapted to own schedule. - Started with mild symptoms.	- Lack of preventive physiotherapy treatment. - Started when symptoms were difficult to resolve with conservative treatment.
	Program satisfaction	- General personal satisfaction. - Nice attention from physiotherapist. - The feeling of being listened to and attended to.	
Program efficacy	Pelvic floor physical symptoms	- Lower leakage. - Lower heaviness sensation. - Not feeling a vaginal bulge. - Improvement of pelvic-perineal pain. - Sexual improvement. - Control of urinary urgency.	- Not a complete cure.
	Secondary physical symptoms	- Improved lower back pain. - Abdominal reduction. - Abdominal muscle strength.	- Back pain when performing exercises.
	Well-being	- Improved self-esteem. - Feeling of well-being.	
	Functional improvement	- Returning to sports routines. - Not fearing to cough, laugh, sneeze or lift weight.	
	Knowledge	- Self-control of symptoms. - Self-control of risk factors. - Awareness of treatment importance. - Being capable of taking responsibility for own dysfunction. - What to do when symptoms worsen. - Who to turn to when symptoms worsen.	

for the exercises (the type of exercise, posture, the demanded conditions of the exercise) and the perceived efficacy of one over another, influenced the adherence.

PFMTI4: "I only practice the maintenance exercise, because I think that to gain force it's ok".

3.4. Intrinsic Factors

The self-perceived symptoms, the self-perceived treatment efficacy, and the ability to reproduce exercises efficiently as well as to correct themselves were important in adherence. Moreover, the participants' beliefs, their immediate environment and the normalization of symptoms of urinary leakage in society affected adherence.

PFMTG3: "Some of my friends do hypopressive exercises, and I'd like to be in the hypopressive group, because I think that they're really good".

The newly acquired awareness of responsibility changed the women from passive agents to active agents in the improvement of their condition.

HEI3: "Now the responsibility is mine, if I don't do anything ... there is no magic".

3.5. Extrinsic Factors

Regular contact with the PT, the use of biofeedback devices and mirrors, and the posterior assessments were named as motivating factors.

PFMTI8: "The gynecology gave me a paper with some exercises. But I didn't understand them, nor fancy doing them. When I came here, I saw the importance they have".

Nevertheless, finishing the continuous physiotherapy treatment required some women to withdraw from the weekly PFM training. The evaluation and feedback provided by other health professionals also was a condition of adherence to the exercises.

4. Discussion

This study shows the adherence of women with PFD to the exercises recommended by their physiotherapist 3 to 6 months after an intensive treatment. To our knowledge, this is the first qualitative research that interviewed women with different mild forms of PFD, who underwent an individualized treatment based on PFM guided exercises with biofeedback and/or hypopressive exercises. Five categories emerged from the thematic analysis that explained the adherence-modifying factors: the exercise program, the program efficacy, the personal experience with exercises, patient's intrinsic aspects and extrinsic factors. Each theme contained related codes, from which positive and negative aspects for adherence were extracted.

Other qualitative studies emerged from randomized clinical trials. Our study is consistent with the study by Hyland et al. [24]. They presented the interviews of five women with POP between 5 and 24 months after participating in prescribed PFM exercises and selected positive adherence codes related to the ease of performing the exercises anywhere and their association with everyday moments. Family duties were emphasized as a determining aspect of adherence and maintenance of PFM exercise over time, a complicated challenge influenced by the low self-efficacy perception. The perception of self-efficacy has been identified as one of the main predictors of adherence to the maintenance of home PFM exercises [25]. To reinforce self-efficacy, the use of motivational interviewing has been proposed [15,26] and agreement reached on individualized goals based on the motivational stage of the patient [27], aspects that were included in the three intervention groups.

Adherence rates in our three study groups were similar. In the PFMT group, 71.9% continued exercising weekly at home, 61.3% in the HE group, and 67.7% in the PFMT+HE group [8]. Hay-Smith et al. [16] focused on PFM exercise comprehension and found that participants had trouble distinguishing the different exercise interventions, which could alter the outcome of their study. In our study, we did not identify confusion by the participants in identifying the different exercises, probably because the PFM exercises and the hypopressive exercises are different in their execution [8]. Our qualitative research showed that women found it difficult to continue a daily home exercise routine, especially if they perceived the exercise to be difficult, exhausting, or incompatible with a simultaneous activity; thus, we were surprised by the high adherence data found in relation to hypopressive exercises. In Spain, hypopressive exercises were popular among women; in fact, a participant from the PFM group revealed in her interview that she would have liked to join the HE group. This social support for an exercise modality could be a significant factor of adherence [28]. Furthermore, the treatment effectiveness perceived by the participants appeared as a positive factor in maintaining its practice at home [29], and in the three intervention groups, the women achieved clinically relevant improvements in their quality of life, which could also explain the similar adherence results.

Women valued the need for a treatment that produced improvements in relation to the symptoms of the pelvic floor, provided them with a feeling of well-being and generated secondary improvements, such as the minimization of low back pain. These findings are in line with the promotion adherence results found by Alewejnse et al. [7], who showed that a well-designed physiotherapy protocol may downplay the addition of a health education program. However, the lack of information and false beliefs have been identified in women with UI [16], assuming educational programs are an essential tool for the health education of these women. In fact, the participants in our study highlighted the knowledge acquired as a positive factor of adherence, finding in other studies how women perceive that it was a useful learning experience for life. The feedback provided by the physiotherapist and the periodic evaluation visits also appeared as facilitating aspects of adherence [30].

Several barriers to adherence were identified based on the experiences of the women in our study. They included difficulty in accessing a pelvic floor physiotherapy service in relation to ignorance of its existence and its high price, as it is not generally integrated into public health services [29–31]; whether treatment is started with advanced symptoms; and failure to achieve complete resolution of the symptoms. Regarding the time when the physiotherapy program should start, the women agreed that around postpartum/first delivery could be a good time. Despite the opinions of women, qualitative studies show that postpartum women are unaware of PFD that may appear after childbirth, and that they believe it is an inevitable consequence and do not know about the treatment alternatives available [31,32]. Grant et al. [33] interviewed 31 women who had given birth in the last 5 years and found that women needed more information and support for proper performance of the MSP exercises, which could also be facilitated by the use of new technologies, such as the creation of an app. Other identified barriers to adherence were related to beliefs about normalization or taboo subjects [31,33], a lack of self-care [34], prioritizing family needs [24], or job obligations [30].

Pakbaz et al. [34] identified feeling ignored by healthcare professionals as an obstacle of attention demand; an assumption in our study was the feeling of gratitude for care as a positive factor for adherence. This appreciation could enable the patients to have good experiences since the physiotherapist who guided the treatment and prescribed the exercises was also the interviewer, which was a possible limitation of the study. To minimize this fact, group interviews were performed by an external physiotherapist who also specialized in women's health. However, to enlist the same intervening physiotherapist for interviews was an advantage because she provided confidence to the interviewed participants, and her knowledge about women was used to interpret the experiences and categorize the information [24]. A strength of our study is that the questions were agreed upon by different health professionals and the process of triangulation and analysis of the information was carried out by five physiotherapist experts in women's health and qualitative research.

The practical implications derived from the present study can be directed first to the planning of effective physiotherapy programs that promote the empowerment of women, and second to the evaluation and management of contextual factors that may be positive or negative. Knowing and exploring both the beneficial factors and the adherence barriers present in each woman would allow the physiotherapist and patient to agree on realistic home exercises [30] and in meaningful environments. For future research, it is considered essential to explore and deepen the experience of women regarding their needs related to improvement in their PFD, their opinions on current management and the possibilities for them to take an active role in their own recovery. Designing mixed-method studies or qualitative studies after intervention research could delve into the personal reasons for adhering or not to a treatment plan, especially important in chronic or long-terms disorders such as PFD.

5. Conclusions

In the present qualitative study on the experience of maintaining home exercises after intensive physiotherapy treatment in women with PFD, five central themes were identified: the exercise program, program efficacy, personal experience with the exercises, intrinsic factors, and extrinsic factors. Interventions with perceived effectiveness and easy exercises suitable for integration into daily life would enhance therapeutic adherence. Providing knowledge so that women recognize their pelvic floor and the importance of PFM exercises as well as take an active role in their self-care process should be a goal of health professionals, also reinforced by professionals.

Author Contributions: Conceptualization, B.N.-B. and M.T.-L.; methodology, F.V.-P. and M.J.Y.-S.; software, B.N.-B. and F.V.-P.; formal analysis, B.N.-B., V.P.-G., F.V.-P., B.S.-S. and M.T.-L.; investigation, B.N.-B. and B.S.-S.; resources, M.T.-L.; data curation, M.J.Y.-S.; writing—original draft preparation, B.N.-B. and F.V.-P.; writing—review and editing, M.T.-L.; visualization, V.P.-G.; supervision, B.S.-S. and M.T.-L. All authors have read and agreed to the published version of the manuscript.

Funding: This research received no external funding.

Institutional Review Board Statement: The study was conducted according to the guidelines of the Declaration of Helsinki and approved by the Clinical Research Committee of the Principe de Asturias Hospital (OE20/2013).

Informed Consent Statement: Written informed consent has been obtained from the patients to publish this paper.

Data Availability Statement: More information on the data presented in this study can be requested from the corresponding author.

Acknowledgments: The authors would like to thank all the women who participated in the study.

Conflicts of Interest: The authors declare no conflict of interest.

References

1. Dumoulin, C.; Pazzoto Cacciari, L.; Mercier, J. Keeping the pelvic floor healthy. *Climacteric* **2019**, *22*, 257–262. [CrossRef]
2. Aoki, Y.; Brown, H.W.; Brubaker, L.; Cornu, J.N.; Daly, J.O.; Cartwright, R. Urinary incontinence in women. *Nat. Res. Dis. Primers* **2017**, *6*, 17042. [CrossRef] [PubMed]
3. Siahkal, S.F.; Iravani, M.; Mohaghegh, Z.; Sharifipour, F.; Zahedian, M.; Nasab, M.B. Investigating the association of the dimensions of genital hiatus and levator hiatus with pelvic organ prolapse: A systematic review. *Int. Urogynecol. J.* **2021**, *32*, 2095–2109. [CrossRef]
4. Maze Good, M.; Solomon, E.R. Pelvic Floor Disorders. *Obstet. Gynecol. Clin. N. Am.* **2019**, *46*, 527–540. [CrossRef]
5. Dumoulin, C.; Cacciari, L.P.; Hay-Smith, E.J.C. Pelvic floor muscle training versus no treatment, or inactive control treatments, for urinary incontinence in women. *Cochrane Database Syst. Rev.* **2018**, *10*, CD005654. [CrossRef]
6. Hagen, S.; Glazener, C.; McClurg, D.; Macarthur, C.; Elders, A.; Herbison, P.; Wilson, D.; Toozs-Hobson, P.; Hemming, C.; Hay-Smith, J.; et al. Pelvic floor muscle training for secondary prevention of pelvic organ prolapse (PREVPROL): A multicentre randomised controlled trial. *Lancet* **2017**, *389*, 393–402. [CrossRef]
7. Alewijnse, D.; Metsemakers, J.; Mesters, I.; van der Borne, B. Effectiveness of pelvic floor muscle exercise therapy supplemented with a health education program to promote adherence among women with urinary incontinence. *Neurourol. Urodynam.* **2003**, *22*, 284–295. [CrossRef] [PubMed]
8. Navarro-Brazález, B.; Prieto-Gómez, V.; Prieto-Merino, D.; Sánchez-Sánchez, B.; McLean, L.; Torres-Lacomba, M. Effectiveness of hypopressive exercises in women with pelvic floor dysfunction: A randomised controlled trial. *J. Clin. Med.* **2020**, *9*, 1149. [CrossRef] [PubMed]

9. Juez, L.; Núñez-Córdoba, J.M.; Couso, N.; Aubá, M.; Alcázar, J.L.; Mínguez, J.A. Hypopressive technique versus pelvic floor muscle training for postpartum pelvic floor rehabilitation: A prospective cohort study. *Neurourol. Urodynam.* **2019**, *38*, 1924–1931. [CrossRef]
10. Soriano, L.; González-Millán, C.; Álvarez Sáez, M.M.; Curbelo, R.; Carmona, L. Effect of an abdominal hypopressive technique programme on pelvic floor muscle tone and urinary incontinence in women: A randomised crossover trial. *Physiotherapy* **2020**, *108*, 37–44. [CrossRef]
11. Dumoulin, C.; Hay-Smith, J.; Frawley, H.; McClurg, D.; Alewijnse, D.; Bo, K.; Burgio, K.; Chen, S.Y.; Chiarelli, P.; Dean, S.; et al. 2014 Consensus statement of improving pelvic floor muscle training adherence: International continence society 2011 state-of-the-science seminar. *Neurourol. Urodynam.* **2015**, *34*, 600–605. [CrossRef] [PubMed]
12. Aguirre, F.; Heft, J.; Yunker, A. Factors associated with Nonadherence to pelvic floor physical therapy referral for the treatment of pelvic pain in women. *Phys. Ther.* **2019**, *99*, 946–952. [CrossRef]
13. Dumoulin, C.; Alewijnse, D.; Bo, K.; Hagen, S.; Stark, D.; Van Kampen, M.; Herbert, J.; Hay-Smith, J.; Frawley, H.; McClurg, D.; et al. Pelvic floor muscle training adherence: Tools, measurements and strategies- 2011 ICS state-of-the-science seminar research paper II of IV. *Neurourol. Urodynam.* **2015**, *34*, 615–621. [CrossRef] [PubMed]
14. Alewijnse, D.; Mesters, I.; Metsemakers, J.; van den Borne, B. Predictors of long-term adherence to pelvic floor muscle exercise therapy among women with urinary incontinence. *Health Educ. Res.* **2003**, *18*, 511–524. [CrossRef]
15. Hay-Smith, E.J.C.; Ryan, K.; Dean, S. The silent, private exercise: Experiences of pelvic floor muscle training in a sample of women with stress urinary incontinence. *Physiotherapy* **2007**, *93*, 53–61. [CrossRef]
16. Pintos-Díaz, M.Z.; Alonso-Blanco, C.; Parás-Bravo, P.; Fernández-de-Las-Peñas, C.; Paz-Zulueta, M.; Fradejas-Sastre, V.; Palacios-Ceña, D. Living with urinary incontinence: Potential risks of women's health? A qualitative study on the perspectives of female patients seeking care for the first time in a specialized center. *Int. J. Environ. Res. Public Health* **2019**, *16*, 3781. [CrossRef] [PubMed]
17. Fernandes, A.C.N.L.; Palacios-Ceña, D.; Hay-Smith, J.; Pena, C.C.; Sidou, M.F.; de Alencar, A.L.; Ferreira, C.H.J. Women report sustained benefits from attending group-based education about pelvic floor muscles: A longitudinal qualitative study. *J. Physiother.* **2021**, *67*, 210–216. [CrossRef]
18. Hay-Smith, J.; Dean, S.; Burgio, K.; McClurg, D.; Frawley, H.; Dumoulin, C. Pelvic-floor-muscle-training adherence "modifiers": A review of primary qualitative studies- 2011 ICS state-of-the-science seminar research paper III of IV. *Neurourol. Urodynam.* **2015**, *34*, 622–631. [CrossRef]
19. Rada, M.P.; Jones, S.; Falconi, G.; Milhem Haddad, J.; Betschart, C.; Pergialiotis, V.; Doumouchtsis, S.K.; CHORUS: An International Collaboration for Harmonising Outcomes, Research and Standards in Urogynaecology and Women's Health. A systematic review and meta-synthesis of qualitative studies on pelvic organ prolapse for the development of core outcome sets. *Neurourol. Urodynam.* **2020**, *39*, 880–889. [CrossRef]
20. Berlanga Fernández, S.; Vizcaya Moreno, M.F.; Pérez Cañaveras, R.M. Percepción de la transición a la maternidad: Estudio fenomenológico en la provincia de Barcelona. *Aten. Primaria* **2013**, *45*, 409–417. [CrossRef]
21. Sandelowski, M. Whatever happened to qualitative description? *Res. Nurs. Health* **2000**, *23*, 334–340. [CrossRef]
22. Buus, N.; Perron, A. The quality of quality criteria: Replicating the development of the Consolidated Criteria for Reporting Qualitative Research (COREQ). *Int. J. Nurs. Stud.* **2020**, *102*, 103452. [CrossRef]
23. Babatunde, F.; MacDermid, J.; MacIntyre, N. Characteristics of therapeutic alliance in musculoskeletal physiotherapy and occupational therapy practice: A scoping review of the literature. *BMC Health Serv. Res.* **2017**, *17*, 375. [CrossRef]
24. Hyland, G.; Hay-Smith, J.; Treharne, G. Women's experiences of doing long-term pelvic floor muscle exercises for the treatment of pelvic organ prolapse symptoms. *Int. Urogynecol. J.* **2014**, *25*, 265–271. [CrossRef]
25. Messer, K.L.; Hines, S.H.; Raghunathan, T.E.; Seng, J.S.; Diokno, A.C.; Sampselle, C.M. Self-efficacy as a predictor to PFMT adherence in a prevention of urinary incontinence clinical trial. *Health Educ. Behav.* **2007**, *34*, 942–952. [CrossRef]
26. McGrane, N.; Galvin, R.; Cusack, T.; Stokes, E. Addition of motivational interventions to exercise and traditional physiotherapy: A review and meta-analysis. *Physiotherapy* **2015**, *101*, 1–12. [CrossRef] [PubMed]
27. Alewijnse, D.; Mesters, I.; Metsemakers, J.; Bart, H.W.; van den Borne, B. Program development for promoting adherence during and after exercise therapy for urinary incontinence. *Patient Educ. Couns.* **2002**, *48*, 147–160. [CrossRef]
28. Alewijnse, D.; Mesters, I.; Metsemakers, J.; van den Borne, B. Predictors of intention to adhere to physiotherapy among women with urinary incontinence. *Health Educ. Res.* **2001**, *16*, 173–186. [CrossRef]
29. Frawley, H.C.; McClurg, D.; Mahfooza, A.; Hay-Smith, J.; Dumoulin, C. Health professionals' and patients' perspectives on pelvic floor muscle training adherence- 2011 ICS state-of-the-science seminar research. *Neurourol. Urodynam.* **2015**, *34*, 632–639. [CrossRef] [PubMed]
30. Milne, J.L.; Moore, K.N. Factors impacting self-care for urinary incontinence. *Urol. Nurs.* **2006**, *26*, 41–51.
31. Salmon, V.E.; Hay-Smith, E.J.C.; Jarvie, R.; Dean, S.; Terry, R.; Frawley, H.; Oborn, E.; Bayliss, S.E.; Bick, D.; Davenport, C.; et al. Implementing pelvic floor muscle training in women's childbearing years: A critical interpretive synthesis of individual, professional, and service issues. *Neurourol. Urodynam.* **2020**, *39*, 863–870. [CrossRef] [PubMed]
32. Encabo-Solana, N.; Torres-Lacomba, T.; Vergara-Pérez, F.; Sánchez-Sánchez, B.; Navarro-Brazález, B. Percepción de las puérperas y de los profesionales sanitarios sobre el embarazo y el parto como factores de riesgo de las disfunciones del suelo pélvico. Estudio cualitativo. *Fisioterapia* **2016**, *38*, 142–151. [CrossRef]

33. Grant, A.; Currie, S. Qualitative exploration of the acceptability of a postnatal pelvic floor muscle training intervention to prevent urinary incontinence. *BMC Women's Health* **2020**, *20*, 1–8. [CrossRef] [PubMed]
34. Pakbaz, M.; Persson, M.; Löfgren, M.; Mogren, I. 'A hidden disorder until the pieces fall into place'—A qualitative study of vaginal prolapse. *BMC Women's Health* **2010**, *10*, 1–9. [CrossRef] [PubMed]

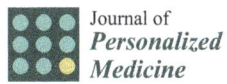

Journal of Personalized Medicine

Article

Functional Profile of Older Adults Hospitalized in Convalescence Units of the National Network of Integrated Continuous Care of Portugal: A Longitudinal Study

Ana Ramos [1], César Fonseca [2,3], Lara Pinho [2,3,*], Manuel Lopes [2,3], Henrique Oliveira [4] and Adriana Henriques [1,5]

1. Nursing Research, Innovation and Development Centre of Lisbon (CIDNUR), Nursing School of Lisbon (ESEL), 1600-096 Lisbon, Portugal; ramos.anafilipa@gmail.com (A.R.); ahenriques@esel.pt (A.H.)
2. Escola Superior de Enfermagem de São João de Deus, Universidade de Évora, 7000-801 Evora, Portugal; cfonseca@uevora.pt (C.F.); mjl@uevora.pt (M.L.)
3. Comprehensive Health Research Centre (CHRC), Universidade de Évora, 7000-801 Evora, Portugal
4. Instituto de Telecomunicações, 1049-001 Lisbon, Portugal; hjmo@lx.it.pt
5. Instituto de Saúde Ambiental (ISAMB), Faculdade de Medicina, Universidade de Lisboa, 1649-028 Lisbon, Portugal
* Correspondence: lmgp@uevora.pt

Abstract: Aim: To evaluate the evolution of the functional profile of older adults admitted to a health unit in Portugal; to relate the functional profile of these individuals with age, sex, education level and emotional state; and to evaluate the probability of the degree of dependence as a function of age and sex. Methods: longitudinal, retrospective study with a sample of 59,013 older adults admitted to convalescence units of the National Network of Integrated Continuous Care of Portugal. Results: In the first 75 days of hospitalization, activities of daily living, mobility and cognitive state improved, but there was a decline after 75 days of hospitalization. The ability to perform instrumental activities of daily living improved in the first 15 days of hospitalization, stabilized until 45 days and then began to worsen. Women had a higher probability of having a severe/complete dependence three years earlier than men (88 years to 91 years). A higher education level and stable emotional state were protective factors against functional decline. Conclusions: The functional profile of older adults improved during the length of stay recommended for hospitalization in convalescence units (30 days). It is critical for health systems to adopt strategies to prevent declines in the emotional state of frail individuals.

Keywords: older adults; functional status; health care; hospitalization; activities of daily living

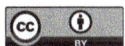

1. Introduction

With the increasing aging of the population and the increase in life expectancy, it is necessary to pay greater attention to the health of older adults. The European Pathway Association states that for care pathways to be successful, they must obey a set of principles, among which the following stand out: (a) the definition of clear care goals, based on scientific evidence, the best clinical practices and the expectations and characteristics of the person being cared for; (b) the facilitation of communication among all those involved; (c) effective coordination; (d) the correct monitoring and evaluation of results; and (e) the identification of the appropriate resources for the individual and the clinical situation [1]. In this sense, a care pathway should be based on both the integration of care and the continuity of care [2].

The integration of care is considered by the World Health Organization (WHO) to be the result of multifaceted efforts made to promote integration, with benefits for people [3]. It has been considered an international priority in health policy and health management research [4]. Recent data confirm that integrated care models have had benefits in improving the health-related quality of life and functionality of people with multimorbidity and frailty [5]; in reducing hospitalization and readmission rates [6]; in reducing polypharmacy [7]; and in improving patient satisfaction, perceived quality of care and access to services [8].

In Portugal, the National Network of Integrated Continuous Care (RNCCI, acronym in Portuguese) was created in 2006 through Decree Law no. 101/2006, which is intended for people who, regardless of age, are functionally dependent. The RNCCI was developed as an integrated Health and Social Security response that mobilizes the public, private and social sectors. Its intervention objectives are the rehabilitation, readaptation and reintegration of frail individuals who no longer require acute hospital care [9]. The RNCCI is focused on community outreach services and includes hospitals, health centers, district and local social security services, the Solidarity Network and local authorities. There are several types of care provided in the RNCCI, which includes inpatient units (convalescence units; medium-term and rehabilitation units; long-term and maintenance units; and level 1 pediatric integrated inpatient units) and outpatient units (mental health integrated continuous care units; day and autonomy promotion units; pediatric outpatient units and integrated continuous care teams) [9].

Convalescence Units (CUs) are intended for individuals with a potentially recoverable transitory loss of autonomy, and their purpose is clinical stabilization and functional rehabilitation. These units have their own facilities and are connected to an acute care hospital to ensure health care 24 h a day over a total length of hospitalization of 30 days [9].

As the purpose of CUs is functional rehabilitation, it seems clear to us the importance of assessing the functionality of patients to better evaluate health outcomes. The WHO developed the International Classification of Functioning, Disability and Health (ICF) to standardize the international assessment of functioning and disabilities related to the health-disease process, taking into account the body's structures and functions and environmental factors [10]. Studies indicate that the evaluation of functionality is crucial in care models for older adults [11,12].

The performance of self-care behavior is considered extremely important for the individual person and for the health system, due to the benefits associated with it [13]. The gains from the development of self-care health behavior are related to reduced risk of complications, healthcare expenditures, hospital readmission rates, increased satisfaction with care, feelings of responsibility, control, independence, and autonomy, adoption of effective coping strategies, improved well-being, functional capacity, quality of life, symptom control, and pain [14–16]. In the care process, we seek to assess dependence in self-care skills (mobility, basic and instrumental activities of daily living, and cognitive status) [17,18], with the purpose of maintaining life, healthy functioning and personal development. The self-care deficit presents itself in degradé, as it can fluctuate in different levels, from mild to complete/severe [15]. The WHO report for the 2021–2030 decade emphasizes the importance of implementing actions that improve the functional ability of older adults, presenting four areas of action for this purpose: a) changing the way we think, feel and act toward age and aging; b) ensuring that communities foster the abilities of older people; c) providing integrated person-centered care and services that meet the needs of older people; and d) providing access to long-term care for older people who need it [19]. One of the strategies defined in the same report to accelerate the implementation of functional ability is to strengthen data, research and innovation [19]. Thus, the aim of the present study is to assess the functional trajectory of older adults hospitalized in CUs of the RNCCI of Portugal. For this purpose, the following objectives were defined: (1) to evaluate the evolution of the functional profile of older adults hospitalized in CUs; (2) to relate the functional profile of these individuals with age, sex, education level and emotional state; and (3) to evaluate the probability of the degree of dependence as a function of age and sex.

2. Materials and Methods

2.1. Study Type and Sample

This was a longitudinal, retrospective study with a sample of 59,013 older adults aged 65 or older hospitalized in health units belonging to CUs of the RNCCI of Portugal.

2.2. Instrument

To evaluate the functional profile, variables of the International Classification of Functioning, Disability and Health (ICF), which contains the ICF components: Body Functions (Mental Functions) and Activities and Participation (Mobility, Self-care, Communication, Domestic Life, Main life areas), were used. The ICF items were transformed into a Likert scale so that they could be analyzed (no problem = 1; mild or moderate problem = 2; severe problem = 3; complete problem = 4). The global Cronbach's $\alpha = 0.951$ is obtained, which means excellent internal consistency.

2.3. Data Collection

The data were collected from the records made by health workers and entered in the RNCCI portal. To trace the sociodemographic profile, data related to the first evaluation of each hospitalization episode occurring between 1 January 2010, and 27 February 2017, were selected.

Subsequently, the evolution of the functional profile was evaluated through the analysis of biweekly evaluations of older adults hospitalized in CUs who were targets of a set of structured professional interventions (objective 1).

To meet the second objective, which was to relate the functional profile with the variables age, sex, education level and emotional state, principal component analysis of each of the instrument domains (mobility, ADL, IADL, and cognitive state), was combined with cluster analysis. This procedure presented the advantage of reducing the number of input variables in the cluster analysis, thus helping to simplify the characterization of the upstream clusters [20].

To meet the third objective, the probabilities of each class as a function of age and by sex were evaluated.

2.4. Statistical Analysis

To analyze the four components of self-care capacity, over the days of hospitalization, a longitudinal analysis was performed, based on parametric tests (One-way ANOVA and t-Student test) (objective 1).

The exploratory analysis of clusters was performed using the hierarchical method (Analyze Classify Hierarchical Cluster). Since it is big data, it was necessary to perform a random partition of the database, to create a sub-sample with approximately 20% of the data, so that it was possible to process the information by SPSS. When obtaining the agglomeration coefficients (Ward's method), a graphic projection was performed, of the highest (last 30), to visualize their distances, where it was possible to verify that the best solution resided in the retention of 3 clusters. Consecutively, the cluster analysis was carried out using the non-hierarchical optimization method available in IBM SPSS: K-means (objetive 2).

Ordinal regression with the probit link function was used to assess whether age and sex had a significant effect on the probabilities related to the type of dependence (objective 3). The link function was chosen based on the frequency distribution criteria of the classes of the dependent variable "degree of dependence" [21].

2.5. Ethical Procedures

The study was conducted in accordance with the guidelines of the Declaration of Helsinki and was approved by the Ethics Committee of Scientific Research in the Areas of Human Health and Welfare of the University of Évora (report number, 17036; date of approval, 26 April 2017).

3. Results

3.1. Sociodemographic and Clinical Characteristics

The mean age of the sample was 78.93 years (SD = 7.28), with an age range of 65 to 109 years. The majority of older adults admitted to CUs were in the age group of 75 to 84 years (47.2%), followed by 65 to 74 years (29.0%), and last, people aged 85 or older (23.8%). Most of the sample was female (61.5%), had a partner (44.7%), had less than 6 years of schooling (60.4%), and had an unskilled professional level at working age (70.3%). Table 1 provides the sociodemographic characterization of the sample.

Table 1. Sociodemographic characterization of older adults hospitalized in convalescence units by sex (2010–2017).

Sociodemographic Variables	n (%)
Age (years)	
65–74	15,320 (29.0)
75–84	24,987 (47.2)
≥85	12,578 (23.8)
Sex	
Female	32,535 (61.5)
Male	20,350 (38.5)
Marital status	
Single	6193 (13.2)
Married	20,763 (44.4)
Domestic partnership	454 (0.3)
Divorced	2018 (4.3)
Widowed	17,578 (37.6)
Unknown	109 (0.2)
Education (years)	
No education	8244 (31.5)
1 to 6	15,802 (60.4)
7 to 12	1087 (4.2)
≥13	1047 (4.0)
Professional Level	
Unskilled	18,379 (70.3)
Skilled	6191 (23.7)
Intermediate	1139 (4.4)
Specialist	453 (1.7)
Cohabitation	
Lives alone	7192 (27.5)
Lives with other (s)	18,988 (72.5)
Region of Portugal	
Alentejo	4913 (9.7)
Algarve	3659 (7.2)
Center	11,937 (22.6)
Lisbon and Vale do Tejo	11,362 (22.4)
North	18,805 (37.1)

3.2. Evolution of the Functional Profile during Hospitalization

Figure 1 shows the evolution of the functional profile of the sample throughout hospitalization, over time, with the evaluation performed every 15 days since admission. There were significant differences in each of the components: dependence in mobility ($F_{(65.161954)} = 143.337$; $p < 0.001$), ADLs ($F_{(65.166854)} = 479.340$; $p < 0.001$), IADLs ($F_{(53.42791)} = 9.271$; $p < 0.001$) and cognitive state ($F_{(65.161945)} = 34.303$; $p < 0.001$).

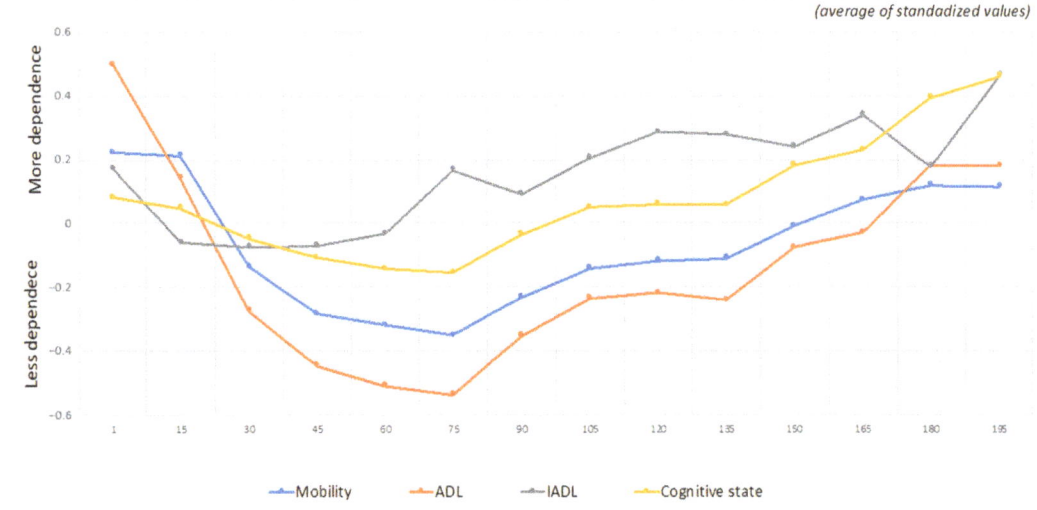

Figure 1. Components: mobility, activities of daily living (ADL), instrumental activities of daily living (IADL) and cognitive status in convalescence units (standardized mean values).

3.3. Dependence Clusters

The nonhierarchical exploratory method of cluster grouping was used, yielding the following partition: Cluster 1—29.6% (n = 11,248); Cluster 2—52.1% (n = 19,785); and Cluster 3—18.3% (n = 6932). These clusters differed significantly in the dimensions mobility ($F_{(2.37962)} = 0.162$; $p < 0.001$), ADLs ($F_{(2.37962)} = 0.734$; $p < 0.001$), IADLs ($F_{(2.37962)} = 0.905$; $p < 0.001$) and cognitive state ($F_{(2.37962)} = 0.811$; $p < 0.001$).

In general terms, the three clusters were quite distinct, with the following configuration, presented in Figure 2:

(1) Cluster 1: Older adults with a higher degree of dependence (severe/complete self-care deficit);
(2) Cluster 2: Older adults with an intermediate degree of dependence (moderate self-care deficit);
(3) Cluster 3: Older adults with a lower degree of dependence (mild self-care deficit).

Figure 3 shows the differences among the three clusters and the variables sex, age group, education, sad/depressed emotional state and anxious emotional state.

(1) Cluster 1 (severe/complete dependence) is composed of a higher percentage of males, aged 85 years or older, older adults who did not attend school and who have been feeling depressed and anxious for a long time;
(2) Cluster 2 (moderate dependence) encompasses a greater percentage of females, aged between 65 and 84 years, with 1 to 6 years of education and who have felt sad or anxious for a short time;
(3) Cluster 3 (mild dependence) is predominantly composed of males aged 65 to 74 years, with more years of schooling (7 or more) and who feel depressed or anxious for a short time.

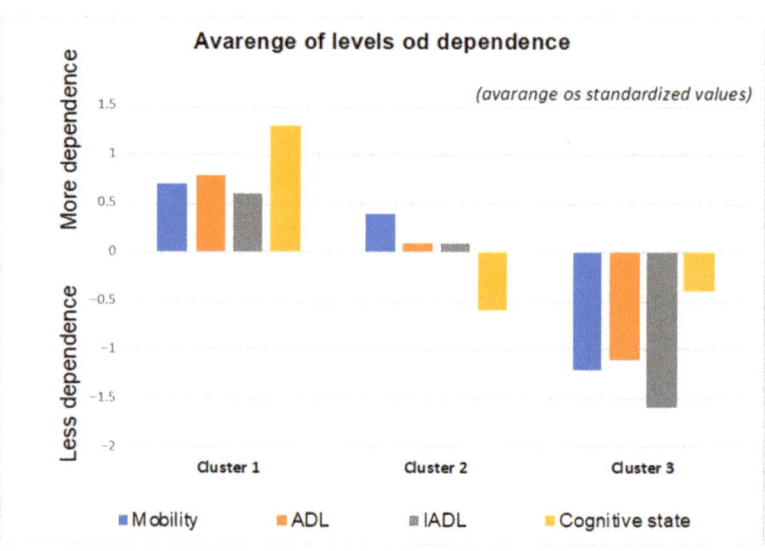

Figure 2. Mean dependence levels for Cluster 1, Cluster 2 and Cluster 3 in the convalescence units.

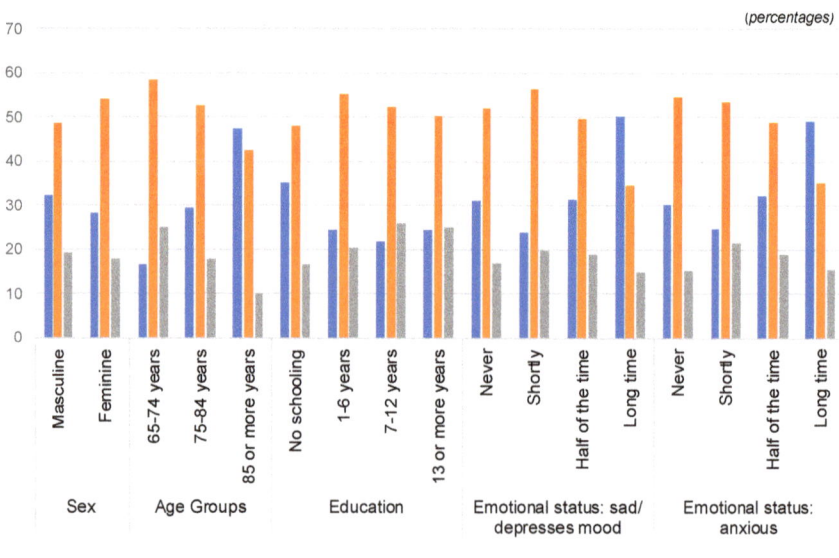

Figure 3. Distribution of people aged 65 years or older in the convalescence units by sex, age group, education level, emotional state: sad/depressed and emotional state: anxious, per cluster.

3.4. Degree of Dependence as a Function of Age and Sex

The assumption of the slope homogeneity model was validated ($\chi^2(2) = 4.531$; $p = 0.104$).

The model was considered highly significant ($\chi^2(2) = 274.822$; $p < 0.001$), although the effect size was small ($R^2_{MF} = 0.096$; $R^2_N = 0.132$; $R^2_{CS} = 0.129$). In the ordinal regression model, the link function "Probit" was adopted ($\Phi^{-1}(P[Y \leq k]) = \alpha_k - (0.043 \times Age + 0.101 \times Sex_{Female})$, where Φ is the standard normal distribution $\mathcal{N}(0,1)$), because this function is recommended when the latent variable presents a normal distribution. The coefficients and statistical significance of the adjusted ordinal model are shown in Table 2.

Table 2. Estimates and significance of the adjusted "Probit" model.

Parameters		Estimate	Standard Error	χ^2_{Wald}	df	p Value	95% Confidence Interval
Thresholds	Mild	$\alpha_{Mild} = 2.439$	0.065	1421.020	1	<0.001	[2.312; 2.566]
	Moderate	$\alpha_{Moderate} = 3.946$	0.066	3559.323	1	<0.001	[3.816; 4.075]
Localization	Age	$b_{Age} = 0.043$	0.001	2684.676	1	<0.001	[0.041; 0.044]
	Sex (Female)	$b_{Sex(Female)} = 0.101$	0.012	69.659	1	<0.001	[0.078; 0.125]

The results obtained suggest that with advancing age, the probability of observing higher-order classes, i.e., the probability of observing a higher degree of dependence, increases ($b_{Age} = 0.043$; $p < 0.001$). Regarding sex, the results obtained suggest a higher probability of observing a higher dependence type in women than in men ($b_{Sex(Female)} = 0.101$; $p < 0.001$); however, this difference is moderate.

The evaluation of the probabilities of each of the classes as a function of age and by sex is shown in Figure 4. The analysis revealed that a) for both women and men, the probability of a dependence profile of "mild" is always inferior to any of the other two profile types; b) for women, starting at 88 years of age, the dependence profile that most likely occurs is "severe/complete"; for men, the same occurs, but starting at 91 years of age (three years later); c) by year of age, the ratio of the probability of observing profiles of lower dependence, compared to the probability of observing profiles of greater dependence, decreases by 4.2% (1-exp(-0.043)); and d) the odds ratio of lower dependence (mild) relative to higher dependence (severe/complete) decreases by 9.6% (1-exp(-0.101)) from males to females.

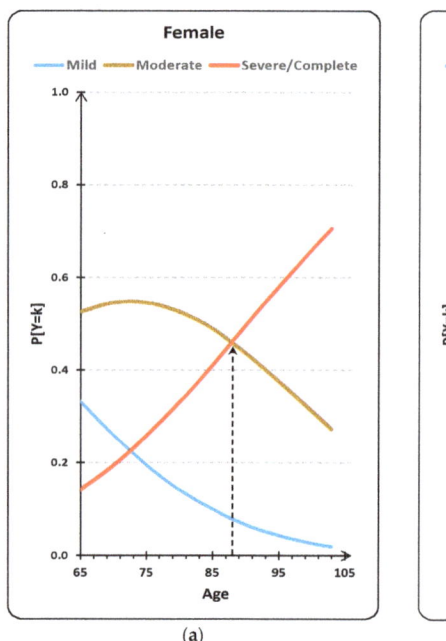
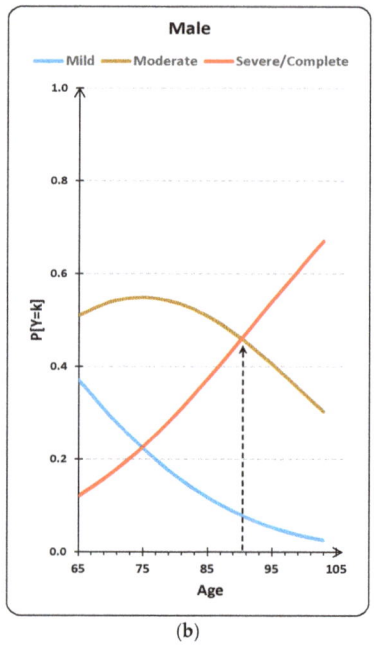

Figure 4. Evaluation of the probabilities for mild, moderate and severe dependence for women (**a**) and men (**b**) ($\chi^2(2) = 274.822; p < 0.001; R^2_{MF} = 0.096; R^2_N = 0.132; R^2_{CS} = 0.129$).

4. Discussion

This study evaluated the evolution of the functional profile of older adults hospitalized in CUs of the RNCCI, related it to the variables discussed below and evaluated the probability of the degree of dependence as a function of age and sex.

Regarding the evolution of self-care components throughout hospitalization, in the first 75 days of hospitalization, ADLs, mobility and cognitive state improved, but there was a decline after 75 days of hospitalization. In contrast, the ability to perform IADLs improved in the first 15 days of hospitalization, stabilized up to 45 days, and worsened thereafter. Considering that IADLs include tasks such as preparing meals, washing clothes, and housework, activities that are not performed by patients during hospitalization, it would be expected that with the lack of practice, the ability to perform these tasks would begin to decrease earlier than would ADLs, mobility or cognitive state because the tasks related to these components are maintained throughout hospitalization. However, at 75 days of hospitalization, the ability to perform these activities also begins to decline. One study reports that 30 to 60% of older adults experience a functional decline in ADL during hospitalization [22]. Low mobility during hospitalization and functional and physical changes can lead to functional deficits in ADLs and cognitive impairments [23]. However, 80% of cases are preventable with effective health care [24,25]. Importantly, individuals who are hospitalized for more than 30 days in CUs are those with less potential for rehabilitation or without family support to provide continuity of rehabilitation at home; the length of hospitalization recommended for individuals referred to CUs is 30 days, which may explain these results. Thus, it is concluded that most individuals stay for the recommended time and experience reductions in acquired deficits in all dimensions.

Regarding age, as would be expected, most individuals older than 85 years are in the severe/complete dependence cluster, the age group of 65 and 84 years is mostly in the moderate dependence cluster, and most individuals in the age group of 65 to 74 years old are in the mild dependence cluster. Other authors have also concluded that the older the age, the worse the functionality [26].

When analyzing the clusters by sex, we found that there was a higher percentage of males in the severe/complete dependence cluster and in the mild dependence cluster and a higher percentage of females in the moderate dependence cluster. However, when analyzing the probability of the degree of dependence as a function of age and sex, for women, starting at 88 years of age, the type of dependence profile that most likely occurs is "severe/complete", while for men, the same occurs only after 91 years of age (three years later). This finding should be interpreted with caution because studies are conflicting, as some report that women have a higher degree of dependence than do men and others report that there are no differences. A literature review revealed that the incidence of functional disability was identical between sexes [27]. However, the results from two Portuguese studies with older adults indicated that the functional profile is worse in women than in men [26], regardless of age [28]. Another study that analyzed data from Spain, Portugal and Italy found that compared with men, women after 65–70 years of age had a higher risk of suffering from severe functional limitations. The same study added that in the age group of 75–80 years of age, women were 3.3% more likely than men to have severe functional limitations and that in the age group of 80 years or older, this probability increased to 15.5% [29]. The results from another study indicated that there are significant differences between sexes regarding the probability of occurrence of disability, with a higher probability for women in the following countries: United States, Korea, Southern Europe, Mexico and China. However, these differences do not exist in Northern, Central and Eastern Europe, England, and Israel. The authors conclude that gender inequality in society at the macro level is significantly associated with the probability of women developing disabilities [30]. A European study concluded that there are differences between sexes in relation to some important health indicators and that these differences are higher in Southern and Eastern Europe than in Western and Northern Europe. The same study warns that the presence of a sex difference in health cannot be considered a universal factor because, depending on the indicator and the country, the difference tended to increase, decrease or even reverse with age [31]. It should be noted that neither of the two previous studies included Portugal.

With regard to education, several studies are consistent in indicating that the lower the educational level, the worse the functional profile and the greater the degree of dependence [26,28,32] and that a lower education level is associated with worse physical and mental health outcomes [33–35]. In addition, a study showed that the impact of multimorbidity on ADLs was three times higher at the lowest education level than at the highest education level [36]. Another study added that after 65 years of age, the average probability of severe functional limitations for individuals with a low education level increased to more than 40% at age 80 years and older, while it was 26% in the higher education category [29]. The results of the present study are in line with those described in the literature, with a predominance of individuals who did not attend school in the severe/complete dependence cluster; those who studied for 1 to 6 years were predominant in the moderate dependence cluster, and those with a higher education level (7 or more years) were mostly in the mild dependence cluster. Thus, it is confirmed that in individuals admitted to CUs, the higher the educational level is, the lower the likelihood of dependence; additionally, education is extremely important for health and for active and healthy aging.

Regarding the analysis of emotional state, in the severe/complete dependence cluster, there was a predominance of individuals who felt depressed and anxious for a long time, and in the moderate dependence and mild dependence clusters, there was a predominance of older adults who felt sad or anxious for a short time. In fact, in a literature review, depression was considered one of the main risk factors for functional disability in older adults [27]. Another recent study that analyzed several combinations of multimorbidity concluded that those that included depression were the only consistent predictors of disability [37]. Another study followed the same direction, with the results indicating that depression and/or cognitive deficit was associated with a substantially greater potential disability than combinations composed exclusively of somatic diseases [38].

The strengths of the present study include the relatively large sample size and the heterogeneity of the participants.

The limitations of the present study include the lack of an analysis of the time period after 2017 and the inclusion of only some of the determinants identified in the literature as influencing functional ability (e.g., emotional state).

5. Conclusions

The recommended length of hospitalization in CUs of the RNCCI of Portugal is 30 days, although some individuals remain longer. During this period, there was a significant improvement in the functional profile of older adults hospitalized in these units, and there was a decline in those who remained beyond 75 days. More studies are needed to understand the reason for the observed decline after this cutoff point.

Women hospitalized in CUs were more likely to have a severe degree of/complete dependence three years earlier than men (88 years compared to 91 years of age, respectively). The higher the education level and the better the emotional state was, the lower the degree of dependence. This study confirms the importance of the education level and emotional state in functional ability in older adults. It is necessary that future studies evaluate the effectiveness of interventions that seek to prevent declines in the emotional state of individuals so that they are applied in clinical practice when a situation occurs that threatens the independence of such individuals, as is the case of people referred to CUs. In addition, the importance of strategies that promote literacy in the population is reinforced.

Author Contributions: Conceptualization, M.L. and C.F.; methodology, A.R. and H.O.; validation, M.L., C.F. and A.H.; formal analysis, A.R. and H.O.; investigation, M.L. and C.F.; resources, A.R. and L.P.; data curation, A.R. and H.O.; writing—original draft preparation, A.R. and L.P.; writing—review and editing, all authors; supervision, M.L., C.F. and A.H.; project administration, M.L.; funding acquisition, M.L. and C.F. All authors have read and agreed to the published version of the manuscript.

Funding: This research was funded by FEDER. Programa Interreg VA España-Portugal (POCTEP), grant number 0499_4IE_PLUS_4_E. This research received an external funding for the PhD scholarship from the Foundation for Science and Technology, grant number SFRH/BD/140865/2018, Portugal (of the one of the authors Ana Ramos).

Institutional Review Board Statement: The study was conducted according to the guidelines of the Declaration of Helsinki, and approved by the Ethics Committee of Scientific Research in the Areas of Human Health and Welfare of the University of Évora (report number 17036 and date of approval 26 April 2017).

Informed Consent Statement: Not applicable.

Data Availability Statement: Data are available from the authors upon reasonable request and with permission of University of Évora.

Conflicts of Interest: The authors declare no conflict of interest.

References

1. European Pathway Association. Care Pathways. 2019. Available online: http://e-p-a.org/care-pathways/ (accessed on 31 July 2021).
2. Lopes, M.J. *Desafios de Inovação em Saúde: Repensar os Modelos de Cuidados*; Universidade de Évora: Évora, Portugal, 2021.
3. World Health Organization. *Integrated Care Models: An Overview: WHO Regional Office for Europe*; World Health Organization, Ed.; World Health Organization: Geneva, Switzerland, 2016; Available online: https://www.euro.who.int/en/health-topics/Health-systems/health-services-delivery/publications/2016/integrated-care-models-an-overview-2016 (accessed on 31 July 2021).
4. Goddard, M.; Mason, A.R. Integrated Care: A Pill for All Ills? *Int. J. Health Policy Manag.* **2016**, *6*, 1–3. [CrossRef]
5. Hopman, P.; de Bruin, S.R.; Forjaz, M.J.; Rodriguez-Blazquez, C.; Tonnara, G.; Lemmens, L.C.; Onder, G.; Baan, C.A.; Rijken, M. Effectiveness of comprehensive care programs for patients with multiple chronic conditions or frailty: A systematic literature review. *Health Policy* **2016**, *120*, 818–832. [CrossRef]

6. Agerholm, J.; de Leon, A.P.; Schön, P.; Burström, B. Impact of Integrated Care on the Rate of Hospitalization for Ambulatory Care Sensitive Conditions among Older Adults in Stockholm County: An Interrupted Time Series Analysis. *Int. J. Integr. Care* **2021**, *21*, 22. [CrossRef]
7. Fanciullo, G.J.; Washington, T. Best practices to reduce the risk of drug-drug interactions: Opportunities for managed care. *Am. J. Manag. Care* **2011**, *17* (Suppl. 1), S299–S304.
8. Baxter, S.; Johnson, M.; Chambers, D.; Sutton, A.; Goyder, E.; Booth, A. The effects of integrated care: A systematic review of UK and international evidence. *BMC Health Serv. Res.* **2018**, *18*, 350. [CrossRef]
9. Pereira, C.; Fonseca, C.; Pinho, L. A Rede Nacional de Cuidados Continuados Integrados em Portugal. In *Os Cuidados de Saúde Face Aos Desafios do Nosso Tempo: Contributos para a Gestão da Mudança*; Lopes, M., Sakellaridesm, C., Eds.; Universidade de Évora: Évora, Portugal, 2021; pp. 36–47.
10. World Health Organization. *The International Classification of Functioning, Disability and Health (ICF)*; World Health Organization, Ed.; World Health Organization: Geneva, Switzerland, 2001.
11. Morgado, B.; Fonseca, C.; Lopes, M.; Pinho, L. *Components of Care Models that Influence Functionality in People Over 65 in the Context of Long-Term Care: Integrative Literature Review BT Gerontechnology III*; García-Alonso, J., Fonseca, C., Eds.; Springer International Publishing: Cham, Switzerland, 2021; pp. 324–335.
12. Lesende, I.M.; Crespo, L.I.M.; Manzanares, S.C.; Otter, A.-S.D.; Bilbao, I.G.; Rodríguez, J.P.; Pérez, I.N.; Azcoaga, I.S.; Fernández, M.J.D.L.R. Functional decline and associated factors in patients with multimorbidity at 8 months of follow-up in primary care: The functionality in pluripathological patients (FUNCIPLUR) longitudinal descriptive study. *BMJ Open* **2018**, *8*, e022377. [CrossRef] [PubMed]
13. Narasimhan, M.; Kapila, M. Implications of self- care for health service provision. *Bull. World Health Organ* **2019**, *97*, 76A. [CrossRef] [PubMed]
14. Romeyke, T.; Stummer, H. Clinical pathways as instruments for risk and cost management in hospitals—A discussion paper. *Glob. J. Health Sci.* **2012**, *4*, 50–59. [CrossRef]
15. Narasimhan, M.; Allotey, P.; Hardon, A. Self care interventions to advance health and wellbeing: A conceptual framework to inform normative guidance. *BMJ* **2019**, *365*, l688. [CrossRef]
16. Romeyke, T.; Noehammer, E.; Stummer, H. Ensuring Quality in Interdisciplinary Inpatient Chronic Care. *SAGE Open* **2020**, *10*, 1–10. [CrossRef]
17. Ramos, A.; Lopes, M.; Fonseca, C.; Henriques, A. Sociodemographic Profile of People Aged 65 or Over in Long-Term Care in Portugal: Analysis of a Big Data. In *Gerontechnology III. IWoG 2020. Lecture Notes in Bioengineering*; García-Alonso, J., Fonseca, C., Eds.; Springer: Cham, Switzerland, 2021; pp. 438–446. Available online: https://doi.org/10.1007/978-3-030-72567-9_40 (accessed on 31 July 2021). [CrossRef]
18. Ramos, A.; Fonseca, C.; Henriques, A. Developing and Managing Health Systems and Organizations for an Aging Society. In *Handbook of Research on Health Systems and Organizations for an Aging Society*; Fonseca, C., Mendes, D., Mendes, F., García-Alonso, J., Eds.; IGI Global: Hershey, PA, USA, 2020; pp. 62–68. [CrossRef]
19. World Health Organization. *Decade of Healthy Ageing: Baseline Report*; World Health Organization: Geneva, Switzerland, 2020; Available online: https://www.who.int/publications/i/item/9789240017900 (accessed on 31 July 2021).
20. Brites, R. *Análise de Dados com IBM SPSS®: Mix Essencial para Relatórios Profissionais e Teses Académicas, Módulo I—Básico*; ISEG, Ed.; ISEG: Lisboa, Portugal, 2015.
21. Marôco, J. *Análise Estatística com o SPSS Statistics v18–v27*, 8th ed.; Pêro Pinheiro: Lisboa, Portugal, 2021.
22. Lafont, C.; Gérard, S.; Voisin, T.; Pahor, M.; Vellas, B. Reducing "iatrogenic disability" in the hospitalized frail elderly. *J. Nutr. Health Aging* **2011**, *15*, 645–660. [CrossRef] [PubMed]
23. Cuevas-Lara, C.; Izquierdo, M.; de Asteasu, M.L.S.; Ramírez-Vélez, R.; Zambom-Ferraresi, F.; Zambom-Ferraresi, F.; Martínez-Velilla, N. Impact of Game-Based Interventions on Health-Related Outcomes in Hospitalized Older Patients: A Systematic Review. *J. Am. Med. Dir. Assoc.* **2021**, *22*, 364–371. [CrossRef] [PubMed]
24. Gill, T.M.; Allore, H.G.; Gahbauer, E.A.; Murphy, T.E. Change in disability after hospitalization or restricted activity in older persons. *JAMA* **2010**, *304*, 1919–1928. [CrossRef]
25. Luchetti, M.; Cutti, A.G.; Verni, G.; Sacchetti, R.; Rossi, N. Impact of Michelangelo prosthetic hand: Findings from a crossover longitudinal study. *J. Rehabil. Res. Dev.* **2015**, *52*, 605–618. [CrossRef]
26. Fonseca, C.; de Pinho, L.G.; Lopes, M.J.; Marques, M.D.C.; Garcia-Alonso, J. The Elderly Nursing Core Set and the cognition of Portuguese older adults: A cross-sectional study. *BMC Nurs* **2021**, *20*, 108. [CrossRef]
27. Rodrigues, M.A.P.; Facchini, L.A.; Thumé, E.; Maia, F. Gender and incidence of functional disability in the elderly: A systematic review. *Cad. Saude Publica* **2009**, *25* (Suppl. 3), S464–S476. [CrossRef]
28. Lopes, M.J.; Pinho, L.G.; de Fonseca, C.; Goes, M.; Oliveira, H.; Garcia-Alonso, J.; Afonso, A. Functioning and Cognition of Portuguese Older Adults Attending in Residential Homes and Day Centers: A Comparative Study. *Int. J. Environ. Res. Public Health* **2021**, *18*, 7030. [CrossRef]
29. Serrano-Alarcón, M.; Perelman, J. Ageing under unequal circumstances: A cross-sectional analysis of the gender and socioeconomic patterning of functional limitations among the Southern European elderly. *Int. J. Equity Health* **2017**, *16*, 175. [CrossRef]
30. Lee, J.; Meijer, E.; Phillips, D.; Hu, P. Disability Incidence Rates for Men and Women in 23 Countries: Evidence on Health Effects of Gender Inequality. *J. Gerontol. A Biol. Sci. Med. Sci.* **2021**, *76*, 328–338. [CrossRef] [PubMed]

31. Schmitz, A.; Lazarevič, P. The gender health gap in Europe's ageing societies: Universal findings across countries and age groups? *Eur. J. Ageing* **2020**, *17*, 509–520. [CrossRef] [PubMed]
32. Coutinho, A.T.D.Q.; Vilela, M.B.R.; Lima, M.L.L.T.D.; Silva, V.D.L. Social communication and functional independence of the elderly in a community assisted by the family health strategy. *Rev. CEFAC* **2018**, *20*, 363–373. [CrossRef]
33. Abalo, E.M.; Mensah, C.M.; Agyemang-Duah, W.; Peprah, P.; Budu, H.I.; Gyasi, R.M.; Donkor, P.; Amoako, J. Geographical Differences in Perceived Health Status Among Older Adults in Ghana: Do Gender and Educational Status Matter? *Gerontol. Geriatr. Med.* **2018**, *4*, 2333721418796663. [CrossRef]
34. Cui, S.; Wang, R.; Lu, L.; Wang, H.; Zhang, Y. Influence of Education Level on Mental Health and Medical Coping Modes: A Correlation Analysis in the Elderlies. *Am. J. Nurs. Sci.* **2019**, *8*, 324. [CrossRef]
35. Quach, A.; Levine, M.E.; Tanaka, T.; Lu, A.T.; Chen, B.H.; Ferrucci, L.; Ritz, B.; Bandinelli, S.; Neuhouser, M.L.; Beasley, J.; et al. Epigenetic clock analysis of diet, exercise, education, and lifestyle factors. *Aging* **2017**, *9*, 419–446. [CrossRef]
36. Chen, Y.H.; Karimi, M.; Rutten-van Mölken, M.P.M.H. The disease burden of multimorbidity and its interaction with educational level. *PLoS ONE* **2020**, *15*, e0243275. [CrossRef]
37. McClellan, S.P.; Haque, K.; García-Peña, C. Diabetes multimorbidity combinations and disability in the Mexican Health and Aging Study, 2012–2015. *Arch. Gerontol. Geriatr.* **2021**, *93*, 104292. [CrossRef] [PubMed]
38. Quiñones, A.R.; Markwardt, S.; Thielke, S.; Rostant, O.; Vásquez, E.; Botoseneanu, A. Prospective Disability in Different Combinations of Somatic and Mental Multimorbidity. *J. Gerontol. A Biol. Sci. Med. Sci.* **2018**, *73*, 204–210. [CrossRef] [PubMed]

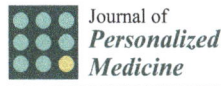

Journal of Personalized Medicine

Article

Exploring the Social Networks of Women Bereaved by Stillbirth: A Descriptive Qualitative Study

Tosin Popoola *, Joan Skinner and Martin Woods

School of Nursing, Midwifery and Health Practice, Victoria University of Wellington,
Wellington 6012, New Zealand; Joan.Skinner@vuw.ac.nz (J.S.); Martin.Woods@vuw.ac.nz (M.W.)
* Correspondence: Tosin.Popoola@vuw.ac.nz

Abstract: The loss of a baby to stillbirth is a traumatic experience and can lead to secondary losses, such as the loss of social relationships. In Nigeria, stillbirths are a common public health problem. However, limited attention has been given to the social ramifications of stillbirths. This study describes the social networks of women who have experienced a stillbirth and the factors influencing their social networks. Interviews and social network diagrams were used to collect data from 20 women about their social networks before and after stillbirth. Findings suggest that the experience of shame, unmet expectation of support, and a lack of trust led to relationship changes after stillbirth. Most participants met bereavement needs with their existing social networks before stillbirth, but many participants also experienced relationship losses (even among family networks). Information from social network analysis can reveal the risks and strengths inherent in social networks, which can be helpful for the provision of tailored/personalized bereavement care.

Keywords: drawings; Nigeria; perinatal loss; social networks; stillbirth; stillborn

Citation: Popoola, T.; Skinner, J.; Woods, M. Exploring the Social Networks of Women Bereaved by Stillbirth: A Descriptive Qualitative Study. *J. Pers. Med.* **2021**, *11*, 1056. https://doi.org/10.3390/jpm11111056

Academic Editors: Riitta Suhonen, Minna Stolt and David Edvardsson

Received: 28 September 2021
Accepted: 19 October 2021
Published: 21 October 2021

Publisher's Note: MDPI stays neutral with regard to jurisdictional claims in published maps and institutional affiliations.

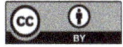

Copyright: © 2021 by the authors. Licensee MDPI, Basel, Switzerland. This article is an open access article distributed under the terms and conditions of the Creative Commons Attribution (CC BY) license (https:// creativecommons.org/licenses/by/ 4.0/).

1. Introduction

The loss of a baby to stillbirth is a devastating and traumatic experience for women [1,2]. However, women do not just lose a baby when they experience stillbirth. When a child is lost to stillbirth, women often lose their emerging social status as an 'expecting mother' [3,4], leading to shame and low self-esteem [5] The experience of shame after stillbirth often leads to social withdrawal, loneliness, and relationship deterioration [5,6], which may lead to prolonged or complicated grief [4].

Generally, bereaved people experience changes in their social networks [7,8], and this is no different for mothers of stillborn babies [9,10]. However, in stillbirth bereavement, mothers may feel unsupported and isolated [9,11]. As a result of social withdrawal due to stigma, women's social networks may become smaller, disconnected, or under-resourced [10–12] and their family may emerge as the primary source of support [1,2]. However, the social ramifications of stillbirths extend beyond the family [1,13]. Even if the family was supportive, the bereaved mother would need others outside the family to successfully reintegrate back into society [4]. However, there is limited focus on the social networks of women bereaved by stillbirths.

Social networks, understood here as the people and institutions through which an individual receives and gives social support, is important in stillbirth bereavement. After a stillbirth, women turn to their social networks to seek and receive social support [4]. However, many factors determine whether social support will be exchanged. For example, in spousal bereavement, Morrigan et al. [8] found that unmet expectations of support led to relationship loss and changes. Similarly, Aoun et al. [7] found that the amount, timing, function, and structure of social support influenced bereaved peoples' perception of the helpfulness or unhelpfulness of their social networks. However, research continues to favor the individual and psychological aspects of stillbirth bereavement over social dimensions of stillbirth loss.

In Nigeria, stillbirths are a significant public health problem. In 2019 alone, 171,428 babies were stillborn in Nigeria [14]. Dated but important studies on perinatal loss in Nigeria suggest that social support protects against depression and anxiety [15,16]. However, social norms have also been reported to prevent new social relationships after stillbirth in Nigeria [17]. For example, research suggests that Nigerian women have little to no opportunities to connect with their social networks after stillbirth due to the absence of rituals and funerals for stillborn babies [17,18]. Despite this, no research has examined the social ramifications of stillbirth loss in Nigeria.

Women's social networks hold social resources such as thew emotional, financial, and psychological support needed for a healthy grieving. As a result, it is crucial to identify the social networks that women bereaved by stillbirth have access to or do not have access to. This research seeks to describe the social networks of a sample of Nigerian women who have experienced the loss of a baby through stillbirth and the factors influencing their social networks.

2. Method

This study utilized a descriptive qualitative design. After obtaining ethical approvals from the Ethical Review Committee of the Saki Baptist Medical Centre and the Human Ethics Committee of the Victoria University of Wellington (#23450), women bereaved by stillbirth were recruited. Twenty women aged 22 to 44 years (mean = 33.5) were recruited through snowballing from Saki, a town predominantly occupied by the Yoruba ethnic group in southwest Nigeria (Table 1). The sociocultural norms and attitudes of the Yoruba people about stillbirth have been described elsewhere (Popoola et al., 2021b). Potential participants who expressed interest in discussing their stillbirth experience were contacted by the first author (TP) who also happens to be a native of Saki town. Since the focus of the research was on the participants' social networks, eligibility was limited to women whose stillbirth was more than six months but less than three years ago. The eligibility criterion was intended to minimize distress during the early stages of grief and allow a timeframe where mothers could still remember those who played a role in their adjustment to loss.

Table 1. Demographic characteristics of the study participants.

	N = 20
Age in years	
Mean (range)	33.5 (22–44)
Educational level	
No education	7
Primary/secondary/Tertiary	3/2/8
Marital status	
Married or cohabiting	15
Single	4
Widowed	1
Time of death of baby	
Intrapartum (during childbirth)	17
Antepartum (before childbirth)	3
Place of birth	
Healthcare facilities	19
Homebirth	1
Gestational age at the time of loss	
37 weeks and above	16
30–36 weeks	4
Gravidity (number of previous pregnancies before stillbirth)	
Primigravida	8
Multigravida	12

2.1. Data Collection

All women who participated in this study signed written informed consent before data were collected with face-to-face semi-structured interviews and social network diagrams in 2017 (Table 2). Most of the participants ($n = 19$) were interviewed in their homes based on their preferences. Interviews preceded social network diagrams since we wanted to build rapport and ease the participants into talking about a traumatic loss. The drawings were made on a Livescribe A5 notebook with the Livescribe pen since it allowed digital capturing of the diagrams and recording of the interviews.

Table 2. Interviews and diagrams' instructions.

Semi-Structured Interview Guide	Social Network Diagrams
1. What was your relationship with friends, neighbors, colleagues, family and others like after loss?	1. I would like you to draw an image of yourself.
2. Could you tell me how the loss of your child impacted on your relationship with others?	2. I would like you to add images of people (friends, neighbors, partner, extended families, colleagues) that come to mind when you think of the loss of your child.
3. What are those things that you can say assisted you to deal with your loss and where did you receive those from?	3. I would like you to add images of any social/environmental systems (hospital, church, mosque, midwife/nurse/doctor, school, work, child support agency) that played either positive or negative roles in your experience of loss.
4. How well would you say you were supported by your relatives, friends, colleagues and others after the loss of your baby?	4. Please join yourself to the people you have added to your drawing with a maximum of three lines and a minimum of one line, depending on how you perceive the person's support.

The instructions that guided the creation of the diagrams were adapted from Pienaar et al.'s [19] communication mapping methodology, an approach that is embedded in communicative ecology models. Broad et al. [20] defined communicative ecologies as the network of connections individuals or groups depend upon to achieve their goals. Thus, from a communicative ecology perspective, the different people who are involved in an ecology, their relationships, and the social institutions and structures that connect them are the focus of analysis [21]. Visually representing social networks through diagrams has been found to facilitate meaningful discussions about social networks and the social context in which giving and receiving social support occurs [22]. In this study, eliciting information through social network drawings was important since women bereaved by stillbirth often perceive that their grief is not real and may be reluctant to discuss their experience publicly [4].

To construct the social network diagram, each participant was asked to draw a picture of herself on the Livescribe A5 notebook. After that, the participant was then asked to add her social networks to the image. Each participant was also asked to join herself with each social network using a maximum of three lines to show the quality of relationships. To identify the changes that might have occurred to the social networks after stillbirth, each participant was asked to look at the diagram and draw another one showing her social networks before stillbirth. After drawing the social network diagrams, the participants were invited to reflect on the changes in their social networks. The participants' reflections on their drawings were validated against the interview data and any discrepancies were discussed and clarified. The collection of two drawings per participant means 40 diagrams were produced in total. The interviews averaged 45 min.

2.2. Analysis

The data collection processes included audio-recordings and digital capture of the diagrams, using a Livescribe A5 notebook/pen. The interviews that were conducted in the Yoruba language were translated to English during transcribing. A back-translation to Yoruba was conducted to ensure translation accuracy, and a second native Yoruba speaker verified this. The back-translation had to consider the challenge presented by the use of metaphors by the participants. Consistent with the nature of the data, we adopted both quantitative and qualitative methods of analysis. Raw images from the participants were used to present their social networks. However, a simple statistical analysis was used to analyze the number of people in the social networks and relationships (such as family). A qualitative analysis (thematic) was performed to explain the factors influencing the participants' social networks. Starting with data familiarization, the dataset was read repeatedly to identify statements relevant to the participants' social networks and the factors that determined why a participant turned to someone for help or not. Based on the significant statements identified from the data, the authors jointly developed a codebook and used it to group the significant statements into themes.

2.3. Rigor

The criteria for ensuring rigor in qualitative research by Lincoln and Guba (cited in Connelly [23]) was followed in this study. The first author (TP) collected all of the data, and this enhanced the consistency of the data collection procedure. The first author also had the advantage of cultural insights, which enhanced the quality of the data interpretation. The use of culturally appropriate probes also assisted with the achievement of prolonged engagement with the participants. Participants also had opportunities to confirm the accuracy of interview transcripts/summaries and those who did ($n = 7$) made no changes. A reflective journal was kept during the project's data collection phase, which was used to debrief the co-authors. The findings are grounded in participants' narratives and all the authors agreed with the final thematic schemata. Pseudonyms SK# was used to present quotations.

3. Results

Before stillbirth, the total number of people found in the social network diagrams of the 20 participants was 127. For individual participants, the lowest social network was 2, while the highest social network was 15 (average = 6.35) before stillbirth. After stillbirth, the total number of people found in the social network diagrams of the 20 participants reduced to 99. For individual participants, the lowest social network after stillbirth was 2, while the highest social network was 8 (average = 4.95). The social network analysis revealed six types of social relationships: family, friends, acquaintances, colleagues, neighbors, and healthcare providers. Family networks (consanguineous and affinal kin) accounted for more than half of participants' social networks before and after stillbirth, while healthcare providers were the least represented (Table 3).

The social network of most of the participants was stable, with 11 participants experiencing no loss or gain in social relationships after stillbirth. This suggests that the majority of the participants met the needs of bereavement with their existing social networks. Eight participants experienced relationship losses after stillbirth, with the most remarkable loss being amongst family relationships, where a total of 15 family members were dropped after stillbirth. Compared to the loss of family networks, the relationship loss in other domains was minimal: acquaintance = 4, friends = 4, colleagues = 4, neighbor = 1. Only one participant gained new social networks (from 2 to 6), with the new additional social networks being acquaintances from the place of worship. Table 3 presents the descriptive statistical analysis of the participants' social networks before and after stillbirth.

Table 3. Description of the participants' social networks.

	Before Stillbirth N = 20 Diagrams	After Stillbirth N = 20 Diagrams
Social networks		
Total network size	127	99
Range	2–15	2–8
Mean	6.35	4.95
Composition of social networks		
Family	65	50
Friends	34	30
Acquaintance	16	12
Colleagues	7	3
Neighbors	4	3
Healthcare providers	1	1
Gender composition of social networks		
Female	98	69
Male	29	30

3.1. Findings Regarding Women's Social Networks and the Factors Influencing It

The factors that influenced the participants' social networks are presented in three categories: the perception of shame, expectation of support, and trust.

3.1.1. The Perception of Shame

> "After I put to bed [gave birth], I hid the loss from people because I was ashamed that people might call me a failure ... " (SK1)

> "Whenever I saw someone who knew I was pregnant, my heart would skip [nervous] and I always tried to scurry away as if I had done something wrong ... I felt like I had some impediments that I needed to be ashamed of". (SK5)

As indicated in the above quotes, participants tried to conceal the loss by avoiding social interactions. All participants experienced self-shame, with some likening the shame of stillbirth to other socially stigmatizing events such as incarceration. For example, one participant who concealed the loss by misleading others about her whereabouts used a metaphor about incarceration to discuss how stillbirth had devalued her. The participant said "kini idunu elewon ton'so ago mo owo [what pride does an ex-convict have to raise shoulders in the community]" (SK10).

The participants concealed the loss by engaging in two types of strategies. The first strategy used to avoid shame was the observance of a protracted period of mourning. Most participants exceeded the culturally stipulated period of mourning (40 days) since they were unsure how people would interpret their demeanor and conduct.

> "Grieving as a mother whose child passed away is very tricky and challenging. On the one hand, you cannot move on too quickly because people expect a lengthy and genuine portrayal of soberness from you ... your conduct should convince people that the loss truly and deeply pained you. On the other hand, you also cannot dwell on it for too long because people expect you to be grateful for your own life ... So, grieving a stillborn child is like a performance; the timing of your re-entrance into the society, the way you carry yourself and your countenance must genuinely reflect your sadness but also your gratitude ... Performing this role is hard". (SK13)

The second type of behavior that the participants used to avoid shame was relocating from their familiar environment. One participant even implied that "*suicide was better than facing shame [iku ya ju esin lo] (SK15)*". To avoid facing the shame of stillbirth, some participants relocated from their homes for up to six months, thinking that the passage of time would make people forget about the pregnancy. One participant who relocated for over six months said, "ki oju ma ri ibi, gbogbo ara lo gun e [in order for my eyes not to see shame, I had to flee with all my body]" (SK18).

Both strategies employed to avoid shame resulted in relationship loss or inhibited the formation of new social networks. As illustrated in Figure 1, efforts to conceal the loss from others mean the family was more likely to be left in the social network after stillbirth, making the family a critical support network.

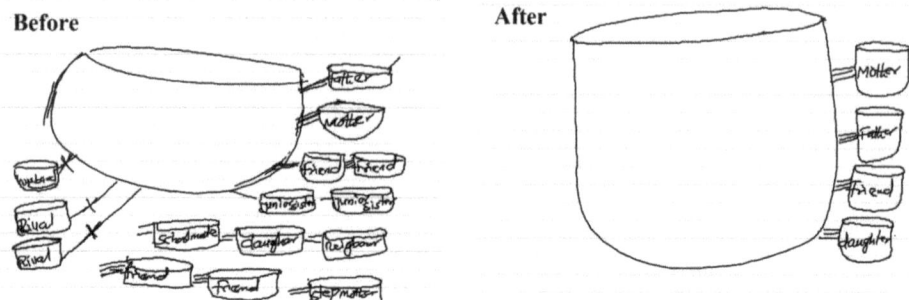

Figure 1. Iku ya ju j'esin lo [death is more preferable to shame] (SK15).

Supportive social interactions tend to counteract the negative impact of shame, as one participant described.

"When it happened [stillbirth], it felt like I was alone and I felt like there was nothing good about me anymore. But with the support of my mother, my level of shame started to reduce, and I started to become more comfortable in the presence of others". (SK13)

3.1.2. Expectation of Support

After the stillbirth, participants evaluated their relationships based on the perception of received/expected support and the level of interest shown by others in the grief. Using the metaphor below, some participants said they realized that some people in their social networks were fair-weather friends and could not be relied on for support.

"owo epo ni araye n'banila, won ki n'banila t'eje [people want to taste part of the oil (palm oil) in your hands, but not the blood]". (SK12)

All relationships were evaluated for their worth and usefulness, but it seemed that women were more critical of family members and close friends in terms of expected support. Unlike other relationships, participants were more likely to describe the support they expected or received from family members as a form of obligation.

"The person [child's father] who was supposed to help and support me was nowhere to be found. Everything he was supposed to do as a spouse and the father of the child, he did not do". (SK12)

"I would have loved my mother-in-law to be there for me, but she ended up disappointing me". (SK17)

"I did not feel that those around me understood my grief. Even though people surrounded me, I felt alone . . . Everyone was saying the same thing and doing the same thing, but I had other needs that nobody cared about". (SK14)

As seen in Figure 2, family or close social relationships that did not meet the mothers' expectations tend to be removed from the social network after stillbirth. Single women also tend to have the lowest social network after stillbirth. The highest number of people in single women's social networks was four (ranged from two to four) and the quality of relationships also tend to be fragile.

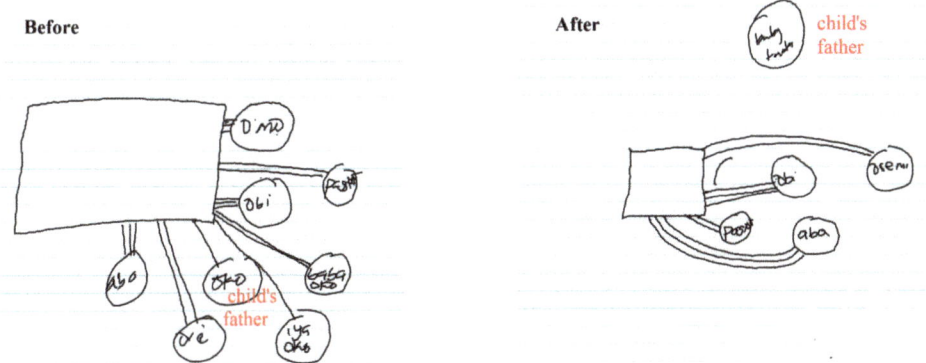

Figure 2. Owo epo ni araye n'banila, won ki n'banila t'eje [people will help you lick your fingers if drenched in palm oil, but not when it is drenched in blood] (SK12).

When social networks met the expectation of support, the quality of the relationship between women and their social networks strengthened. As seen in Figure 3, a participant dropped her sister from her social network after stillbirth. However, the quality of the relationship increased with her mother and husband since they met the participants' emotional needs.

"My mum was very supportive . . . she moved closer to me and listened to my views about how I felt about the whole situation. During that time, I needed someone to talk to, not just people who would tell me it will be alright". (SK9)

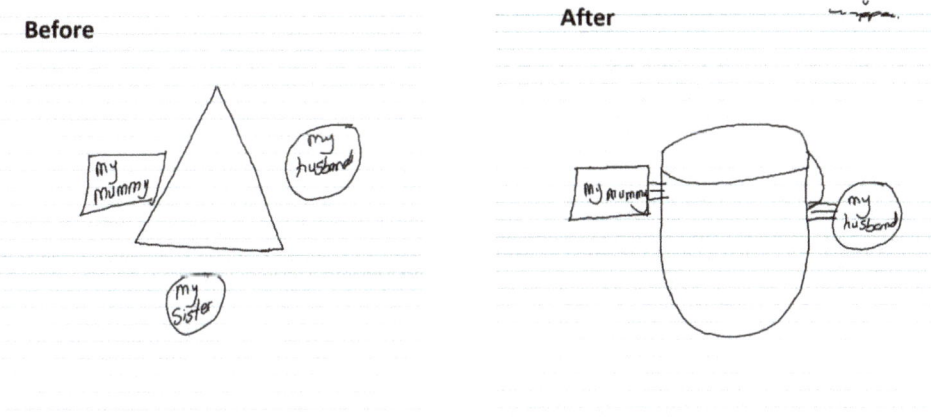

Figure 3. Ti aja ba ni eni lehin, a pa obo [with the support of others, a person can survive any challenges] (SK9).

3.1.3. Trust

A lack of trust between participants and their social relations also prevented the formation of new relationships. Certain behaviors such as gossiping, blaming and insensitive comments created distrust and hindered mothers from engaging with others.

"When it happened, I felt like some people thought I deserved to lose the child because I had a home birth. Whenever I walk past, they gossip about me and I sometimes overhear them saying, 'look at the woman who did not value the life of a child' ... I came out of the experience as a very introverted and paranoid person". (SK17)

"After the incident, the doctors and the nurses did not even give me the chance to gather myself together before they started asking how we were going to pay the hospital bills ... they did not show any human feeling and I did not trust them to look after me". (SK10)

While a lack of trust prevented the formation of social relationships, participants bonded with those who were deemed trustworthy in their social network. The majority of the participants received the most support from their spouses and found them trustworthy.

"From my experience, I think the greatest gift you can receive when you lose a child is a true friend that you can trust with your pains ... My husband was the one who really stood by me. He didn't go to work until two weeks after the incident ... ". (SK2)

4. Discussion

The findings of this study confirm earlier studies that have reported that bereavement leads to relationship changes [7,8,10]. The factors that influenced relationship changes in this study: shame [5,13], the unmet expectation of support [2] and mistrust [2,10] have been confirmed separately by other studies. Of the three factors that influenced the participants' social networks, shame/stigma has received the most attention in stillbirth research. In response to perceived/anticipated shame, women may try to conceal the loss [5,13], leading to relationship changes [2,10]. Consistent with earlier studies [5,6], we found that our participants employed strategies such as relocating or observing prolonged mourning to avoid shame, but this resulted in relationship loss or stagnancy. While concealment strategies might provide temporary salve for mothers, Pollock et al. [5] note that such strategies might heighten the risk of internalized grief and guilt, which may worsen bereavement outcomes in the long term.

In times of loss and crisis, people commonly turn to their social network for support [4]. However, being embedded within a network of relationships does not guarantee support for bereaved people [7]. Factors that determine whether support will be perceived as helpful or unhelpful have been explored from the size or quality of social networks but with conflicting results. For example, among people who have experienced traumatic events, Platt et al. [24] found that heterogeneous social network, not perception of strong social support, was more protective against post-traumatic stress disorder. In contrast, Ferlander et al. [25] found that a homogenous social network comprising of immediate family was more protective against depression for Russian women. Limited studies on bereavement, including stillbirths, suggest that type, size, and quality of social networks are essential for bereavement outcomes [7,26].

The needs of bereaved people are often complex and multifaceted [7,8]. Common needs during stillbirth bereavement, such as rebuilding identity, planning funerals, resolving psychological trauma, planning future reproductive health, and meeting financial needs, may be best met by a combination of intrapersonal and interpersonal social networks [1,27]. In this study, the participants' social networks did not include stillbirth support groups and there was an under-representation of health personnel. In addition, the participants who were single also tend to have smaller social networks and this echoes earlier studies that have reported that unmarried women have limited support after stillbirth [26,28]. This finding highlights that single women and those whose social networks are devoid of stillbirth support groups and health professionals may have limited support and feel socially isolated.

Similar to earlier studies [2,10], our findings also suggest that women rely more on family networks than any other types of relationships. In stillbirth bereavement, women may have no other choice but to rely on their family and existing social networks due to stigma and lack of social recognition of stillbirth loss. However, while the family may not be able to meet all the bereavement needs, Cacciatore et al. [26] found that family support is the only type of support that predicted anxiety and depression. Our findings replicate previous studies that family support is not a guarantee in stillbirth bereavement [2,6]. Previously, it has been reported separately that incongruent grieving styles, migration and insensitive comments from family members lead to family breakdown after stillbirth [2,6,29]. Our study adds that moral obligations within family relationships can play dual roles in bereavement; it can guarantee support for mothers, but also increase the likelihood of family breakdown. Family crises pose a severe threat to mothers' wellbeing and bereavement outcomes, especially in low and middle-income countries where social support groups, trained counsellors, and psychiatrists may not always be available [27]. Therefore, health personnel must recognize that the family network may be under pressure to meet bereavement needs, especially when external support is limited.

In this study, the mean social network of mothers after stillbirth was 4.95 (range 2–8). This is smaller compared to women in general, where an average number of 10 people has been reported among women's social networks [30–32]. The paucity of evidence on the social network of mothers of stillborn babies means we cannot compare the size of social networks that we found with other studies. However, it is important for those caring for women bereaved by stillbirth to know whether they should focus their interventions on social networks' size/quality, or structure/contents. Future studies are needed to increase our understandings of aspects of social networks that influence bereavement outcomes.

5. Strength and Limitations

This study employed a creative and novel method to facilitate dialogue about a tabooed and challenging subject. The use of drawings permitted metaphors, which unlocked the barriers posed by language and social norms around the issue. The use of dual media of interviews and drawings allowed the participants to express feelings that may have been difficult in words. The limitations in this study are related to the methodological decisions taken. First, the participants' social network may be more extensive than we found if this study was conducted immediately after stillbirth. Second, the network size that we found may differ if the participants were asked to list or estimate their social networks instead of drawings (see Morrigan et al. [8], for instance). Third, time since loss might have resulted in the under-estimation of the social networks, but we did not notice any significant difference between participants based on time since the loss. Fourth, real-life relationships are intertwined and conceptually distinguishing them by the nature of relationships might overlook some nuances in the way people experience their social relationships. Fifth, due to the small sample size and the fact that all the participants belonged to the same Yoruba ethnic group, the transferability/generalizability of the findings to other contexts need to be assessed carefully. However, while the social networks that we found in this study might not represent all possible ties and relationships, it presents the social network that the participants identify as significant for themselves after stillbirth.

6. Conclusions and Practice Recommendations

The loss of social networks and the inability to form new social networks after stillbirth suggests that mothers of stillborn babies may feel unsupported, isolated and miss out on critical bereavement support. Our study adds to the emerging literature on social networks of bereaved people [7,8] by suggesting that bereaved mothers' social networks can be influenced by shame, mistrust and unmet expectation of support.

The use of drawings to capture the social networks of mothers proved to be useful in analyzing the social relationships and the risk factors for social isolation. Since the experience of grief is unique and individual, the social network technique used in this study can help health personnel to provide personalized/person-centered bereavement care. When diagrams are used to elucidate the social relationships of women bereaved by stillbirth, health personnel may find that mothers' social networks are conflictive, broken or fragmented and may be tempted to want to fix such broken relationships. However, Sanicola [33] argued that the goal of care is not to remedy broken ties but to facilitate collective caregiving. This means that healthcare providers can achieve better bereavement outcomes if they locate bereavement care within the context of supportive and reliable relationships.

Despite the loss of family networks, the family was still a reliable source of support for the participants. However, the vulnerabilities of family relationships to breakdown cannot be overlooked in clinical care. Family breakdown can negatively impact the bereavement outcome, especially in Nigeria, where there is no external support for mothers after stillbirth [11,17]. Due to the risk that stillbirth presents to women and their families, healthcare providers need to approach stillbirth bereavement from a family-centered perspective. Healthcare providers can help mothers and their families discuss expectations and link the family with appropriate and supportive resources.

Author Contributions: Conceptualization T.P.; data acquisition T.P., data analysis and interpretation T.P., J.S. and M.W.; manuscript drafting T.P.; critical revisions T.P., J.S. and M.W. All authors have read and agreed to the published version of the manuscript.

Funding: The research was funded by the Victoria University of Wellington, grant number 400348.

Institutional Review Board Statement: The protocol for this study was granted ethical approvals by Victoria University of Wellington Human Ethics Committee and Saki Baptist Medical Centre Ethical Review Committee.

Informed Consent Statement: Written informed consent was obtained from all participants involved in the study.

Data Availability Statement: The de-identified transcripts of interviews and diagrams are still held by the primary author and can be provided upon reasonable request and sound methodological justification.

Conflicts of Interest: The authors declare no conflict of interest.

References

1. Avila, M.C.; Medina, I.M.F.; Jiménez-López, F.R.; Granero-Molina, J.; Hernández-Padilla, J.M.; Sánchez, E.H.; Fernández-Sola, C. Parents' Experiences About Support Following Stillbirth and Neonatal Death. *Adv. Neonatal. Care* **2020**, *20*, 151–160. [CrossRef]
2. Mills, T.; Ayebare, E.; Mukhwana, R.; Mweteise, J.; Nabisere, A.; Nendela, A.; Ndungu, P.; Okello, M.; Omoni, G.; Wakasiaka, S.; et al. Parents' experiences of care and support after stillbirth in rural and urban maternity facilities: A qualitative study in Kenya and Uganda. *BJOG: Int. J. Obstet. Gynaecol.* **2021**, *128*, 101–109. [CrossRef]
3. Hill, P.W.; Cacciatore, J.; Shreffler, K.M.; Pritchard, K.M. The loss of self: The effect of miscarriage, stillbirth, and child death on maternal self-esteem. *Death Stud.* **2017**, *41*, 226–235. [CrossRef]
4. Markin, R.D.; Zilcha-Mano, S. Cultural processes in psychotherapy for perinatal loss: Breaking the cultural taboo against perinatal grief. *Psychother.* **2018**, *55*, 20–26. [CrossRef] [PubMed]
5. Pollock, D.; Pearson, E.; Cooper, M.; Ziaian, T.; Foord, C.; Warland, J. Voices of the unheard: A qualitative survey exploring bereaved parents experiences of stillbirth stigma. *Women Birth* **2020**, *33*, 165–174. [CrossRef] [PubMed]
6. Fernández-Basanta, S.; Van, P.; Coronado, C.; Torres, M.; Fernández, M.J.M. Coping After Involuntary Pregnancy Loss: Perspectives of Spanish European Women. *Omega-J. Death Dying* **2021**, *83*, 310–324. [CrossRef] [PubMed]
7. Aoun, S.M.; Breen, L.; Rumbold, B.; Christian, K.M.; Same, A.; Abel, J. Matching response to need: What makes social networks fit for providing bereavement support? *PLoS ONE* **2019**, *14*, e0213367. [CrossRef] [PubMed]
8. Morrigan, B.; Keesing, S.; Breen, L.J. Exploring the Social Networks of Bereaved Spouses: Phenomenological Case Studies. *Omega-J. Death Dying* **2020**, 1–17. [CrossRef]
9. Ayebare, E.; Lavender, T.; Mweteise, J.; Nabisere, A.; Nendela, A.; Mukhwana, R.; Wood, R.; Wakasiaka, S.; Omoni, G.; Kagoda, B.S.; et al. The impact of cultural beliefs and practices on parents' experiences of bereavement following stillbirth: A qualitative study in Uganda and Kenya. *BMC Pregnancy Childbirth* **2021**, *21*, 1–10. [CrossRef]
10. Das, M.K.; Arora, N.K.; Gaikwad, H.; Chellani, H.; Debata, P.; Rasaily, R.; Meena, K.R.; Kaur, G.; Malik, P.; Joshi, S.; et al. Grief reaction and psychosocial impacts of child death and stillbirth on bereaved North Indian parents: A qualitative study. *PLoS ONE* **2021**, *16*, e0240270. [CrossRef] [PubMed]

11. Popoola, T.; Skinner, J.; Woods, M. 'Every woman wants to know what came out of her body': Grief experiences of women after stillbirth in Nigeria. *OMEGA—J. Death Dying*. (In Press)
12. De Bernis, L.; Kinney, M.V.; Stones, W.; ten Hoope-Bender, P.; Vivio, D.; Leisher, S.H.; Lancet Ending Preventable Stillbirths Series study group. Stillbirths: Ending preventable deaths by 2030. *Lancet* **2016**, *387*, 703–716. [CrossRef]
13. Testoni, I.; Bregoli, J.; Pompele, S.; Maccarini, A. Social Support in Perinatal Grief and Mothers' Continuing Bonds: A Qualitative Study with Italian Mourners. *Affil.* **2020**, *35*, 485–502. [CrossRef]
14. UNICEF. *Hidden Tragedy: A Neglected Tragedy: The Global Burden of Stills*; UNICEF: New York, NY, USA, 2020.
15. Adewuya, A.O.; Ola, B.A.; Aloba, O.O.; Dada, A.O.; Fasoto, O.O. Prevalence and correlates of depression in late pregnancy among Nigerian women. *Depress. Anxiety* **2006**, *24*, 15–21. [CrossRef]
16. Adeyemi, A.; Mosaku, K.; Ajenifuja, O.; Fatoye, F.; Makinde, N.; Ola, B. Depressive Symptoms in a Sample of Women Following Perinatal Loss. *J. Natl. Med Assoc.* **2008**, *100*, 1463–1468. [CrossRef]
17. Adebayo, A.; Liu, M.; Cheah, W. Sociocultural Understanding of Miscarriages, Stillbirths, and Infant Loss: A Study of Nigerian Women. *J. Intercult. Commun. Res.* **2018**, *48*, 91–111. [CrossRef]
18. Popoola, T.; Skinner, J.; Woods, M. Beliefs and strategies for coping with stillbirth: A qualitative study in Nigeria. *Bereave. Care*, in press.
19. Pienaar, A.; Swanepoel, Z.; Van Rensburg, H.; Heunis, C. A qualitative exploration of resilience in pre-adolescent AIDS orphans living in a residential care facility. *Sahara-J J. Soc. Asp. HIV/AIDS* **2011**, *8*, 128–137. [CrossRef]
20. Broad, G.M.; Ball-Rokeach, S.J.; Ognyanova, K.; Stokes, B.; Picasso, T.; Villanueva, G. Understanding Communication Ecologies to Bridge Communication Research and Community Action. *J. Appl. Commun. Res.* **2013**, *41*, 325–345. [CrossRef]
21. Foth, M.; Hearn, G. Networked individualism of urban residents: Discovering the communicative ecology in inner-city apartment buildings. *Inf. Commun. Soc.* **2007**, *10*, 749–772. [CrossRef]
22. De Morais, R.D.C.M.; de Souza, T.V.; dos Santos Oliveira, I.C.; de Moraes, J.R.M.M. Structure of the social network of mothers/caregivers of hospitalized children. *Cogitare Enferm* **2018**, *23*, e50456.
23. Connelly, L.M. Trustworthiness in Qualitative Research. *Medsurg Nurs. Off. J. Acad. Med-Surg. Nurses* **2016**, *25*, 435–436.
24. Platt, J.; Keyes, K.M.; Koenen, K.C. Size of the social network versus quality of social support: Which is more protective against PTSD? *Soc. Psychiatry Psychiatr. Epidemiol.* **2014**, *49*, 1279–1286. [CrossRef] [PubMed]
25. Ferlander, S.; Stickley, A.; Kislitsyna, O.; Jukkala, T.; Carlson, P.; Mäkinen, I.H. Social capital—A mixed blessing for women? A cross-sectional study of different forms of social relations and self-rated depression in Moscow. *BMC Psychol.* **2016**, *4*, 37. [CrossRef] [PubMed]
26. Cacciatore, J.; Schnebly, S.; Froen, J.F.F. The effects of social support on maternal anxiety and depression after stillbirth. *Health Soc. Care Community* **2009**, *17*, 167–176. [CrossRef]
27. Shakespeare, C.; Merriel, A.; Bakhbakhi, D.; Blencowe, H.; Boyle, F.M.; Flenady, V.; Gold, K.; Horey, D.; Lynch, M.; Mills, T.A.; et al. The RESPECT Study for consensus on global bereavement care after stillbirth. *Int. J. Gynecol. Obstet.* **2020**, *149*, 137–147. [CrossRef]
28. Gold, K.J.; Treadwell, M.C.; Mieras, M.E.; Laventhal, N. Who tells a mother her baby has died? Communication and staff presence during stillbirth delivery and early infant death. *J. Perinatol.* **2017**, *37*, 1330–1334. [CrossRef]
29. Romney, J.; Fife, S.T.; Sanders, D.; Behrens, S. Treatment of Couples Experiencing Pregnancy Loss: Reauthoring Loss from a Narrative Perspective. *Int. J. Syst. Ther.* **2021**, *32*, 134–152. [CrossRef]
30. Asrese, K.; Adamek, M.E. Women's social networks and use of facility delivery services for uncomplicated births in North West Ethiopia: A community-based case-control study. *BMC Pregnancy Childbirth* **2017**, *17*, 441. [CrossRef]
31. McLaughlin, D.; Vagenas, D.; Pachana, N.; Begum, N.; Dobson, A. Gender Differences in Social Network Size and Satisfaction in Adults in Their 70s. *J. Heal. Psychol.* **2010**, *15*, 671–679. [CrossRef]
32. Smith, K.; Wilson, J.; Strough, J.; Parker, A.; De Bruin, W.B. Social support network size and gender composition across the adult life span. *Innov. Aging* **2018**, *2* (Suppl. 1), 999–1000. [CrossRef]
33. Sanicola, L. Caring for the relationship. *J. Med. Person* **2009**, *7*, 129–138. [CrossRef]

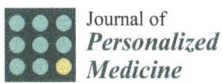

Article

Use of Digital Educational Technologies among Nursing Students and Teachers: An Exploratory Study

Fernanda Loureiro [1,*], Luís Sousa [2] and Vanessa Antunes [1]

1 Centro de Investigação Interdisciplinar Egas Moniz (CiiEM), Escola Superior de Saúde Egas Moniz, 2829-551 Almada, Portugal; vanessa2em@gmail.com
2 Comprehensive Health Research Centre (CHRC), Nursing Department, Universidade de Évora, 7004-516 Évora, Portugal; lmms@uevora.pt
* Correspondence: floureiro@egasmoniz.edu.pt

Abstract: The emergence of digital educational technologies (DET) raises questions regarding the personalization of both teaching and care. DET use implies profound changes with consequences in nursing care and in nursing teaching-learning process. With the purpose of contributing to the improvement of the teaching-learning process through the use of DET, an exploratory-descriptive, cross-sectional, and observational study, with a quantitative approach (descriptive and inferential statistics), was developed. Online questionnaires were applied (n = 140 students and n = 23 teachers) after ethics committee approval. Results point to low cost and access without time/space limits as the main benefits, and decreased interaction, less physical contact, and technical difficulties as constraints. Globally, there was no difference between students and teachers in the use of DET. Still, men report more constraints than women. In this sample, the use of DET is still at an early stage. Both students and teachers are still unfamiliar with the scope and possibilities of these tools, not taking full advantage of the potential they have to offer. The impact of DET used in personalized nursing care is still yet to be understood.

Keywords: education; distance; education; learning; digital

Citation: Loureiro, F.; Sousa, L.; Antunes, V. Use of Digital Educational Technologies among Nursing Students and Teachers: An Exploratory Study. *J. Pers. Med.* **2021**, *11*, 1010. https://doi.org/10.3390/jpm11101010

Academic Editors: David Edvardsson, Minna Stolt and Riitta Suhonen

Received: 7 September 2021
Accepted: 5 October 2021
Published: 8 October 2021

Publisher's Note: MDPI stays neutral with regard to jurisdictional claims in published maps and institutional affiliations.

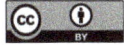

Copyright: © 2021 by the authors. Licensee MDPI, Basel, Switzerland. This article is an open access article distributed under the terms and conditions of the Creative Commons Attribution (CC BY) license (https://creativecommons.org/licenses/by/4.0/).

1. Introduction

Digital educational technologies (DET) have been used increasingly in recent years due to technological evolution. It implies profound changes in teaching practices with consequences in the teaching-learning process [1]. The use of platforms not only for providing academic content, but also for distance learning, have a great impact on both teachers and students: in the format of the contents that are made available, in the language used, class duration, time management, methods and hours of study, and in communication strategies. The recent public health pandemic emphasized the need for digital technologies use to maintain activity with social distance. In this context, DET represents an added value since they increase the interactivity and promote additional space for knowledge construction [2]. DET can be used in an asynchronous or a synchronous way. When used in its asynchronous form, it offers as added benefits: the possibility of a flexible schedule, the availability of quality material at low cost, and the potential to reach a high number of students without geographical limits [3]. However, issues on humanization of education and knowledge systematization are raised and, additionally, although DETs offer a wide range of possibilities, they do not guarantee learning quality [4]. Still, there is some reluctance in its use, particularly by teachers, as DETs break with traditional education, placing the emphasis on the student as the protagonist of the teaching-learning process [5].

As technology evolves, it has been integrated into different areas where education is included. Having this in mind, DET can be defined as the use of technological resources to improve teaching and learning, promote educational development and access to data and material [1]. It implies the use of virtual scenarios, online platforms, and digital resources, among others. Historically, educational sciences have used DET as a resource to improve teaching since the 80s, but in nursing its use is more recent. Benefits can be pointed out from its use, such as improved interaction and content integration [2,4], easy access, more dynamism and interaction with students outside a physical school space [1]. However, constrains can also be pointed to, namely financial (adopting state-of-the-art technology can be expensive) and personal (teachers may be reticent to change traditional educational methods). It is not integrated in any theory of learning, but it fits a diverse theoretical framework. A major element of this theoretical frameworks is socio-constructivism that underlines the role of social processes in individuals' learning [6]. Social constructivism-based theory understands learning as a process that occurs through supportive collaboration with other people and leads to knowledge and evolution [7].

In nursing, the use of DET is seen as a resource that is complementary to traditional teaching [4] with increasing use and good results such as enhanced nursing students' problem-solving skills [6]. An example of the use of DET with other educational strategies is its use combined with case studies improving its benefits [8]. However, Chavaglia et al. [9] pointed to the need for greater diversification in the use of DET. In their study with undergraduate nursing students, they concluded that digital power point presentations, email and a google search engine were the predominant digital tools used by students.

A link between the use of DET, nursing education and sustainability is also found in the literature. Education in sustainable development is recognized as important particularly in health professions such as nursing. The use of DET offers an opportunity to reinforce this link since DET are sustainable and can be applied with low environmental impact [10]. Other innovative andragogical approaches are also being used, such as augmented reality and virtual simulation. Foronda et al. state that results from the use of these technologies are encouraging, since they suggest efficacy in improving nursing students learning outcomes [11].

However, some caution is required in the implementation of DET, especially by teachers. They have to be conscious of factors that influence the success in DET's application, and a minimum quality requirement has to be assured [10]. Usually, the types of DETs used by teachers are limited to those available in their institution and with easy access [12], which limits the quality of teaching and consequently the quality of the learning process. On the other hand, there has been a greater trend towards personalization of care and patient-centeredness. The use of this type of technology in teaching and its impact on care is still unknown. However, it seems to be consensual that DET may expand nursing education and consequently improve patient outcomes [11].

For the present study non-presential classroom was considered as classes that occur without physical presence in the same room of both students and teachers. The purpose of this study is to contribute to the improvement of the teaching-learning process in the nursing undergraduate degree through the use of DET in non-presential classroom teaching. The objective is to evaluate the use of DET in non-presential classroom teaching, benefits, constraints, and implications for teaching-learning process in nursing students. The following questions were defined: how is the use DET fulfilled in non-presential classroom teaching in nursing? What are the benefits and constrains to the use of DET? What are the implications for teaching-learning process of nursing students with the use of DET?

2. Materials and Methods

2.1. Study Design

An exploratory-descriptive, cross-sectional, and observational study was outlined. The research design fits into the quantitative paradigm with the use of surveys as a data collection technique.

The study was approved by the school board as well as by the school ethics committee. It was an independent study not integrated in any course or curricular unit. The study was applied to 230 inquiries and invitation to participate in the study was sent by email with a survey link attached. Prior to fill the survey information regarding framework, aim, confidentiality, ethical issues and researchers contacts was provided. Consent was obtained prior to data collection. Participants had to mandatorily give their consent to advance with participation.

2.2. Sample and Setting

The population consists of all nursing students and teachers who lecture the undergraduate nursing course at a private nursing school in Lisbon, Portugal. The sample is therefore of simple non-probabilistic type. Students from all academic years were invited to participate (n = 205). Teachers who teach classes of any type (n = 25) were selected and teachers involved solely in clinical nursing were excluded.

2.3. Instrument

The online survey designed for this study includes 60 items based on previously published literature [13–16]. It had two parts: first part with sociodemographic data such as sex, age, and type of experience in the use of DET. Additional data collected included academic year for students' and professional experience and type of employment for teachers. The second part of the survey had questions related to the use of DET, selected and adapted from a previous literature review.

Types of DET [13] included it a 5-point Likert scale with 23 items within 5 dimensions (organizational tools, communications tools, presentation tools, learning assessment tools and identity transformation tools). Benefits of using DET include 10 dichotomous items and were retrieved from Kokol et al. [14]. These authors applied a survey to 125 nursing students' study and identified benefits and challenges of online education. Constraints of using DET was adapted from Lloyd et al. [15] and comprise 13 dichotomous items. The original scale included 22 items and authors performed exploratory factor analysis for validity and Cronbach alpha for reliability. Four factors were extracted that had high reliabilities (0.892; 0.806; 0.805; 0.870). In our study, we adapted the items for our context. Finally, implications in the use of DET include 14 dichotomous items adapted from an integrative review on digital technologies in the teaching of nursing skills by Silveira and Cogo [16].

Before its application, the surveys were sent to 5 experts. Content validity index was calculated as described by Polit and Becket [17] to verify the extend of expert agreement. A value of 0.90 was obtained which is considered adequate by the same authors.

Additionally, for instrument validity, to understand how types of DET were related and to favor statistical analysis, exploratory principal components factor analysis with varimax rotation was performed on the 23 items that addressed types of DET. The Kaiser-Meyer-Olkin measure verified the sampling adequacy for the analysis, KMO = 0.759. Additionally, Bartlett's sphericity test indicated that correlations between items were sufficiently large, X^2 = 1146.772, $p < 0.001$.

Initially, for the first-dimension sevens factors were identified that explained 64.9% of variance. However, two item (calendars and electronic portfolio) had correlations <0.3. By removing them and forcing analysis to the initial 5 factors that were identified in the literature, a 53.8% of the variance was obtained as explained on Table 1. Regarding communalities values ≥ 0.4 were considered. We also included the item: "Instant messages" although h^2 value is 0.386 because it is a marginal value and due to its conceptual importance in the context of this study.

Table 1. Exploratory factorial analysis for types of DET.

Types of DET	Factors					h² *
	1	2	3	4	5	
Discussion Forums	0.466					0.533
Blogs	0.653					0.490
Avatars	0.715					0.606
Virtual Scenarios	0.709					0.599
Immersive Technology	0.744					0.649
Videocalls		0.580				0.470
Web conference		0.429				0.415
Audio		0.762				0.655
Video		0.763				0.645
Slides			0.715			0.587
Tutorials			0.481			0.526
Image sharing			0.593			0.556
Bibliography sharing			0.653			0.597
Activities			0.540			0.590
Tests			0.611			0.613
Online Schedule				0.713		0.545
Mind maps or graphic organizers				0.703		0.579
File and management store				0.531		0.515
Instant messages					0.543	0.386
Research					0.697	0.589
Social network					0.730	0.665
Eigenvalues	2.80	2.47	2.38	2.11	2.04	
% of variance	13.35	11.77	11.34	10.06	9.72	
Cronhbach Alpha	0.739	0.667	0.715	0.602	0.594	

*-h²: communalities.

For reliability assessment the Cronbach Alpha coefficient as well as the Kuder-Richardson formula were determined. Regarding types of DET, the alpha Cronbach values range between 0.594 in factor 5 and 0.739 in factor 1 as shown in Table 1. For benefits, constraints and implications thar are dichotomous items in the Kuder-Richardson formula indicated the following values: 0.670 (benefits); 0.502 (constrains) and 0.584 (implications). The values obtained are considered satisfactory [18], and additionally, it must be taken into consideration that it is a first attempt to use this instrument.

2.4. Procedure

Participant's recruitment was performed by email. Since this was an independent study, not integrated in any course or discipline, researchers contacted students and professors through email addresses. An email was sent to all the participants inviting them to participate in the study. This email contained a survey link that allowed access to the online instrument. It was available for 1 week, and after that time, a reminder was sent, and the survey was available for one week more. The number of answered surveys were monitored by the researchers at the end of each week. After two weeks had passed the link was removed and data was transferred for analysis. All surveys were fully completed by participants.

2.5. Data Analysis

Descriptive and inferential statistics were used for data analysis. Statistical analyses was performed with SPSS statistical package, 27.0 version (SPSS, Inc., Chicago, IL, USA). Categorical variables are presented as percentages. All variables followed a non-normal distribution so nonparametric test namely Mann-Whitney U test was used for comparisons between groups. To verify association between categorical variables Phi/Cramer V was used. A p value of 0.05 or less was considered statistically significant.

3. Results

3.1. Sample Characteristics

Of the study population, 163 subjects (140 students and 23 teachers) completed and returned the surveys, so the response rate was 70.8%. Most respondents were female (85%; n = 138) and had no training or formal education on DET, only experience as users (86%; n = 140). Sociodemographic characteristics are summarized in Table 2.

Table 2. Sample sociodemographic characteristics.

Variables	n	%
Sex		
Female	138	85
Male	25	15
Age (students)		
<20 years	48	28
21–30 years	84	52
>31 years	8	5
Age (teachers)		
<30 years	2	9
31–50 years	5	22
>51 years	14	61
Curricular Year (students)		
1st	35	25
2nd	33	24
3rd	56	40
4th	16	11
Teaching experience (teachers)		
<5 years	5	22
6–10 years	2	9
11–20 years	10	43
>21 years	6	26
Experience in using DET		
Experience as user	140	86
Did or is doing a course	21	13

3.2. Types of DET

Regarding the type of DET used, they were grouped into the five categories identified in factorial analysis. For presentation data, answers were clustered into two group: very frequently and frequently answers and occasionally, rarely or never answers. Results are summarized in Table 3.

Table 3. Results regarding type of DET used by teachers and students.

Types of DET	Total Sample (n = 163)				Students (n = 140)				Teachers (n = 23)			
	VF and F		O, R or N		VF and F		O, R or N		VF and F		O, R or N	
	n	%	n	%	n	%	n	%	n	%	n	%
Factor 1												
Discussion forums	22	13	141	87	14	10	126	90	8	35	15	65
Bloggs	18	11	145	89	16	11	124	89	2	9	21	91
Avatars	13	8	150	92	11	8	129	92	2	9	21	91
Virtual scenarios	12	7	151	93	10	7	130	93	2	9	21	91
Immersive technology	22	13	141	87	20	14	120	86	2	9	21	91
Factor 2												
Videocalls	121	74	42	26	104	74	36	26	17	74	6	26
Web conferences	78	48	85	52	65	46	75	54	13	57	14	43
Audio	121	74	42	26	107	76	33	24	14	61	9	39
Video	113	69	50	31	100	71	40	29	13	57	10	43
Factor 3												
Slides	145	89	18	11	123	88	17	12	22	96	1	4
Tutorials	63	39	100	61	52	37	88	63	11	48	12	52
Image sharing	120	74	43	26	102	73	38	27	18	78	5	22
Bibliography sharing	107	66	56	34	87	62	53	38	20	87	3	13
Activities	109	67	54	33	91	65	49	35	18	78	5	22
Tests *	109	67	54	33	96	69	44	31	13	57	10	43
Factor 4												
On-line schedule	42	26	121	74	30	21	110	79	12	52	11	48
Mind maps or graphic organizers	46	28	117	72	41	29	99	71	5	22	18	78
File and management store	110	67	53	33	92	66	48	34	18	78	5	22
Factor 5												
Instant messages and chats	137	84	26	16	119	85	21	15	18	78	5	22
Research	118	72	45	28	108	77	32	23	10	43	13	57
Social network	98	60	65	40	95	68	45	32	3	9	20	91

VF—very frequently; F—frequently; O—occasionally; R—rarely; N—never; * significant at $p < 0.05$.

Mann-Whitney U test was used to assess if there were association between student's sample and teachers sample and the use of DET. No significative association was found except on the item "tests" (U = 2094.5; $p = 0.016$).

As to technologies used, results show the use of the technologies provided and available in the institution where the survey was applied: Moodle (98.8%; n = 161) and Microsoft Teams (98.2%; n = 160). Other technologies identified included Zoom (22.1%; n = 36), Mentimeter (4.9%; n = 8), Kahoot (4.3%; n = 7), Skype (2.5%; n = 4) and Google classrooms (1.2%; n = 2).

As to type of classes DET they were mostly used in theoretical class (93%; n = 153). In practical and laboratory classes DET were used less frequently (37% and 28%, respectively).

3.3. Benefits and Constrains in the Use of DET

Regarding benefits and constraints responses are summarized in Table 4.

Table 4. Results regarding benefits and constraints in the use of DET.

	Total Sample (n = 163)		Students (n = 140)		Teachers (n = 23)	
Benefits of using DET	n	%	n	%	n	%
It allows access to educational content without time/space limit;	115	71	51	37	15	65
Low cost;	110	68	21	15	4	17
It allows the integrating of multiple learning tools (pdf, links, app, among others); *	108	66	35	25	9	39
Promotes student accountability; *	96	59	50	36	4	17
Improves the quality of the teaching-learning process;	67	41	33	24	9	39
Enhances multidisciplinary work;	54	33	101	72	14	61
Improves the student's ability to analyze, synthesize and think critically;	45	28	38	27	7	30
Improves students' preparation for applying theoretical content to practice;	44	27	95	68	15	65
Increases students' creativity, motivation, and quality of care;	42	26	86	61	10	43
Improves the presentation of nursing care sensitive results.	25	15	92	66	16	70
Constraints of using DET	n	%	n	%	n	%
Less physical contact with students;	126	77	111	79	15	65
Decreased interaction between students/teachers;	117	72	73	52	13	57
Technical difficulties (network failure, server overload);	109	67	72	51	17	74
Difficulty in obtaining visual feedback;	89	55	99	71	18	78
Depersonalization of teaching;	86	53	11	8	10	43
Moving away from traditional teaching models;	85	52	43	31	10	43
Lack of preparation in the use of DET;	53	33	21	15	5	22
Difficulty in managing time and content;	43	26	99	71	10	43
Lack of infrastructure and technologies;	26	16	8	6	5	22
Lack of regulation in the use of DET;	21	13	39	28	4	17
Constant updating and innovation of DET;	13	8	79	56	6	26
Resistance to the use of DET;	8	5	6	4	2	9
Fear of technology.	7	4	6	4	1	4

* significant at $p < 0.05$.

To assess association between type of inquiries (students or teachers) Phi/Cramer's V was calculated. There were only significant statistical differences between teachers and students in two items: "it allows the integrating of multiple learning tools (pdf, links, app, among others)" and "promotes student accountability". Teachers refer to more benefits in the integration of multiple learning tools (V = 0.170; p = 0.030), and students attribute more benefits in item: "promotes accountability" (V = 0.170; p = 0.030). Regarding constrains, the same procedure was followed; however, no significant statistical differences were found.

3.4. Implications in the Use of DET

The last question of the questionnaire referred to implications in the use of DET. Answers are synthetized in Table 5.

Table 5. Results regarding implications in the use of DET.

Implications in the Use of DET	Total Sample (n = 163)		Students (n = 140)		Teachers (n = 23)	
	n	%	n	%	n	%
Implications—Simulations						
Possibility to repeat simulations until learning, ensuring patient safety;	90	55	78	56	14	61
Possibility of using software in simulation scenarios;	93	57	73	52	16	70
Promotion of meaningful learning;	51	31	30	21	6	26
Ensures better practical performance for the student.	36	22	53	38	11	48
Implications—Stimulation of learning						
Arouses students' curiosity;	47	29	73	52	16	70
Stimulates students' independence;	108	66	95	68	12	52
The existence of multiple tools makes learning more stimulating;	57	35	45	32	3	13
It allows to personalize the teaching;	48	29	33	24	14	61
Improved use of theoretical content.	49	30	48	34	9	39
Implications—Learning skills						
Stimulate self-learning;	115	71	29	21	8	35
It makes learning less monotonous;	39	24	37	26	6	26
Existence of a safe environment allowing errors that lead to improved technical execution;	51	31	18	13	4	17
Decreases anxiety when performing techniques;	44	27	102	73	13	57
Improves performance in the execution of techniques.	22	14	46	33	8	35

Regarding implications also Phi/Cramer's V was calculated to assess association between type of inquiries (students or teachers) and implications. Nevertheless, there were no significant statistical differences between the groups.

Globally, there was no difference between students and teachers in the use of DET. Still, when analysis is performed by gender differences were found regarding Factor 3 in types of DET and constrains.

Women got a higher score concerning the types of DET used (Factor 3) compared to men, that is, women use these resources more than men (U = 1531.5; p = 0.040). Still, men report more constraints than women in the use of DET (U = 2255; p = 0.005).

As stated earlier, all questions had an open space for additional answers; however, there were few answers and those who did respond mentioned aspects already identified.

4. Discussion

This study allowed us to gather evidence related to the use of DET, being a first step to the improvement of the teaching-learning processes in the nursing undergraduate degree. Our results show a scarce use of DET by both teachers and students. Literature points to an increase in the use of DET in nursing teaching [16]. Our results show that there is space for improvement in this area. A possible explanation for this result may be the existence of interpersonal and institutional barriers, training and technological constrains and the lack of cost/benefit analysis [15].

Overall, 86% of our sample had no formal training on DET, which is in line with the literature. However, studies highlight that digital technologies are used both with academic and personal purposes [19]. Probably teachers in this sample do not feel the need for formal education as the day-to-day use of these tools allows them to use them without limitations or constraints. Additionally, digital tools are, naturally intuitive and user friendly. When considering our sample of students, they belong to a generation raised with information technology, internet, and social networks, which make them more confident manipulating new platforms and devices, not really requiring training in the area.

As mentioned in the results chapter, the statistical procedure allowed to group the types of DET in five new factors, categorized as follows: Training and Discussion Tools (factor 1); Communication tools (factor 2); Presentation and assessment tools (factor 3); Organization tools (factor 4); and Complementary learning tools (factor 5).

The training and discussion tools (factor 1) included the following items: discussion forums, blogs, avatars, virtual scenarios, and immersive technology. In this category, results show that avatars and virtual scenarios are poorly used. This types of DET are identified as particularly relevant in nursing education since they may provide a solution to issues such as: faculty shortages, scarcity of clinical placements and limited onsite laboratory space [11]. Additionally, its use allows students to repeatedly simulate procedures and care or even recreate high risk events that they may not contact within clinical context [11,16].

Communication tools category (factor 2) includes: videocalls, web conferences, audio, and video. Videocalls (74%) and audio (74%) are the preferred communication tools for the total sample. Although web conferences can save students time and prevent the inconveniences of traveling, video and audio conferencing provide the benefit of visual aids, allowing participants to make use of multiple senses, improving their concentration levels and increasing their capacity to absorb more information [20,21].

Within the presentation and assessment tools category (factor 3), the following items were identified: slides, tutorials, image sharing, bibliography sharing, activities, and tests. Tutorials got the lowest score (39%). This technology is still underused in our sample, but perhaps the changes in the lifestyle of today's society could lead to a greater need and recognition of its use in this setting. The traditional classroom can restrict daily life, as it requires anticipated planning. Otherwise, the tutorial can be paused, rewound or fast-forwarded, and the lecture can be heard as many times as needed. These characteristics fit the current generation of students that crave the digital world and are extreme consumers of technology [22]. On the other hand, slides got the most representative score, as it is used by 89% of our sample. The use of DET to share slides can be framed as a simplistic and traditional use of this type of technologies.

In this category, it is also possible to verify an association between gender and the use of presentation and assessment tools, as women got a higher score compared to men ($U = 1531.5$; $p = 0.040$). Additionally, men report more constraints than women in the use of DET ($U = 2255$; $p = 0.005$). These results are quite interesting, as there is the general idea that women are outnumbered in informatics. Nevertheless, literature shows that the very first computer programmers and IT users were women, and that technology are more frequently used in female-dominated areas [23], such as teaching and nursing. Cai et al. [24] found that there are no significant gender differences in the attitudes toward technology. However, these authors argue that in the academic context, women are more prepared for technology use than the general female population.

In types of DET, factor 4 covers the following organization tools: online schedule, mind maps or graphic organizers, and file and management store. This last one is the most used by 67% of our sample. It is a more cost-effective system, as it reduces organization bureaucracy and saves space. Students can easily search, access, and share files. Additionally, support for decision-making and knowledge discovery can be achieved in an effectively way through the use of massive amounts of data that can be easily stored [24].

Instant messages and chats, research, and social network were considered as complementary learning tools (factor 5). Instant messages and chats (84%) are the mostly used by both students and teachers in our sample. They may be more relevant because they are one of the oldest communication tools, and usually a quick option when network failures occur. Within this category, the results also demonstrate that DET are used for research by 72% of the sample. These results are aligned with literature that shows that traditional libraries are being partially replaced by digital search, specially by students who prefer it because they are easy and quick to search [25].

More than half of our sample identified the following benefits of using *DET*: the integration of multiple learning tools (66%), low cost (68%) and access without time or space limits (71%). Pinto and Leite [19] also mention that the use of DET has effects on the interaction time between students and teachers extending it beyond the traditional academic period. This access 24/7 can also be seen as a constraint and reduce teacher's quality of life. However, considering the students' perspective, it can be a major benefit. Männistö et al. [6] reported that the use of DET in nursing teaching enhances motivation for learning. When used in nursing education DET can improve the learning experience particularly in clinical learning settings [26]. Regarding low cost, there is no robust evidence that e-learning is a more cost-effective way to deliver knowledge when compared to traditional methods [27]. Yet, for students and teachers it may prove to be a more economical option as it avoids travel or food expenses.

Still regarding the benefits, no significant associations were identified between the teacher and student groups, except for the items: it allows the integrating of multiple learning tools (pdf, links, app, among others)" and "promotes student accountability". These results are quite surprising because, given the age difference between the two groups in our sample, a more pronounced association would be expected. Literature shows that older adults are less likely to use technology that younger adults [28,29].

Our results show that constraints had greater statistical evidence than benefits. The more relevant were: the decreased interaction between students/teachers (72%), the less physical contact (77%), and the technical difficulties (67%). These aspects are pointed as the main barriers to the use of DET in literature and in fact, digital technologies can be used to enhance education, but they cannot completely replace face-to-face teaching [26]. Regarding technical difficulties, Naveed et al. [30] showed that efficient technology, infrastructure readiness and system reliability are some of the main critical success factors in implementing DET. To overcome these constrains several measures can be taken such as the use of combined methodologies (both presential and non-presential), a balanced and flexible schedule that maintains physical contact between students and teachers and permanent technical support available for users.

Implications identified by more than half of our sample include both the possibility of using software in simulation scenarios (57%) and the possibility to repeat simulations until learning, ensuring patient safety (55%). Overall, 66.9% of our sample consider that DET stimulates students' independence (66%) and stimulate self-learning (71%). In nursing, the possibility to repeat simulations is identified as important and relevant for learning [31]; additionally, it is a significant factor for patient safety. Nevertheless, in our sample, only 14% considered that the use of DET improves performance in the execution of techniques. This could be due to a broader interpretation of the DET concept, as the technology by itself does not improve the practical skills required for nurses. Rather, the use of specific technology tools, such as clinical virtual simulation, can be used as a complementary strategy to DET, improving clinical reasoning skills [31].

The impact of DET on nursing care and patient outcomes is still poorly explored. Although there seems to be a link between improved nursing education and improved patient outcomes, this issue must be further explored. Additionally, there is a trend towards more centered and personalized models of care and the use of massive forms of education may not be suitable to this trend. It should be noted that some of the digital tools used in education are used in the health area, also with the aim of personalizing and, in this case, improving care. With regard to students, DET may be adapted to their educational and personal needs, which translates into a more student-centered teaching. Additionally, due to its positive impact, these technologies are being implemented in continuing education and professional development. A good example is the use of immersive technologies that allow nurses to have dynamic experiences with patients and be more prepared for real-world clinical settings. Nevertheless, the impact of DET on nursing care and patient outcomes is still poorly explored. Although, there seems to be a link between improved nursing education and improved patient outcomes, this issue should be further studied.

It is also worth exploring if more student-centered teaching is later reflected in more people-centered nursing care.

Palvia et al. [32] state that e-education is advancing and is here to stay all around the world, which brings implications such as the need for improvement of telecommunications infrastructure, the acknowledgement of online education as equivalent to traditional face to face education and the globalization of e-education, which is inevitable, similar to the globalization of email or e-commerce. This authors also state that both online (virtual) and offline education must be combined so the virtues of both can be used.

It is necessary to have a more in-depth knowledge on this subject and a greater investment, both by teachers and educational institutions. Additionally, to understand the impact of the use of these technologies on nursing students learning, both in academic and clinical contexts, is needed. Nursing schools must invest in updated information technologies appropriate to the nursing curriculum, as well as providing training on their use to teachers and students. In our study, we verify that both teachers and students use mainly the tools made available by the school. Therefore, one way to improve the use of DET is to make more tools available. Additionally, in our setting the current teacher's generation is more familiar with the first tools that were created and used as DET so those are the ones they mostly use. In our sample, most teachers do not have formal education on the use of DET and this should be included in the annual training program.

As to limitations this study was applied after the first lockdown that occurred in Portugal which triggered an exponential growth in the use of DET. As more periods of lockdown occurred both teachers and students were forced to improve the use of DET. Therefore, we consider that if the application of this study had occurred after these periods the results would have been different. Study design and type of sample are also limitations since our exploratory-descriptive study used a convenience sample and therefore results cannot be generalized.

5. Conclusions

Our results show that the use of DET in this sample is it is still at an early stage. Both students and teachers are still unfamiliar with the scope and possibilities of these tools, not taking full advantage of the potential they have to offer. The integration of multiple learning tools, low cost, and access without time or space limits are considered the main benefits of DET. On the other hand, the decreased interaction between students/teachers, the less physical contact, and the technical difficulties, are seen as the greater constraints. The main implications of DET are the possibility of using software in simulation, and the possibility to repeat simulations until learning, ensuring patient safety. It is also considered as a method that stimulates students' independence and self-learning.

Although distance education through DET is a few years old, as far as nursing education is concerned, this concept is still very recent. Globalization and, more recently, the pandemic context that forced social isolation, have further boosted the introduction of DET in nursing education. Distance education thus becomes an effective strategy to reach people who want or need to be qualified, but who, for different reasons, cannot depart from their context of life and work [2]. Nevertheless, this constitutes a challenge to the nursing traditional teaching-learning methods, which have a predominantly practical and proximity component [27]. The distance between students and teachers, should be used to its potential, involving students dynamically in the learning process, respecting independence, and autonomy, establishing links between learning and life and professional experience. On the one hand, it is necessary to provide teachers with skills to establish a link with students and stimulate their learning and engagement. It is also recommended that schools select the appropriate DET methods for teaching nursing, namely investing in robust digital platforms and state-of-the-art simulated practice technology [32]. The link between improved nursing education and its implication on nursing care must also be further explored.

Author Contributions: Conceptualization, F.L., L.S. and V.A.; methodology, F.L., L.S. and V.A.; software, F.L., L.S. and V.A.; validation, F.L., L.S. and V.A.; formal analysis, F.L., L.S. and V.A.; investigation, F.L. and V.A.; resources, F.L., L.S. and V.A.; data curation, F.L., L.S. and V.A.; writing—original draft preparation, F.L.; writing—review and editing, L.S. and V.A.; visualization, F.L., L.S. and V.A.; supervision, F.L., L.S. and V.A.; project administration, F.L. and V.A.; funding acquisition, F.L., L.S. and V.A. All authors have read and agreed to the published version of the manuscript.

Funding: This work is financed by national funds through the FCT—Foundation for Science and Technology, I.P., under the project UIDB/04585/2020. The researchers would like to thank the Centro de Investigação Interdisciplinar Egas Moniz (CiiEM) for the support provided for the publication of this article.

Institutional Review Board Statement: The study was conducted according to the guidelines of the Declaration of Helsinki, and approved by the Institutional Review Board and Ethics Committee of Escola Superior de Saúde Egas Moniz (reference number 881/2020).

Informed Consent Statement: Informed consent was obtained from all subjects involved in the study.

Conflicts of Interest: The authors declare no conflict of interest.

References

1. Damascena, S.C.C.; Santos, K.C.B.; Lopes, G.S.G.; Gontijo, P.V.C.; Paiva, M.V.S.; Lima, M.E.S.; Alves, J.M.F.; Campos, R.S. Use of Digital Educational Technologies as a Teaching Tool in the Nursing Teaching Process. *Braz. J. Dev.* **2019**, *5*, 29925–29939. [CrossRef]
2. Andrade, D.C.M.; Brum, A.K.R.; Neves, R.P.S.; de Melo Calvo, D.D.G.; de Lima Silva, D.M. Use of Interactive Digital Tools in Meeting to Teach Patient Safety. *Braz. J. Health Rev.* **2020**, *3*, 1531–1541. [CrossRef]
3. Parulla, C.D.; Galdino, D.M.; Pai, D.D.; Azzolin, K.D.O.; Cogo, A.L.P. Nursing assessment: The elaboration and development of a massive open online course. *Rev. Gaúcha Enferm.* **2020**, *41*, e20190199. [CrossRef] [PubMed]
4. Barboza, V.S.; Azevedo, S.L.D.; Lindolpho, M.D.C.; Reis, L.B.D.; Chaves, W.B.; Chrizóstimo, M.M.; Wisnesky, U.D.; Silva, J.V.L.D. Website in the Teaching-Learning Process of Physical Examination: The Construction of Knowledge in Undergraduate Nursing. *Braz. J. Health Rev.* **2020**, *3*, 1881–1892. [CrossRef]
5. Chaves, M.J.C.; Barbosa, E.D.S.; Nóbrega-Therrien, S.M. Facebook as a Virtual Learning Environment in Nursing Course. *Educ.-Rev. Multidiscip. Educ.* **2020**, *7*, 143–164. [CrossRef]
6. Männistö, M.; Mikkonen, K.; Kuivila, H.; Virtanen, H.; Kyngäs, H.; Kääriäinen, M. Digital collaborative learning in nursing education: A systematic review. *Scand. J. Caring Sci.* **2020**, *34*, 280–292. [CrossRef]
7. Danish, J.A.; Gresalfi, M. Cognitive and Sociocultural Perspectives on Learning. In *International Handbook of the Learning Sciences*; Fischer, F., Hmelo-Silver, C.E., Goldman, S.R., Reimann, P., Eds.; Routledge: New York, NY, USA, 2018; pp. 34–43. [CrossRef]
8. Hara, C.Y.N.; Aredes, N.D.A.; Fonseca, L.M.M.; Silveira, R.; de Camargo, R.A.A.; de Goes, F.S.N. Clinical case in digital technology for nursing students' learning: An integrative review. *Nurse Educ. Today* **2016**, *38*, 119–125. [CrossRef]
9. Chavaglia, S.R.R.; Barbosa, M.H.; Santos, A.D.S.; Duarte, R.D.; Contim, D.; Ohl, R.I.B. Estratégias Didáticas Identificadas Junto a Graduandos de Enfermagem. *Cogitare Enferm* **2018**, *23*, 53876. [CrossRef]
10. Álvarez-Nieto, C.; Richardson, J.; Parra-Anguita, G.; Linares-Abad, M.; Huss, N.; Grande-Gascón, M.L.; Grose, J.; Huynen, M.; López-Medina, I.M. Developing digital educational materials for nursing and sustainability: The results of an observational study. *Nurse Educ. Today* **2018**, *60*, 139–146. [CrossRef]
11. Foronda, C.L.; Alfes, C.M.; Dev, P.; Kleinheksel, A.J.; Nelson, D.A.; O'Donnell, J.M.; Samosky, J.T. Virtually Nursing. *Nurse Educ.* **2017**, *42*, 14–17. [CrossRef]
12. García-Barrera, A. Assessment of Technological Teaching Resources through E-Rubrics. *Rev. Educ. Distancia* **2016**, 1–13. [CrossRef]
13. Manning, S.; Johnson, K.E. *The Technology Toolbelt for Teaching*; Jossey-Bass, Ed.; Cambridge University Press: San Francisco, CA, USA, 2011.
14. Kokol, P.; Blazun, H.; Micetić-Turk, D.; Abbott, P. e-Learning in nursing education–Challenges and opportunities. *Stud. Health Technol. Inform.* **2006**, *122*, 387–390.
15. Lloyd, S.A.; Byrne, M.M.; Mccoy, T.S. Faculty-Perceived Barriers of Online Education. *MERLOT J. Online Learn. Teach.* **2012**, *8*. Available online: https://jolt.merlot.org/vol8no1/lloyd_0312.htm (accessed on 1 April 2020).
16. Silveira, M.D.S.; Cogo, A.L.P. The Contributions of Digital Technologies in the Teaching of Nursing Skills: An Integrative Review. *Rev. Gaúcha Enferm.* **2017**, *38*. [CrossRef]
17. Polit, D.F.; Beck, C.T. *Essentials of Nursing Research*, 9th ed.; Lippincott Williams & Wilkins: Philadelphia, PA, USA, 2017.
18. De Souza, A.C.; Alexandre, N.M.C.; Guirardello, E.D.B. Psychometric Properties in Instruments Evaluation of Reliability and Validity. *Epidemiol. Serv. Saude Rev. Sist. Unico Saude Bras.* **2017**, *26*, 649–659. [CrossRef]
19. Pinto, M.; Leite, C. Digital Technologies in Successful Academic Itineraries of Higher Education Non-Traditional Students. *Educ. Pesqui.* **2020**, *46*. [CrossRef]

20. Amin, F.M.; Sundari, H. EFL students' preferences on digital platforms during emergency remote teaching: Video Conference, LMS, or Messenger Application? *Stud. Engl. Lang. Educ.* **2020**, *7*, 362–378. [CrossRef]
21. Correia, A.-P.; Liu, C.; Xu, F. Evaluating videoconferencing systems for the quality of the educational experience. *Distance Educ.* **2020**, *41*, 429–452. [CrossRef]
22. Chicca, J.; Shellenbarger, T. Connecting with Generation Z: Approaches in Nursing Education. *Teach. Learn. Nurs.* **2018**, *13*, 180–184. [CrossRef]
23. Wilson, B.L.; Butler, M.J.; Butler, R.J.; Johnson, W.G. Nursing Gender Pay Differentials in the New Millennium. *J. Nurs. Sch.* **2018**, *50*, 102–108. [CrossRef]
24. Cai, Z.; Fan, X.; Du, J. Gender and attitudes toward technology use: A meta-analysis. *Comput. Educ.* **2017**, *105*, 1–13. [CrossRef]
25. Storey, V.C.; Song, I.-Y. Big data technologies and Management: What conceptual modeling can do. *Data Knowl. Eng.* **2017**, *108*, 50–67. [CrossRef]
26. Abbas, A.; Faiz, A. Usefulness of digital and traditional libraries in higher education. *Int. J. Serv. Technol. Manag.* **2013**, *19*, 149. [CrossRef]
27. Heinonen, A.-T.; Kääriäinen, M.; Juntunen, J.; Mikkonen, K. Nursing students' experiences of nurse teacher mentoring and beneficial digital technologies in a clinical practice setting. *Nurse Educ. Pract.* **2019**, *40*, 102631. [CrossRef]
28. Meinert, E.; Alturkistani, A.; A Foley, K.; Brindley, D.; Car, J. Examining Cost Measurements in Production and Delivery of Three Case Studies Using E-Learning for Applied Health Sciences: Cross-Case Synthesis. *J. Med. Internet Res.* **2019**, *21*, e13574. [CrossRef]
29. Hülür, G.; Macdonald, B. Rethinking social relationships in old age: Digitalization and the social lives of older adults. *Am. Psychol.* **2020**, *75*, 554–566. [CrossRef]
30. Naveed, Q.N.; Qureshi, M.R.N.; Tairan, N.; Mohammad, A.; Shaikh, A.; Alsayed, A.O.; Shah, A.; Alotaibi, F.M. Evaluating critical success factors in implementing E-learning system using multi-criteria decision-making. *PLoS ONE* **2020**, *15*, e0231465. [CrossRef] [PubMed]
31. Padilha, J.M.; Machado, P.P.; Ribeiro, A.; Ramos, J.; Costa, P. Clinical Virtual Simulation in Nursing Education: Randomized Controlled Trial. *J. Med. Internet Res.* **2019**, *21*, e11529. [CrossRef] [PubMed]
32. Palvia, S.; Aeron, P.; Gupta, P.; Mahapatra, D.; Parida, R.; Rosner, R.; Sindhi, S. Online Education: Worldwide Status, Challenges, Trends, and Implications. *J. Glob. Inf. Technol. Manag.* **2018**, *21*, 233–241. [CrossRef]

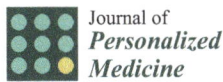

Article

The Impact of the COVID-19 Pandemic on Nursing Care: A Cross-Sectional Survey-Based Study

Marco Clari [1], Michela Luciani [1], Alessio Conti [1,*], Veronica Sciannameo [2], Paola Berchialla [3], Paola Di Giulio [1], Sara Campagna [1] and Valerio Dimonte [1]

[1] Department of Public Health and Pediatrics, University of Torino, 10126 Turin, Italy; marco.clari@unito.it (M.C.); michela.luciani@unito.it (M.L.); paola.digiulio@unito.it (P.D.G.); sara.campagna@unito.it (S.C.); valerio.dimonte@unito.it (V.D.)
[2] Department of Cardiac, Vascular Sciences and Public Health, University of Padova, 35128 Padua, Italy; veronica.sciannameo@unito.it
[3] Department of Clinical and Biological Sciences, University of Torino, 10043 Orbassano, Italy; paola.berchialla@unito.it
* Correspondence: alessio.conti@unito.it; Tel.: +39-0116705823

Abstract: The COVID-19 pandemic has had a severe impact on nursing care. This cross-sectional survey-based study compared aspects of nursing care and nurses' satisfaction with care provided before and during the first wave of the COVID-19 pandemic. A total of 936 registered nurses (RNs) rated the frequency with which they performed fundamental care, nursing techniques, patient education, symptom management, and nurse–patient relationships before and during the pandemic. A recursive partitioning for ordered multivariate response in a conditional inference framework approach was applied. More frequent fundamental cares were associated with their frequency before the pandemic ($p < 0.001$), caring for COVID-19 patients ($p < 0.001$), and workplace reassignment ($p = 0.004$). Caring for COVID-19 patients ($p < 0.001$), workplace reassignment ($p = 0.030$), and caring for ≤ 7.4 COVID-19 patients ($p = 0.014$) increased nursing techniques. RNs in high-intensity COVID-19 units ($p = 0.002$) who educated patients before the pandemic, stopped this task. RNs caring for COVID-19 patients reported increased symptom management ($p < 0.001$), as did RNs caring for more non-COVID-19 patients ($p = 0.037$). Less frequent nurse–patient relationships before the pandemic and working in high-intensity COVID-19 units decreased nurse–patient relationships ($p = 0.002$). Despite enormous challenges, nurses continued to provide a high level of care. Ensuring the appropriate deployment and education of nurses is crucial to personalize care and to maintain nurses' satisfaction with the care provided.

Keywords: COVID-19; nursing care; patient care planning; quality of health care; personalized care; conditional inference trees

Citation: Clari, M.; Luciani, M.; Conti, A.; Sciannameo, V.; Berchialla, P.; Di Giulio, P.; Campagna, S.; Dimonte, V. The Impact of the COVID-19 Pandemic on Nursing Care: A Cross-Sectional Survey-Based Study. *J. Pers. Med.* **2021**, *11*, 945. https://doi.org/10.3390/jpm11100945

Academic Editor: Riitta Suhonen

Received: 30 July 2021
Accepted: 22 September 2021
Published: 23 September 2021

Publisher's Note: MDPI stays neutral with regard to jurisdictional claims in published maps and institutional affiliations.

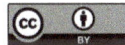

Copyright: © 2021 by the authors. Licensee MDPI, Basel, Switzerland. This article is an open access article distributed under the terms and conditions of the Creative Commons Attribution (CC BY) license (https://creativecommons.org/licenses/by/4.0/).

1. Introduction

From 31 December 2019, when the World Health Organization's China Office reported a case of pneumonia of unknown etiology in Wuhan, the Coronavirus Disease 2019 (COVID-19) started to spread across the globe [1]; on 11 March 2020, COVID-19 was declared a pandemic [2]. Italy was one of the first countries outside of China to report cases [1]. As of July 2021, Italy has reported more than 4,200,000 confirmed COVID-19 cases and more than 128,000 COVID-19 deaths [3]. The COVID-19 pandemic has had a severe impact on healthcare systems around the world, affecting the availability of beds in hospitals and intensive care units [4]. The second and following waves of the COVID-19 pandemic are still challenging healthcare systems and professionals [5].

Nurses have been recognized as fundamental actors in public health crises and have played a major role in the COVID-19 pandemic; however, the pandemic has had a severe impact on nursing care. This is due to the challenges associated with the preparedness and response to emergencies shown by several healthcare systems in different care settings [6,7]. In the face of a heavy workload, nurses have had to wear personal protective equipment (PPE) [4,8] and have been confronted with a lack of PPE [9,10], staff [10,11], and other resources [9,12], all of which have led to decreased mental health and well-being [13,14], occupational satisfaction [15], and high infection rates among nurses [16]. Nurses also reported being reassigned due to changes in human resource allocations, having to quickly learn new skills and competencies, having to work with newly-graduated nurses, and difficulties in communicating with patients and their families due to PPE and isolation. All of the factors mentioned above could have affected personalized care, an essential aspect of nursing, during the COVID-19 pandemic [17]. The concept of personalized health care in nursing is influenced by the care environment and the ability of general nursing care to meet a patient's needs, which were inevitably affected by the emergency, thereby potentially impacting clinical outcomes and satisfaction with care.

However, to the best of our knowledge, no rigorous study exists on how the pandemic has impacted nursing care. In particular, no studies have examined differences in the care provided by nurses who cared for COVID-19 and non-COVID-19 patients, or between those who were reassigned due to the pandemic and those who continued to work in their unit. Moreover, there is still a limited understanding of the factors associated with nurses' satisfaction with the care provided during the pandemic. This information could help decision makers ensure that nurses in a given unit have the appropriate education, skill mix, and patient-to-nurse ratio, thereby improving clinical practice and care personalization during this pandemic [5] and future health emergencies. Hence, this study aimed to identify changes in nursing care by comparing aspects of nursing care and satisfaction with care provided before and during the first wave of the COVID-19 pandemic, examining differences between nurses who cared for COVID-19 and non-COVID-19 patients, and between those who were reassigned and those who continued to work in their unit.

2. Materials and Methods

2.1. Study Design and Participants

This cross-sectional study included registered nurses (RNs) in Italy who delivered nursing care in the 3 months before study enrollment. No restrictions regarding the type of patient nor the setting were applied.

2.2. Procedures

RNs were invited to complete an online questionnaire, which was available between 12 May and 31 July 2020. Invitations were disseminated through ads on social media (Facebook, Twitter, Instagram), informational links on the websites of the Nursing Councils, and through texts and e-mails sent directly to RNs, using contact lists obtained from nursing schools in each of the Italian regions. Every 2 weeks, ads and informational links were reposted, and texts and e-mails were resent to RNs. The response rate (RR) was calculated as the RR2 [18], i.e., the sum of complete (I) and partial (P) questionnaires divided by the sum of complete, partial, non-questionnaires (NC, defined as respondents who logged on to the questionnaire but did not complete any item), and other (O, defined as respondents who could not fit in any of previous classifications; in this study, this category was not present): $RR2 = (I + P)/((I + P) + (NC + O))$. For this study, the RR2 was 81.4%.

2.3. Instruments

The online questionnaire was composed of six sections that covered: (I) changes in nursing care due to the COVID-19 pandemic; (II) changes in work organization; (III) ethics choices; (IV) most challenging case; (V) additional education needed to care for COVID-19 patients; (VI) socio-demographic characteristics. In the present analysis, only sections I, II, and VI were considered.

In section I, RNs reported the frequency with which they carried out the following tasks: fundamental care (i.e., personal hygiene, elimination, nutrition, mobility) [19], nursing techniques (i.e., respiratory support, vascular access, device positioning and management), patient education (i.e., respiratory exercises, medication, education), symptom management (pain, dyspnea, fatigue), and nurse–patient relationships (i.e., personal interactions with patients). These frequencies were reported for two time periods: before the COVID-19 pandemic and during what RNs perceived to be the worst week of the pandemic, using a 5-point Likert-type scale (1 = never; 2 = rarely; 3 = sometimes; 4 = often; 5 = most of the time). For each time period, RNs were also asked to rate their overall satisfaction with the care they provided (1 = very poor; 2 = poor; 3 = fair; 4 = good; 5 = excellent).

In section II, RNs reported the number of patients they cared for before the COVID-19 pandemic, if that number increased, remained stable, or decreased during the pandemic, if they were reassigned to another unit, and, if so, how many times. RNs were also asked if they thought there was enough time to prepare for the pandemic in terms of work organization, education/training, and their personal lives, with responses given on 5-point Likert-type scale (1 = not at all; 2 = not really; 3 = neutral; 4 = somewhat; 5 = very much). Finally, RNs were asked to report the number of patients they personally cared for during their last shift, and those caring for COVID-19 patients were also asked to report the number of patients who required no respiratory support, high-flow oxygen, non-invasive ventilation, and mechanical ventilation. The number of patients was then weighted based on the respiratory support provided, with a higher coefficient for patients with mechanical ventilation and a lower coefficient for those with no support.

2.4. Analysis

Continuous variables were described using medians and interquartile ranges (IQRs), or means and standard deviations (SDs). The Mann–Whitney U test was performed to evaluate differences in quantitative variables, and Chi-square or Fisher's exact test was used for categorical variables as appropriate.

A recursive partitioning for ordered multivariate response in a conditional inference framework approach was applied. Conditional inference trees were constructed to identify the pattern of work organization, nurse education/training, and personal lives associated to the different levels of fundamental care, nursing techniques, patient education, symptom management, and nurse–patient relationships in post COVID-19.

Independent variables were selected and split through multiplicity-adjusted p-values following the Bonferroni's criterion. The split of variables determines a set of rules associated to different values of the dependent variable. In more detail, for each variable, the conditional regression tree determines the optimal split and a partitioning is performed, selecting the input variable with the highest multiplicity-adjusted p-value. Then, a binary split is performed on the selected input variable, and this process is recursively performed until a stopping criterion is reached. The stopping criterion was based on significant results, i.e., splitting continues until the minimum of the adjusted p-values is less than a pre-specified level of significance (0.05) or otherwise stops [20].

In our analysis, a conditional inference tree was constructed for each nursing task as dependent variables (fundamental care, nursing techniques, patient education, symptom management, and nurse–patient relationships). Independent variables included in the trees were: values from before the pandemic for investigated nursing tasks, caring for COVID-19 patients, gender, age, education, geographic area, work experience, working unit, workplace reassignment, preparedness (in terms of work organization, education/training, and personal lives), decrease/increase in number of patients, number of non-COVID-19 patients, a weighted sum of COVID-19 patients with different respiratory support, and type of contract.

We also performed sensitivity analyses using multivariate logistic regression. Likert scores for the investigated nursing tasks before and during the COVID-19 pandemic were dichotomized into never/rarely/sometimes (0) and often/most of the time (1), and odds ratios and 95% confidence intervals were computed. Missing data were deleted listwise. Analyses were performed using R version 3.6.1 [21].

2.5. Ethics

RNs were informed about the study before accessing the online questionnaire, and consent was obtained before they began the questionnaire. RNs were not compensated for their role in the study, and participation was voluntary. All data were collected anonymously, and respondents could leave the questionnaire at any time. The study was approved by the University of Torino Ethics Committee (Approval no. 279061–01/07/2020) and conducted following the Declaration of Helsinki guidelines.

3. Results

A total of 936 RNs completed the online questionnaire (68.2% female); the median age in the sample was 39 years (IQR 30–49), and 40.7% of RNs had a bachelor's degree (Table 1).

Table 1. Participants' characteristics.

Variables [1]	Respondents			p-Values
	Total Nurses (n = 936)	Worked with COVID-19 Patients (n = 722, 77.1%)	Worked with Non-COVID-19 Patients (n = 214, 22.9%)	
Gender, n (%)				
Female	627 (68.2)	474 (66.8)	153 (72.9)	
Male	144 (15.7)	125 (17.6)	19 (9.0)	0.011
Prefer not to say	149 (16.1)	111 (15.6)	38 (18.1)	
Age in years, median (IQR)	39 (30–49)	37 (29–48)	45 (34–51)	<0.001
Educational background, n (%)				
Vocational diploma	191 (24.7)	145 (24.2)	46 (26.7)	
Bachelor's degree	314 (40.7)	257 (42.8)	57 (33.2)	
Professional master's diploma (1st lev)	177 (22.9)	127 (21.2)	50 (29.1)	0.137
Master's degree	71 (9.2)	56 (9.3)	15 (8.7)	
Professional master's diploma (2nd lev)	10 (1.3)	7 (1.2)	3 (1.7)	
PhD	9 (1.2)	8 (1.3)	1 (0.6)	
Geographical area, n (%)				
North Italy	560 (72.0)	422 (69.9)	138 (79.3)	
Lombardy	113 (14.5)	104 (17.2)	9 (5.2)	<0.001
Centre and South Italy	105 (13.5)	78 (12.9)	27 (15.5)	
Work experience in years, median (IQR)	14 (5–25)	11 (4–23)	20 (10–29)	<0.001
Working unit, n (%)				
High-intensity	296 (39.5)	270 (46.1)	26 (16.0)	
Low-intensity	370 (49.4)	275 (46.9)	95 (58.2)	0.157
Primary care	83 (11.1)	41 (7.0)	42 (25.8)	
Workplace change, n (%)				
No	547 (64.1)	387 (58.5)	160 (83.3)	
Yes	306 (35.9)	274 (41.5)	32 (16.7)	<0.001
Preparedness, median (IQR)				
Organizational	2 (1–3)	2 (1–2)	2 (1–2)	0.765
Educational	2 (1–2)	2 (1–2)	2 (1–3)	0.617
Personal	1 (1–2)	1 (1–2)	2 (1–2)	0.073

[1] Presence of missing data.

Most RNs worked in Northern Italy during the pandemic (86.5%). The median work experience was 13 years (IQR 5–25). Most RNs worked in a hospital setting (67.8%), 77.1% cared for COVID-19 patients, 28% worked in a dedicated COVID-19 unit, and 35.9% were reassigned following reorganizations to increase beds for COVID-19 patients. Almost half of RNs reported that they cared for fewer patients during the pandemic (45.8%): the median patient-to-nurse ratio among RNs caring for non-COVID-19 patients was 8 (IQR 3–15), compared to 2.4 (IQR 1–5) among those caring for COVID-19 patients. RNs caring for COVID-19 patients were significantly younger and had less work experience. Furthermore, there was a higher number of male RNs among those caring for COVID-19 patients. Lastly, in areas of high COVID-19 prevalence (i.e., Northern Italy and the Lombardy Region) more RNs were reassigned to COVID-19 hospital units. RNs reported there was little time to prepare for the pandemic in terms of work organization (median 2 (rarely), IQR 1–3), education/training (median 2, IQR 1–2), and their personal lives (median 1 (no time), IQR 1–2) (Table 1).

The highest number of reassigned RNs was observed in the Lombardy Region (19.0% versus 10.1%; $p = 0.003$). Reassigned RNs ($p = 0.042$; median 38, IQR 29–48 versus median 40, IQR 30–50 among those not reassigned) felt poorly prepared in terms of work organization ($p = 0.004$; median 1, IQR 1–2 versus median 2, IQR 1–3) and their personal lives ($p = 0.009$; median 1, IQR 1–2 versus median 1, IQR 1–2) (Table 2).

Table 2. Differences between nurses who changed their work unit.

Variables [1]	Respondents		p-Values
	Reassigned Nurses (n = 306, 35.8%)	Not Reassigned Nurses (n = 547, 64.2%)	
Gender, n (%)			
Female	222 (72.5)	405 (74.0)	
Male	57 (18.6)	87 (15.9)	0.738
Prefer not to say	23 (7.5)	46 (8.4)	
Age in years, median (IQR)	38 (29–48)	40 (30–50)	0.042
Educational background, n (%)			
Vocational diploma	67 (21.9)	124 (22.7)	
Bachelor's degree	103 (33.7)	211 (38.6)	
Professional master's diploma (1st lev)	72 (23.5)	105 (19.2)	NA
Master's degree	29 (9.5)	42 (7.7)	
Professional master's diploma (2nd lev)	4 (1.3)	6 (1.1)	
PhD	4 (1.3)	5 (0.9)	
Geographical area, n (%)			
North Italy	189 (61.8)	370 (67.6)	
Lombardy	58 (19.0)	55 (10.1)	0.003
Centre and South Italy	31 (10.1)	72 (13.2)	
Work experience in years, median (IQR)	12 (3.75–24.5)	14 (5–25)	0.057
Number of patients change, n (%)			
Decreased	134 (43.8)	255 (46.6)	
Stable	78 (25.5)	202 (36.9)	<0.001
Increased	94 (30.7)	90 (16.5)	

[1] Presence of missing data; NA Not available.

Reassigned nurses reported caring for a higher number of patients ($p < 0.001$), and they comprised a higher number of self-employed (9.2% versus 3.8% among those not reassigned; $p = 0.028$) and temporary contract workers (public temporary 3.3% versus 2.6%; private temporary 3.9 versus 2.9). RNs were mostly reassigned from medium–low-intensity facilities, and especially from community care to tertiary care hospitals ($p = 0.003$); RNs reassigned to COVID-19 units were most often transferred from medium–low-intensity facilities to tertiary care hospitals ($p < 0.001$). Conversely, RNs who were not reassigned and did not care for COVID-19 patients were significantly older ($p < 0.001$; median 45.5, IQR 36–51 versus median 37.5, IQR 30–48 among reassigned RNs who did care for COVID-19 patients) and had more work experience ($p < 0.001$; median 20, IQR 10–30 versus median 11, IQR 4–23) (Table 2).

Nursing Tasks

The frequency of fundamental care tasks before the pandemic was associated with the frequency during the pandemic ($p < 0.001$; before: median 3, IQR 2–4; during: median 3, IQR 2–5). In Figure 1, the conditional inference tree with the frequency of fundamental care tasks as a dependent variable, reported at the bottom of the figure as a boxplot, is represented. At the top of Figure 1, we can see that the first split of the decision tree was performed based on the frequency of fundamental care registered in the pre-pandemic period (node 1). RNs who frequently performed fundamental care before the pandemic continued this practice ($p < 0.001$), as we can see in the rightmost branch of the tree. Furthermore, among those who declared to not usually perform fundamental care before the pandemic, caring for COVID-19 patients ($p < 0.001$) or being reassigned ($p = 0.004$) significantly increased the frequency of fundamental care during the COVID-19 pandemic, as expressed in the boxplot on the Likert scale, reported in the bottom of the Figure 1, left part.

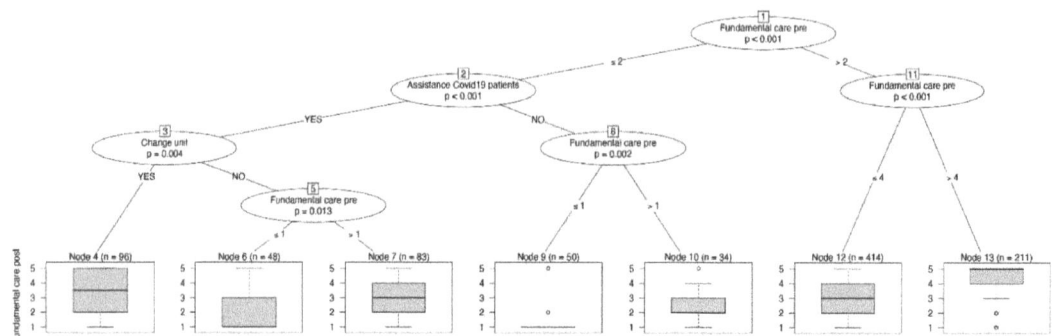

Figure 1. The conditional inference tree with the frequency of fundamental care tasks as dependent variable, reported at the bottom of the figure as boxplot.

In Figure 2, the conditional inference tree about fundamental care is represented. RNs caring for COVID-19 patients who frequently performed nursing techniques before the pandemic continued this practice ($p < 0.001$; before: median 4, IQR 3–5; during: median 5, IQR 4–5), as we can see by following the rightmost branch. RNs who cared for COVID-19 patients ($p < 0.001$), those who were reassigned ($p = 0.030$), and those who assisted ≤ 7.4 patients ($p = 0.014$) significantly increased the frequency of nursing techniques, with a median Likert scale of 5, as shown in the leftmost boxplot (Figure 2).

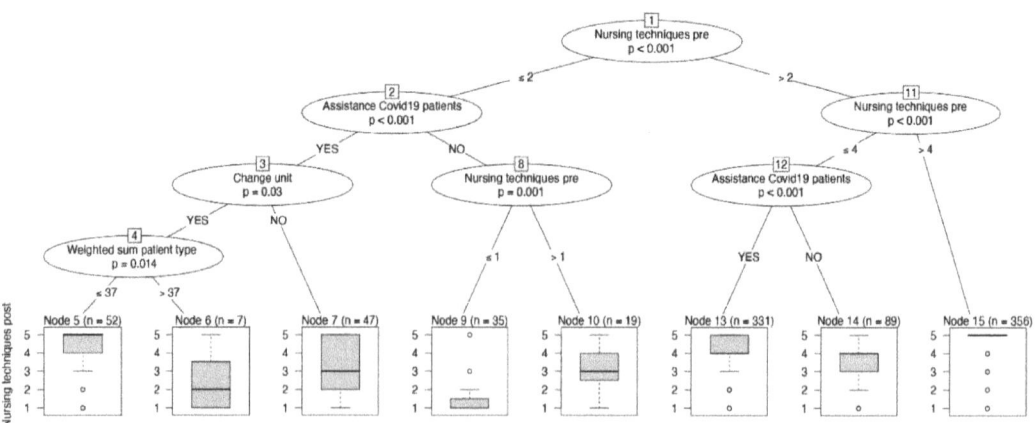

Figure 2. The conditional inference tree with the frequency of nursing techniques as dependent variable, reported at the bottom of the figure as boxplot.

RNs who performed patient education often before the pandemic and worked in high-intensity COVID-19 units ($p = 0.002$) stopped performing this task, as shown in the rightmost branch in Figure 3, while those in other settings continued their usual practice ($p < 0.001$; before: median 3, IQR 2–4; during: median 3, IQR 1–4).

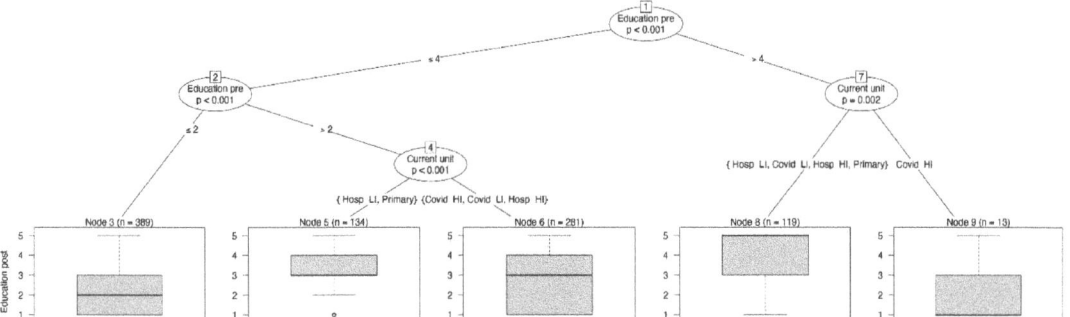

Figure 3. The conditional inference tree with the frequency of patient education as dependent variable, reported at the bottom of the figure as boxplot.

In Figure 4, the decision tree with symptom management as the outcome variable is reported. The frequency of symptom management during the COVID-19 pandemic was similar to that before the pandemic ($p < 0.001$; before: median 4, IQR 3–5; during: median 4, IQR 3–5), but it increased for RNs who cared for COVID-19 patients ($p < 0.001$), as shown in the leftmost branch. Caring for a higher number of non-COVID-19 patients (>6) increased the frequency of symptom management ($p = 0.037$), as reported in the eighth node, with a median Likert scale of 4.

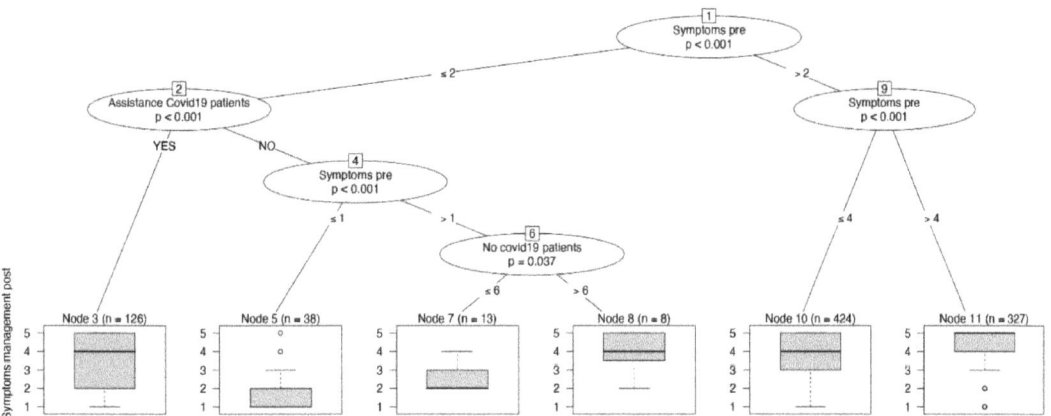

Figure 4. The conditional inference tree with the frequency of symptom management as dependent variable, reported at the bottom of the figure as boxplot.

Nurse–patient relationships before the pandemic were associated with those during the pandemic ($p < 0.001$; before: median 5, IQR 4–5; during: median 4, IQR 2–5), but nurses working in high-intensity COVID-19 units who reported frequent nurse–patient relationships before the pandemic had no chance to relate with patients during the pandemic ($p = 0.002$), as shown in the rightmost branch of the conditional decision tree reported in Figure 5.

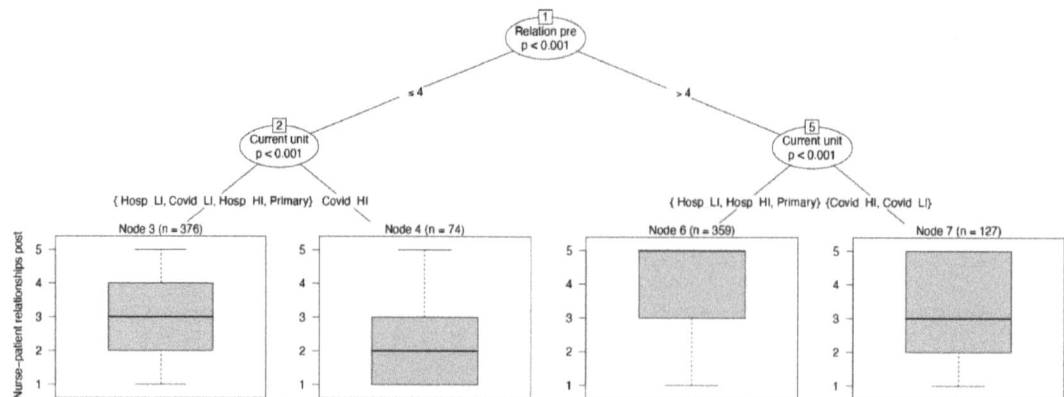

Figure 5. The conditional inference tree with the frequency of nurse–patient relationships as dependent variable, reported at the bottom of the figure as boxplot.

RNs' satisfaction with the care provided remained stable during the pandemic ($p < 0.001$; before: median 4, IQR 3–4; during: median 3, IQR 2–4), but younger nurses (aged ≤27 years) tended to judge their care as poor ($p = 0.047$), with a median Likert scale of 2 (node 12, Figure 6). Similarly, nurses with less work experience (≤13 years) reported a decreased quality of care ($p = 0.032$). RNs who reported high preparedness in terms of education/training showed increased care satisfaction ($p = 0.039$), with a median Likert scale of 4 (node 10, Figure 6).

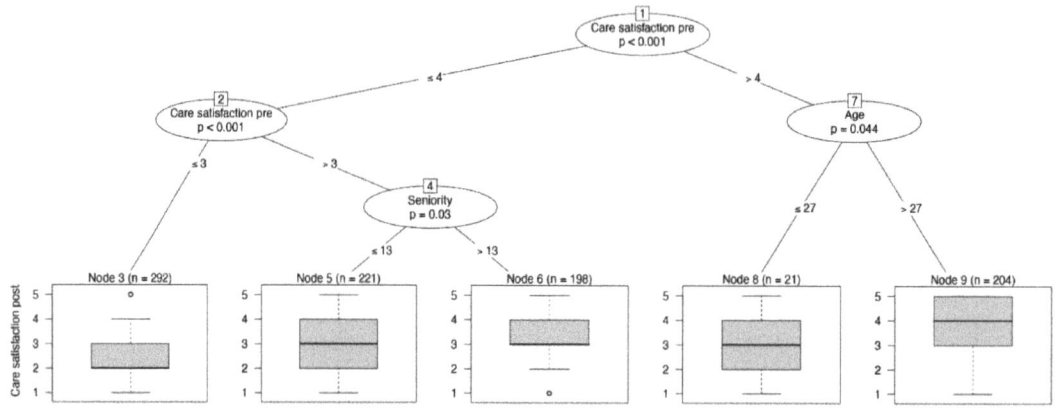

Figure 6. The conditional inference tree with the RNs' satisfaction with the care provided as dependent variable, reported at the bottom of the figure as boxplot.

The results of sensitivity analyses, performed through logistic regressions, confirmed those obtained from the decision trees. In the logistic regression models, the variables associated with the care provided during the COVID-19 pandemic were the same as those identified in the conditional inference trees.

4. Discussion

The present study described how nursing care was affected during the first wave of the COVID-19 pandemic and provided indications as to why nurses changed their practices. The first wave of the COVID-19 pandemic hit healthcare systems hard, affecting all aspects of nursing care; more nursing techniques were performed to care for patients, but the nurse–patient relationship suffered. These changes in nursing care led nurses to report lower satisfaction with the care provided.

The impact of the COVID-19 pandemic on nursing care mainly was felt on a clinical level. COVID-19 is a life-threatening illness that requires complex, clinically-focused, and personalized care; many patients were hospitalized for long periods with unpredictable outcomes. The COVID-19 pandemic was influenced by RNs' previous care habits, indicating the real professional commitment demonstrated by nurses, regardless of the circumstances [22]. Although the pandemic caused high levels of stress among nurses due to the high workload and uncertainty [23], nurses endeavored to guarantee the same level of care they provided before the pandemic to each patient. The prioritization of nursing care provided was affected [24], likely due to the unknown trajectory of the disease, the increase in fundamental care due to high patient dependency, the acquisition of new technical skills, and difficulties in communication and patient education due to infection containment measures.

Nurses who were reassigned to COVID-19 units increased the amount of fundamental care provided. A possible explanation could be that the COVID-19 context often requires many specialized skills, and newly-hired nurses may have preferred to perform more fundamental care while they learned these skills. Conversely, reassigned nurses could have increased the amount of fundamental care simply because COVID-19 patients require more personalized support for their activities of daily living [25].

The physiological needs of COVID-19 patients also required the performance of more nursing techniques. In fact, nurses who cared for COVID-19 patients performed these techniques far more frequently during than before the pandemic. Nurses had to adapt to the needs of these patients, often learning or refreshing techniques such as non-invasive ventilation support and arterial puncture for blood gas analysis [26]. Symptom management was also performed more frequently given the higher number of patients as healthcare systems reached capacity [27].

A biomedical perspective is often predominant in life-threatening situations, but it should be balanced by the value of caring for others and the individualization of care, something on which technical skills should also focus [28]. This is particularly crucial for COVID-19 patients, who have to face an unknown disease without the support of their loved ones and likely without a close relationship with healthcare providers. Education is the most commonly omitted task when resources are strained [29], and nurse–patient relationships and patient education in our study were reduced due to infection prevention measures [30]. Despite these problems, nurses tried to invent new ways to interact with patients, such as drawing on gowns, printing their pictures to show their faces, and writing their names on face shields [31].

Another relevant finding was the lower satisfaction with care provided among RNs from areas of high COVID-19 prevalence and those who worked in high-intensity units. This may be due to the lack of therapeutic solutions and the patients' reduced chance of recovery, especially the elderly, making nurses feel less confident that the care they provided was adequate [32]. Nurses working in primary care were also less satisfied with the care provided, probably due to the exceptional number of patients that were treated at home and in other community settings [33].

The devastating, rapid impact that the pandemic has had on the Italian healthcare system might explain some of the lack of preparedness reported by our respondents. During the first wave, COVID-19 was an unknown disease, and a trial and error approach was often applied, with frequent changes in therapies, use of ventilation, and supination [34]; thus, nurses had to adapt their daily work to rapidly changing guidelines and protocols, individualizing the care they provided. Moreover, in Italy, newly-graduated nurses were hired to work in new community care units specifically dedicated to COVID-19 patients, which aimed to identify those who required medical assistance and those who could stay isolated at home with telephone follow-ups [35]. More experienced community care nurses were also recruited for these units, which led to a decreased availability of nurses for established home care services. These factors could have influenced the preparedness of nurses working in community settings.

The pandemic globally highlighted the nursing shortage and the lack of adequate, coordinated management responses to population health crises [36]. However, contextual factors must be considered when evaluating care outcomes, which should not be merely interpreted quantitatively. In this regard, the patient-to-nurse ratio should not be the only index collected to evaluate staffing needs but, perhaps, environmental and organizational factors should also be considered [37]. Healthcare systems should maintain, and be prepared to implement, plans for pandemic events, and hospital managers should draw up specific emergency plans that define the human resources required in case of a long-term pandemic with recurrent waves, based on competencies, skill mix (e.g., of experienced and novice nurses), and job rotations. Nurse staffing should be proportionate to the clinical complexity of patients and to the organizational complexities to individualize care, minimizing the risk of missed care and patient death [38]. These actions would improve the healthcare system's response and alleviate the stress imposed by crises, although maintaining the highest standard of nursing care delivered.

The present study has a number of limitations. The majority of the respondents were from the areas most affected by the pandemic in Italy, and most worked in hospital settings. Moreover, our sample could not completely represent the Italian nursing population, which consists of around 367,000 individuals. This may have produced some response bias as nurses from hospital settings may have felt more implicated in the pandemic and, thus, may have been more interested in the survey. Moreover, considering that data collected were self-reported, findings may be affected by the respondents' emotional or physical condition. High negative and low positive affect have been associated with an emotional autobiographical memory [39]; in the emotionally-charged pandemic, recall may also have influenced our results. Our findings should be interpreted considering that data were collected during the first wave in Italy, the first European country hit by the pandemic, and the first country that had to reorganize its healthcare system to respond to the emergency. Moreover, the use of a cross-sectional design means that causality cannot be proven. However, the decision tree analysis used, and the sensitivity analyses performed, increased the confidence in the inferences.

5. Conclusions

This study highlighted the impact of the COVID-19 pandemic on nursing care and the differences between nurses who were and were not reassigned. Despite all of the difficulties faced by nurses, they were generally satisfied with the care provided, except for younger nurses and those with limited working experience. Furthermore, in spite of the healthcare reorganization, and the need to educate, prioritize, and individualize their activities to meet the needs of patients with complex clinical conditions, nurses continued to provide a high level of care, individualizing their practices and ensuring the highest quality of care. Nurses who felt more prepared in terms of education and training were more satisfied with the care provided, and an increase in the number of patients decreased the frequency of fundamental care and nurse–patient relationships. Nurses caring for COVID-19 patients performed nursing techniques more often, to the detriment of patient education. Ensuring the appropriate deployment and education of nurses is crucial to personalize care, especially during a pandemic, and to maintain nurses' satisfaction with the care provided. Policy makers should consider these results to create structured plans to address long-term pandemics and ensure appropriate nurse staffing in hospitals and primary care settings.

Author Contributions: Conceptualization, M.C., M.L. and A.C.; methodology, M.C., M.L. and A.C.; validation, V.S. and P.B.; formal analysis, V.S. and P.B.; investigation, V.D.; data curation, M.C., M.L. and A.C.; writing—original draft preparation, M.C., M.L., A.C. and V.S.; writing—review and editing, P.B., P.D.G., S.C. and V.D.; supervision, P.B., P.D.G., S.C. and V.D.; project administration, M.C. All authors have read and agreed to the published version of the manuscript.

Funding: This research received no external funding.

Institutional Review Board Statement: The study was conducted according to the guidelines of the Declaration of Helsinki, and approved by the Ethics Committee of the University of Torino (Approval no. 279061–01/07/2020).

Informed Consent Statement: Informed consent was obtained from all subjects involved in the study.

Data Availability Statement: The data presented in this study are available on request from the corresponding author. The data are not publicly available due to privacy reason.

Acknowledgments: We would like to thank all of the nurses who completed the survey in such difficult times.

Conflicts of Interest: The authors declare no conflict of interest.

References

1. World Health Organization. Coronavirus Disease (COVID-19) Situation Reports. Available online: https://www.who.int/emergencies/diseases/novel-coronavirus-2019/situation-reports (accessed on 29 October 2020).
2. World Health Organization. WHO Director-General's Opening Remarks at the Mission Briefing on COVID-19—12 March 2020. Available online: https://www.who.int/director-general/speeches/detail/who-director-general-s-opening-remarks-at-the-mission-briefing-on-covid-19---12-march-2020 (accessed on 29 October 2020).
3. European Centre for Disease Prevention and Control. COVID-19 Situation Dashboard. Available online: https://qap.ecdc.europa.eu/public/extensions/COVID-19/COVID-19.html#global-overview-tab (accessed on 12 February 2021).
4. Liu, Q.; Luo, D.; Haase, J.E.; Guo, Q.; Wang, X.Q.; Liu, S.; Xia, L.; Liu, Z.; Yang, J.; Yang, B.X. The experiences of health-care providers during the covid-19 crisis in China: A qualitative study. *Lancet Glob. Health* **2020**, *8*, e790–e798. [CrossRef]
5. Cacciapaglia, G.; Cot, C.; Sannino, F. Second wave COVID-19 pandemics in Europe: A temporal playbook. *Sci. Rep.* **2020**, *10*, 15514. [CrossRef]
6. Marshall, V.K.; Chavez, M.; Mason, T.M.; Martinez-Tyson, D. Emergency preparedness during the COVID-19 pandemic: Perceptions of oncology professionals and implications for nursing management from a qualitative study. *J. Nurs. Manag.* **2021**. [CrossRef]
7. Quigley, D.D.; Dick, A.; Agarwal, M.; Jones, K.M.; Mody, L.; Stone, P.W. COVID-19 preparedness in nursing homes in the midst of the pandemic. *J. Am. Geriatr. Soc.* **2020**, *68*, 1164–1166. [CrossRef] [PubMed]
8. Zhang, Y.; Wei, L.; Li, H.; Pan, Y.; Wang, J.; Li, Q.; Wu, Q.; Wei, H. The psychological change process of frontline nurses caring for patients with COVID-19 during its outbreak. *Issues Ment. Health Nurs.* **2020**, *41*, 525–530. [CrossRef]
9. Morley, G.; Grady, C.; McCarthy, J.; Ulrich, C.M. Covid-19: Ethical challenges for nurses. *Hastings Cent. Rep.* **2020**, *50*, 35–39. [CrossRef] [PubMed]
10. Tan, R.; Yu, T.; Luo, K.; Teng, F.; Liu, Y.; Luo, J.; Hu, D. Experiences of clinical first-line nurses treating patients with COVID-19: A qualitative study. *J. Nurs. Manag.* **2020**, *28*, 1381–1390. [CrossRef]
11. Bambi, S.; Iozzo, P.; Lucchini, A. New issues in nursing management during the COVID-19 pandemic in Italy. *Am. J. Crit. Care* **2020**, *29*, e92–e93. [CrossRef] [PubMed]
12. Nouvet, E.; Strachan, P.; Luciani, M.; de Laat, S.; Conti, A.; Oliphant, A.; Monette, E.; Kapiriri, L.; Schwartz, L. *Triaging critical care during COVID-19: Global Preparedness, Socio-Cultural Considerations, and Communication*; Humanitarian Health Ethics Research Group: Hamilton, ON, Canada, 2020; ISBN 978-0-9938354-5-2.
13. Stelnicki, A.M.; Carleton, R.N.; Reichert, C. Nurses' mental health and well-being: COVID-19 impacts. *Can. J. Nurs. Res.* **2020**, *52*, 237–239. [CrossRef]
14. Zerbini, G.; Ebigbo, A.; Reicherts, P.; Kunz, M.; Messman, H. Psychosocial burden of healthcare professionals in times of COVID-19—A survey conducted at the University Hospital Augsburg. *Ger. Med. Sci.* **2020**, *18*, 1–9. [CrossRef]
15. Savitsky, B.; Radomislensky, I.; Hendel, T. Nurses' occupational satisfaction during Covid-19 pandemic. *Appl. Nurs. Res.* **2021**, *59*, 151416. [CrossRef] [PubMed]
16. International Council of Nurses. High Proportion of Healthcare Workers with COVID-19 in Italy Is a Stark Warning to the World: Protecting Nurses and Their Colleagues Must Be the Number One Priority. Available online: https://www.icn.ch/news/high-proportion-healthcare-workers-covid-19-italy-stark-warning-world-protecting-nurses-and (accessed on 3 November 2020).
17. Han, C.J. A Concept analysis of personalized health care in nursing. *Nurs. Forum* **2016**, *51*, 32–39. [CrossRef] [PubMed]
18. Shih, T.-H.; Fan, X. Comparing response rates from web and mail surveys: A meta-analysis. *Field Methods* **2008**, *20*, 249–271. [CrossRef]
19. Feo, R.; Kitson, A.; Conroy, T. How fundamental aspects of nursing care are defined in the literature: A scoping review. *J. Clin. Nurs.* **2018**, *27*, 2189–2229. [CrossRef]
20. Wu, Z.; Su, X.; Sheng, H.; Chen, Y.; Gao, X.; Bao, L.; Jin, W. Conditional inference tree for multiple gene-environment interactions on myocardial infarction. *Arch. Med. Res.* **2017**, *48*, 546–552. [CrossRef] [PubMed]
21. R Core Team. *R: A Language and Environment for Statistical Computing*; R Foundation for Statistical Computing: Vienna, Austria, 2019.

22. Fernandez, R.; Lord, H.; Halcomb, E.; Moxham, L.; Middleton, R.; Alananzeh, I.; Ellwood, L. Implications for COVID-19: A systematic review of nurses' experiences of working in acute care hospital settings during a respiratory pandemic. *Int. J. Nurs. Stud.* **2020**, *111*, 103637. [CrossRef] [PubMed]
23. Simonetti, V.; Durante, A.; Ambrosca, R.; Arcadi, P.; Graziano, G.; Pucciarelli, G.; Simeone, S.; Vellone, E.; Alvaro, R.; Cicolini, G. Anxiety, sleep disorders and self-efficacy among nurses during COVID-19 pandemic: A cross-sectional study. *J. Clin. Nurs.* **2021**, *30*, 1360–1371. [CrossRef] [PubMed]
24. Maves, R.C.; Downar, J.; Dichter, J.R.; Hick, J.L.; Devereaux, A.; Geiling, J.A.; Kissoon, N.; Hupert, N.; Niven, A.S.; King, M.A.; et al. Triage of scarce critical care resources in COVID-19 an implementation guide for regional allocation. *Chest* **2020**, *158*, 212–225. [CrossRef]
25. Lomborg, K.; Bjørn, A.; Dahl, R.; Kirkevold, M. Body care experienced by people hospitalized with severe respiratory disease. *J. Adv. Nurs.* **2005**, *50*, 262–271. [CrossRef]
26. Ambrosi, E.; Canzan, F.; Di Giulio, P.; Mortari, L.; Palese, A.; Tognoni, G.; Saiani, L. L'emergenza covid-19 nelle parole degli infermieri. *Assist. Inferm. Ric.* **2020**, *39*, 66–108. [CrossRef]
27. Bowman, B.A.; Back, A.L.; Esch, A.E.; Marshall, N. Crisis symptom management and patient communication protocols are important tools for all clinicians responding to COVID-19. *J. Pain Symptom Manag.* **2020**, *60*, e98–e100. [CrossRef]
28. Feo, R.; Kitson, A. Promoting patient-centred fundamental care in acute healthcare systems. *Int. J. Nurs. Stud.* **2016**, *57*, 1–11. [CrossRef] [PubMed]
29. Jones, T.L.; Hamilton, P.; Murry, N. Unfinished nursing care, missed care, and implicitly rationed care: State of the science review. *Int. J. Nurs. Stud.* **2015**, *52*, 1121–1137. [CrossRef]
30. Jangland, E.; Carlsson, M.; Lundgren, E.; Gunningberg, L. The impact of an intervention to improve patient participation in a surgical care unit: A quasi-experimental study. *Int. J. Nurs. Stud.* **2012**, *49*, 528–538. [CrossRef]
31. Schlögl, M.; Jones, C. Maintaining our humanity through the mask: Mindful communication during COVID-19. *J. Am. Geriatr. Soc.* **2020**, *68*, E12–E13. [CrossRef]
32. Sun, N.; Wei, L.; Shi, S.; Jiao, D.; Song, R.; Ma, L.; Wang, H.; Wang, C.; Wang, Z.; You, Y.; et al. A qualitative study on the psychological experience of caregivers of COVID-19 patients. *Am. J. Infect. Control* **2020**, *48*, 592–598. [CrossRef] [PubMed]
33. Perlini, S.; Canevari, F.; Cortesi, S.; Sgromo, V.; Brancaglione, A.; Contri, E.; Pettenazza, P.; Salinaro, F.; Speciale, F.; Sechi, G.; et al. Emergency department and out-of-hospital emergency system (112—AREU 118) integrated response to coronavirus disease 2019 in a northern italy centre. *Intern. Emerg. Med.* **2020**, *15*, 825–833. [CrossRef] [PubMed]
34. Zagury-Orly, I.; Schwartzstein, R.M. Covid-19—A reminder to reason. *N. Engl. J. Med.* **2020**, *383*, e12. [CrossRef]
35. Marrazzo, F.; Spina, S.; Pepe, P.E.; D'Ambrosio, A.; Bernasconi, F.; Manzoni, P.; Graci, C.; Frigerio, C.; Sacchi, M.; Stucchi, R.; et al. Rapid reorganization of the milan metropolitan public safety answering point operations during the initial phase of the COVID-19 outbreak in Italy. *J. Am. Coll. Emerg. Physicians Open* **2020**, *1*, 1240–1249. [CrossRef]
36. Propper, C.; Stoye, G.; Zaranko, B. The wider impacts of the coronavirus pandemic on the NHS*. *Fisc. Stud.* **2020**, *41*, 345–356. [CrossRef]
37. Di Giulio, P.; Clari, M.; Conti, A.; Campagna, S. The problems in the interpretation of the studies on the relationship between staffing and patients' outcomes: The case of the RN4CAST studies. *Assist. Inferm. Ric.* **2019**, *38*, 138–145. [CrossRef] [PubMed]
38. Campagna, S.; Conti, A.; Clari, M.; Basso, I.; Sciannameo, V.; Di Giulio, P.; Dimonte, V. Factors associated with missed nursing care in nursing homes: A multicentre cross-sectional study. *Int. J. Health Policy Manag.* **2021**. [CrossRef] [PubMed]
39. Vrijsen, J.N.; Hertel, P.T.; Becker, E.S. Practicing emotionally biased retrieval affects mood and establishes biased recall a week later. *Cognit. Ther. Res.* **2016**, *40*, 764–773. [CrossRef] [PubMed]

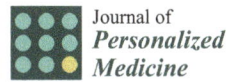

Article

Kinesio Taping vs. Auricular Acupressure for the Personalised Treatment of Primary Dysmenorrhoea: A Pilot Randomized Controlled Trial

Elena Mejías-Gil [1], Elisa María Garrido-Ardila [1,*], Jesús Montanero-Fernández [2], María Jiménez-Palomares [1], Juan Rodríguez-Mansilla [1,*] and María Victoria González López-Arza [1]

[1] ADOLOR Research Group, Department of Medical-Surgical Therapy, Faculty of Medicine and Health Sciences, Extremadura University, 06006 Badajoz, Spain; elenamejias92@gmail.com (E.M.-G.); mariajp@unex.es (M.J.-P.); mvglez@unex.es (M.V.G.L.-A.)

[2] Mathematics Department, Faculty of Medicine and Health Sciences, Extremadura University, 06006 Badajoz, Spain; jmf@unex.es

* Correspondence: egarridoa@unex.es (E.M.G.-A.); jrodman@unex.es (J.R.-M.)

Abstract: Background: Dysmenorrhoea is the medical term for menstrual pain. The World Health Organization estimates that up to 81% of women of childbearing age are affected by this condition, and it is one of the leading causes of absenteeism from work and school among women. Although there are pharmacological treatments available for menstrual-pain relief, they do not respond to all women's needs. Therefore, there is a need to study and develop non-pharmacological alternatives to broaden the individualised treatment options for dysmenorrhea. There are scarce studies published on non-pharmacological treatments, such as kinesio tape and auricular acupressure for the relief of menstrual pain, but the scientific evidence available suggest that these techniques may be beneficial in addressing this problem. The objective of this pilot study was to assess and compare the effectiveness of kinesio tape and auricular acupressure to decrease pain and drug intake in women with primary dysmenorrhoea. Methods: This was a double-blind randomized clinical controlled trial. The period of study was from September 2017 to August 2018. Women enrolled in the University of Extremadura and who had primary dysmenorrhoea were randomized to five groups: control (n = 23), kinesio tape (n = 23), placebo kinesio tape (n = 23), auricular acupressure (n = 23) and placebo auricular acupressure (n = 22). Measures were taken during the pretreatment phase (at four menstrual cycles), during the post-intervention phase (at four menstrual cycles) and during the follow-up phase (at the first and third menstrual cycles after the treatment was completed). The primary outcome measures were mean pain intensity, maximum pain intensity, number of painful days and dose of drug intake during menstruation, measured with the Visual Analogue Scale. The secondary outcome measures were the length of the cycle, the length of menstruation, the drug intake and the type of drug. Results: In all, 108 participants completed the study. The statistical analysis (MANOVA, ANOVA, t-paired and McNemar tests) showed that kinesio tape and auricular acupressure have a beneficial effect on pain relief (mean pain intensity, $p < 0.001$; maximum pain intensity, $p < 0.001$; number of painful days, $p = 0.021$; dose of drug intake, $p < 0.001$). In addition, once the treatments were withdrawn, the auricular-acupressure group maintained lower scores during the first follow-up cycle ($p < 0.001$). Conclusions: Kinesio tape and auricular acupressure decrease pain and drug intake in women with primary dysmenorrhoea. The changes in the auricular-acupressure group seemed to last longer. The results suggest that these techniques could be used as complementary personalised therapies to the pharmacological treatment and not as a substitution.

Keywords: dysmenorrhea; kinesio tape; auricular acupressure; pain

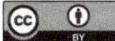

1. Introduction

Dysmenorrhoea is the medical term for menstrual pain. It is a cramping sensation felt in the supra pubic area of the abdomen and can be accompanied by muscle pain, headache and nausea [1,2]. It is classified as primary or secondary according to the absence or presence of underlying pathologies that trigger the pain respectively [2,3].

The World Health Organization estimates that 81% of the female population can be affected by this condition. However, the percentage can vary in different countries [4]. This implies that more than half of the female population of childbearing age experiences this type of pain at least once a month. It has been observed that dysmenorrhoea has a negative impact on the academic, work, sport and social life of women, who can also see their quality of life affected [2,4,5].

Although there are pharmacological treatments available for menstrual-pain relief, they do not respond to all women's needs. Allergies to drugs, lack of effectiveness or refusal to use medication (for personal, religious or social reasons) leave part of these women with no effective treatment for their symptoms [2,6–11].

Therefore, non-pharmacological treatments which provide person-centred and individualised care, such as those proposed in Physiotherapy and Traditional Chinese Medicine, can be very useful. Many publications have focused their studies on the relief of various types of pain through the use of non-pharmacological therapies, such as kinesio tape, thermotherapy, electrotherapy, massage, acupuncture and auricular acupressure obtaining encouraging results [12–16]. In particular, kinesio taping and auricular acupressure are treatment techniques that have been used for a long time in the management of pain from different causes. However, there is very little scientific evidence of the effectiveness of these techniques for primary dysmenorrhoea. Four studies that analyzed the use of kinesio taping in primary dysmenorrhoea can be found in the literature [17–20]. Their results suggested an improvement of menstrual pain. Similarly, the three articles that studies the effectiveness of auricular acupressure in primary dysmenorrhoea showed a pain-relief effect [21–23]. These results would point towards the possible benefits of the use of these non-pharmacological treatment for the management of dysmenorrhoea.

The application of kinesio taping is based on its proprioceptive and skin receptor stimulation effects. When applied correctly, it influences muscle tone and can induce muscle relaxation. In addition, part of the analgesic effect of this technique is based on its ability to decrease interstitial pressure [24,25]. This causes a reduction of the stimulus received by nociceptors and normalizes local blood and lymphatic circulation, thus also eliminating mediators of pain and inflammation [24,25]. Moreover, the literature also suggests the use of mechanisms related to the Gate Control theory, whereby a tactile sensory stimulus interferes with the perception of pain intensity [26].

Although the mechanism of action of auricular acupressure is still under study, the research conducted by using functional magnetic resonance imaging (fMRI) and positron emission tomography (PET) has revealed the presence of brain activity in the areas corresponding to the structure represented by the point on which the stimulus is applied [27–29]. This stimulus has also been shown to trigger specific responses in brain regions related to pain inhibition and to influence the release of endorphins, melatonin and serotonin [27,28].

The objective of this pilot study was to assess the effectiveness of kinesio taping and auricular acupressure improving pain and decreasing drug intake in women with primary dysmenorrhoea, comparing both treatment approaches between them.

2. Materials and Methods

2.1. Study Design

This pilot study was a single-blind randomized clinical controlled trial. The study took place within the University of Extremadura (Spain), in an outpatient setting. The period of study was from September 2017 to August 2018. The study protocol was approved by the Bioethical Commission of the University of Extremadura in Spain (registration number: 58/2017). The trial was registered with the ClinicalTrials.gov registry (Study

Identifier: NCT04400968). All participants signed a written informed consent. The data were guaranteed to be protected and anonymous. The CONSORT statements were used to conduct and report the trial.

2.2. Participants and Procedures

The target population was women enrolled in the University of Extremadura who had primary dysmenorrhoea. Participants were recruited in September 2017. The inclusion criteria were women between 18 and 30 years old affected by primary dysmenorrhoea grade 2 and 3 of Andersch and Milsom classification [30], to have attended gynecologist consultation for a general revision in the last 2 years, to have menstrual pain, to have regular menstrual cycles of 21 to 38 days, and to not have an intrauterine device or to be on oral contraceptive treatment. The exclusion criteria were to have been diagnosed with a condition that could influence menstrual-pain perception and to know or have been previously treated with techniques used in the interventions and pregnancy.

In the first place, an interview was conducted at the begging of the academic year (2017/2018) in order to select the sample. Once the participants were recruited, they were assigned an alphanumeric identifier and randomized into the five study groups, using the SPSS statistical program. The program selected the participants to be included in each group equally. Since the sample was not fully divisible among the five groups, the order of preference to complete the groups was allocated by randomly assigning in a ranking from 1 to 5.

Then a pretreatment phase of 4 menstrual cycles started. During this period, the participants completed the questionnaires at their home to collect information regarding the symptoms experienced in each menstrual cycle. The questionnaires were codified by an identifier number assigned to each participant to ensure masking of identity and group allocation and, therefore, to ensure blinding of the data-collection process and analysis.

Once the pretreatment phase was completed, a four menstrual cycles treatment phase commenced. During this phase the participants continued with the same protocol to collect data and received the treatments assigned to their group. After each cycle finished, the treatments were discontinued, and the follow-up phases started. In the first and second follow-up phase, the data corresponding to the first and the third cycle after the treatments were finished was collected respectively.

Due to the nature of the treatments, participants knew whether they belonged to one of the kinesio-taping or auricular-acupressure groups. However, they did not know whether the technique applied was the placebo or the real one. The therapist in charge of applying the treatments could not be blinded in order to apply the treatments correctly.

The primary outcome measures were four in total: Mean pain intensity for the 3 first days of menstruation, maximum pain intensity, number of painful days and dose of drug intake. Pain intensity was measured with the Visual Analogue Scale (VAS). This scale measure pain in a scale from 0 to 10, where 0 means no pain and 10 means maximum and excruciating pain [31]. All outcome measures were registered at the initial interview and every day during the bleeding period in the pretreatment, treatment and follow-up phases. As the pretreatment and the treatment phases consisted of four periods each, there were ten measures in all.

The secondary outcome measures included the length of the cycle, the length of menstruation, the drug intake and the type of drug. The epidemiological data of the sample (age, body height, body weight, age of menarche and age of first pain) were collected at the baseline measurement.

The sample consisted of 114 participants who were randomly allocated to a control group, a kinesio-tape group, a placebo kinesio-tape group, an auricular-acupressure group and a placebo auricular-acupressure group (Figure 1). Details of the intervention following the Template for Intervention Description and Replication (TIDieR) [32] guidelines are provided in Supplemental Materials Table S1.

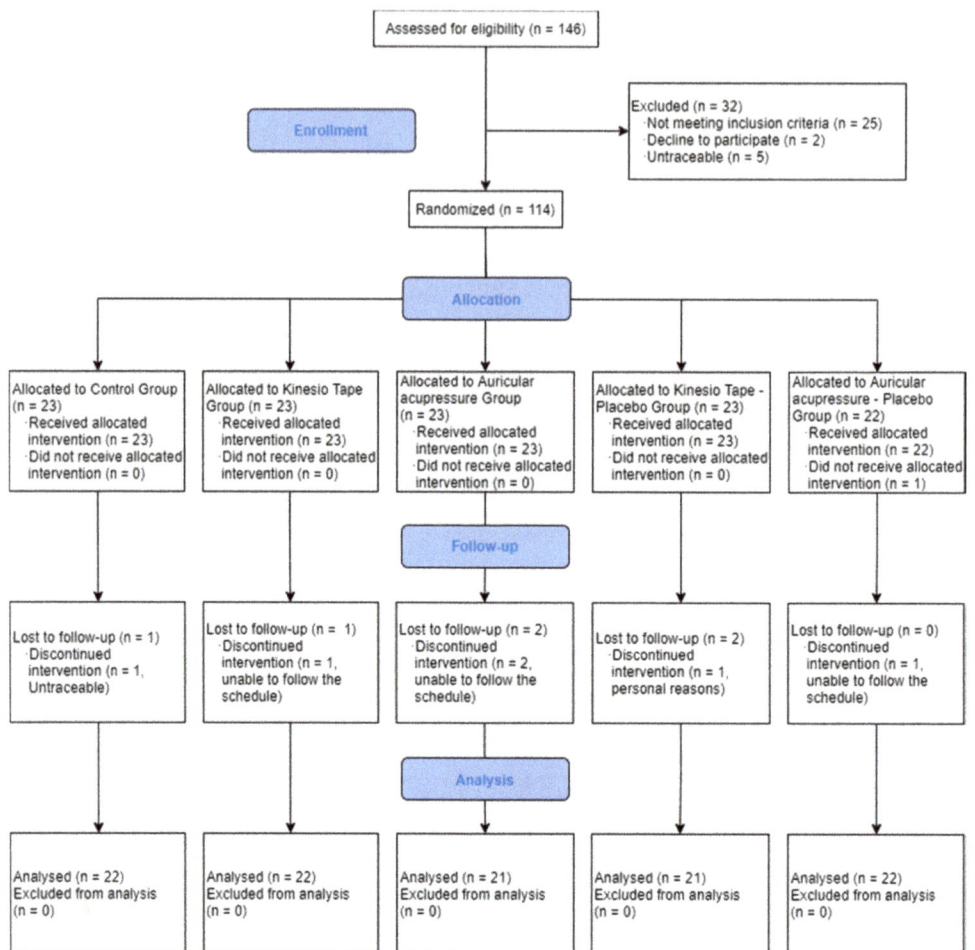

Figure 1. CONSORT flow diagram.

The therapy and the placebo treatments were always placed within 4 h from the beginning of the menstrual cycle and were maintained during 72 h. When the adhesive tapes lost fixation and became detached, the treatment material was replaced as soon as possible (never later than 2 h from detachment). The cases that could not receive the treatments on the scheduled time were excluded.

The participants received the necessary information in order to correctly maintain the tapes and adhesives. All groups received the same information, not differentiating between treatment and placebo groups, to ensure blinding. All participants committed to maintain secret their experiences and not to comment with the rest of women during the study period.

As it was considered unethical, the drug intake was not forbidden if pain relief was necessary. However, all subjects were asked to delay the intake until the appearance of symptoms. In order to control the influence of the medication, the questionnaires included sections where the intake was registered.

The control group did not receive any treatment. However, the controls completed all the questionnaires to collect the information regarding their symptoms in order to observe their progress with no intervention.

2.3. Statistical Analysis

The obtained data were analyzed through the IBM SPSS Statistics 22.0 version (Statistical Package for the Social Sciences). A descriptive analysis of all the outcome measures was performed. Changes on drug intake were analyzed by the McNemar test. In order to assess the primary outcome measures, we distinguished between two steps. Firstly, for each single outcome we applied a one-way multivariate ANOVA considering the ten measurements and the five groups, so that we could contrast the existence of global influence of the treatment. Moreover, drug intake was included as a second factor in the model in order to detect a possible bias due to this circumstance. In the following step, we focused on analysing just the average between the four periods considered during the pretreatment and during treatment stages. This way, the number of phases got reduced to four (average pretreatment, average treatment, follow-up 1 and follow-up 2) for each primary outcome measures. Then, a more exhaustive analysis was performed for each one. On the one hand, we assessed the inter-group differences at each phase by a one-way ANOVA F test or Kruskal–Wallis's H test (depending on the level of skewness or symmetry of the distribution of the different outcomes). On the other hand, we analyzed separately the within-group changes of the outcome measures during the intervention as compared with the pretreatment scores by a t-paired test or Wilcoxon's W test.

The sample size does not respond to a previous calculation. However, as many participants as possible were first recruited and posteriorly randomly allocated into five equal groups of 25 women. Finally, according to Cohen's d, the groups sample size lead to a statistical power of 80% for a 2-sided level 5% t-test to detect an effect size of 0.8.

3. Results

Figure 1 shows the study flow diagram. Except for the auricular-acupressure placebo group, which had no loses, all groups had similar drop-outs rates. This was 5.6% of the total initial sample.

The average duration of the first cycle was 30.26 ± 0.31 days, with 5.63 ± 1.05 days of menstruation. These values hardly changed along the ten menstruations that were followed up. All the participants reported regular drug intake for pain relief. In fact, 88% of women took medication during the first period previous to the application of the treatments. Nevertheless, we observed that this proportion decreased along the treatment phase to 62% during the last menstruation ($p < 0.001$), since 33 participants stopped taking medication. Most of them (namely 29) belonged to the auricular-acupressure and the kinesio-tape groups. This percentage increased progressively after the treatment during the follow-up phases.

Tables 1 and 2 include descriptive statistics of the rest of secondary outcomes and the primary ones, respectively.

Table 1. Epidemiological data and secondary outcome measures.

	CG (n = 22)	KT (n = 22)	KT-P (n = 21)	AP (n = 21)	AP-P (n = 22)
Height (m)	1.63 ± 0.04	1.61 ± 0.05	1.62 ± 0.06	1.61 ± 0.04	1.60 ± 0.04
Weight (Kg)	56.59 ± 6.44	55.69 ± 6.35	54.53 ± 4.78	54.03 ± 6.23	54.54 ± 5.55
Age (years)	20.91 ± 1.26	20.64 ± 1.05	20.95 ± 1.32	20.95 ± 1.85	21.14 ± 0.99
AM (years)	12.14 ± 1.17	11.86 ± 1.45	12.57 ± 1.12	11.81 ± 1.28	12.64 ± 1.33
AFP (years)	13.68 ± 1.32	14.14 ± 1.75	13.57 ± 1.25	13.48 ± 1.63	13.86 ± 1.12
DC (days)	29.04 ± 1.73	30.09 ± 2.68	29.71 ± 3.01	29.09 ± 1.99	30.36 ± 2.57
DM (days)	5.45 ± 1.22	5.22 ± 0.75	5.52 ± 0.67	5.14 ± 1.42	5.27 ± 0.88

CG, control group; KT, kinesio-tape group; KT-P, kinesio-tape placebo group; AP, auricular-acupressure group; AP-P, auricular-acupressure placebo group; AM, age of menarche; AFP, age of first menstrual pain; DC, duration of the cycles; DM, duration of menstruation.

Table 2. Changes (mean ± SD) of the primary outcome measures by groups along the four phases. SD: standard deviation.

	Mean Pain Intensity			
	P-T	T	FU-1	FU-2
CG	4.85 ± 1.13	4.62 ± 1.02 [a]	4.93 ± 0.95 [a]	4.93 ± 0.82
KT	5.18 ± 0.95	**3.40 ± 1.04** [b]	4.59 ± 1.18 [a]	5.24 ± 1.07
KT-P	4.62 ± 1.11	4.63 ± 1.00 [a]	4.52 ± 0.91 [a]	4.58 ± 0.95
AP	4.94 ± 0.88	**3.19 ± 1.18** [b]	**3.28 ± 1.18** [b]	4.74 ± 1.15
AP-P	4.63 ± 1.12	4.60 ± 0.85 [a]	4.45 ± 1.08 [a]	4.68 ± 0.88
F test	$p = 0.373$	$p < 0.001$	$p < 0.001$	$p = 0.204$
	Maximum pain intensity			
	P-T	T	FU-1	FU-2
CG	7.60 ± 0.70	7.65 ± 0.72 [a]	7.86 ± 1.03 [a]	7.72 ± 0.82
KT	7.62 ± 1.02	**6.09 ± 1.44** [b]	7.00 ± 1.11 [a]	7.81 ± 0.95
KT-P	7.78 ± 1.14	7.85 ± 1.02 [a]	7.57 ± 1.02 [a]	7.66 ± 1.01
AP	7.34 ± 0.96	**5.83 ± 1.39** [b]	**5.66 ± 1.68** [b]	7.38 ± 1.20
AP-P	7.61 ± 0.94	7.61 ± 0.84 [a]	7.59 ± 0.90 [a]	7.72 ± 0.82
F test	$p = 0.687$	$p < 0.001$	$p < 0.001$	$p = 0.644$
	Painful days			
	P-T	T	FU-1	FU-2
CG	3.11 ± 0.97	3.05 ± 0.93 [a]	3.09 ± 0.87 [a,b]	3.09 ± 0.81
KT	3.56 ± 0.88	2.63 ± 0.74 [a,b]	3.27 ± 0.77 [a]	3.45 ± 0.67
KT-P	3.03 ± 1.00	2.98 ± 0.93 [a,b]	3.14 ± 0.91 [a,b]	3.10 ± 1.04
AP	3.34 ± 0.78	2.37 ± 0.57 [b]	2.48 ± 0.68 [b]	3.19 ± 0.60
AP-P	3.00 ± 0.83	2.98 ± 0.60 [a,b]	3.00 ± 0.87 [a,b]	2.95 ± 0.72
F test	$p = 0.195$	$p = 0.021$	$p = 0.024$	$p = 0.298$
	Dose of drug intake			
	P-T	T	FU-1	FU-2
CG	1.78 ± 1.02	1.76 ± 1.04 [a]	1.68 ± 1.04 [a]	1.6 ± 0.90
KT	1.84 ± 1.26	**0.89 ± 1.12** [b]	1.59 ± 0.96 [a]	1.72 ± 1.03
KT-P	1.69 ± 1.18	1.61 ± 1.10 [a]	1.62 ± 1.07 [a,b]	1.52 ± 0.87
AP	1.94 ± 1.54	**0.60 ± 0.58** [b]	0.90 ± 1.51 [b]	1.62 ± 1.47
AP-P	1.95 ± 1.04	1.83 ± 0.91 [a]	1.73 ± 0.94 [a]	1.77 ± 0.87
H test	$p = 0.847$	$p < 0.001$	$p = 0.009$	$p = 0.864$

P-T, pretreatment phase; T, treatment phase; FU-1, follow-up 1 phase; FU-2, follow-up 2 phase; CG, control group; KT, kinesio-tape group; KT-P, kinesio-tape placebo group; AP, auricular-acupressure group; AP-P, auricular-acupressure placebo group. Post-hoc results are expressed by letters as follow: for each column, there are significant differences between groups whose letter is different.

A one-way multivariate ANOVA showed the overall changes and influence of the treatment for all the primary outcome measures ($p < 0.001$ in the four of them). When including drug intake as the secondary factor in the model, neither interaction ($p > 0.05$) nor drug intake ($p < 0.05$) was significant. Therefore, there was no evidence of bias due to drug intake. Table 2 also includes the evolution of the primary outcome measures during the study in the following way: between-group comparisons were performed by a one way ANOVA F test or by Kruskal–Wallis's H test, and their p-values are shown in the table. Post hoc results are expressed by letters, as usual. Pretreatment within-group comparisons were performed by t-paired or Wilcoxon test. A mean value is marked in bold if it implies a significant improvement in relation to both pretreatment (within-group) and the control group, the placebo auricular-acupressure group and the placebo kinesio-tape group (between-group).

From the analysis of Table 2, firstly, it can be observed that baseline values of the four primary outcome measures were similar for the five experimental groups (second column of Table 2), as expected. Secondly, the most remarkable is the fact that the auricular-acupressure group achieved the best results in mean, both during the treatment and follow-up one phases, for all the primary outcome measures (mean pain intensity, maximum pain intensity, number of painful days and dose of drug intake). In a deeper analysis and taking into account within-group comparisons, these results showed significant improvements in comparison with the pretreatment phase. Regarding the between-group comparison, we observed that, for the mean pain and maximum pain intensity, the auricular-acupressure group achieved significant improvements during both phases (treatment and follow-up one) in relation to the rest of the groups. In the kinesio-tape group, the results obtained from the treatment phase were similar to those from the auricular-acupressure group. During the first follow-up phase, the auricular-acupressure group performed significantly better.

In addition, we can also say that, regarding the dose of drug intake, the auricular-acupressure and kinesio-tape groups performed significantly better than the control group and both placebo groups. With regard to the number of painful days, the auricular-acupressure group achieved results significantly better than the control group at the treatment phase and significantly better than the kinesio-tape group at the first follow-up phase.

4. Discussion

This pilot study contributes to the scientific literature with the evidence of the effectiveness of two non-pharmacological treatment approaches, kinesio tape and auricular acupressure for the individualised and person-centred management of primary dysmenorrhoea. In addition, it shows, for the first time, a comparative assessment of both techniques.

Our results add new data from a sample of over 100 women to the few studies previously conducted that analyze the effectiveness of these techniques. In addition, the pre- and post-treatment comparisons' accuracy of our study was improved by the extended period of time used to observe the symptoms in the pretreatment phase. Another strength that of the present clinical trial is the presence of a control group and a placebo group for each treatment technique. Participants were blind at all times in relation to the group they were included in (treatment or placebo) and during the data collection.

Only four previous studies that applied kinesio tape for menstrual-pain relief were found in the literature [17–20]. In relation to the application of auricular acupressure in this condition, three studies were the result of the literature review [21–23]. In comparison to these studies, it can be observed that our study has a longer period of intervention.

Our results regarding the mean and the maximum pain-intensity levels in the kinesio-tape group and the auricular-acupressure group coincide with the improvements found by different authors that applied these techniques [17–23]. We were not able to contrast our results in relation to the number of painful days, days of the menstrual cycle and days of the menstruation, as there were no studies found in the literature that analyzed those variables. Although there were no statistically significant changes in the number of days of the menstrual cycle and menstruation after the treatments, we consider that the observation of these variables is important. This is because these variables are risk factors for dysmenorrhoea and can influence the results of the interventions [4].

The scientific evidence available on other non-pharmacological therapies show a great diversity of techniques used for the management of primary dysmenorrhoea, especially related to the field of Physiotherapy and Traditional Chinese Medicine. These include, for example, thermotherapy, massage therapy, electrotherapy, spinal manipulation, Kegel exercises, acupuncture and moxibustion in all its forms (acupressure, electro-acupuncture, laser acupuncture, etc.) [33,34]. However, as in the specific cases of kinesio taping and auricular acupressure, the number of studies published that analyze the effectiveness of these non-pharmacological techniques applied to primary dysmenorrhoea is low. All of these techniques show encouraging results, but, in general, there has been little research on their application to menstrual pain [2,15,33–39]. A remarkable advantage of kinesio taping and auricular acupressure over the other non-pharmacological techniques mentioned is that they are low-cost techniques, self-applicable after proper training and simple and quick to apply. In addition, the patient can keep the tape or the seeds on and continue with her daily routine, without having to travel to a clinic or invest too much time and money and, therefore, without affecting her rhythm of life.

Although we found no evidence of bias in the pilot study in relation to drug intake, we are not in a position to assess the opposite. Indeed, since most participants took medication during the study, the sample size was big enough for this ambitious statistical task. Nearly 10% of the participants stopped taking medication during all the treatment phase. The dose of drug intake was significantly reduced in the kinesio-tape group (kinesio tape–control = −0.9; kinesio tape–kinesio-tape placebo = −0.81), as well as in the auricular acupressure group (auricular acupressure–control = −1.19; auricular acupressure–auricular ac-pressure placebo = −1.36). The study conducted by Tomás-Rodríguez et al. in 2015 is the only study found that analyzed the drug intake. They assessed the between-group differences and found a difference of 1,09 drug units between the kinesio tape and the placebo groups. Asher et al., in 2010 [40], also found that there are studies on auricular acupressure that have shown a decrease on drug intake for pain relief in other conditions, such as surgery or chronic pain.

This decrease in drug consumption coincides with the improvement of pain levels and suggests that both treatment approaches could be beneficial for the management of primary dysmenorrhoea.

The comparisons between the kinesio-tape and the auricular-acupressure groups did not show statistically significant differences during the treatment phase. Nevertheless, when comparing these groups during the follow-up phases, the auricular-acupressure group maintained the improvements achieved during a longer period. These results could not be contrasted, as our study is the first one comparing these treatment techniques. When auricular acupressure has been used for the treatment of other conditions, such as menstrual headache, the results have revealed a reduction of plasma arginine vasopressin and prostaglandine F2α [41]. The most recent research suggests that the cause of primary dysmenorrhoea is the excess of endometrial prostaglandins E2 and F2α, which increase uterine contractions and painful sensation [1]. The longer duration of pain relief maintained by the auricular-acupressure group could be justified by the decrease of prostaglandins F2α and the secretion of pain-inhibiting agents that, according to Wu et al. (2007) [22] and Alimi et al. (2002) [28], this technique achieves.

The results of the present pilot study can have important implications in the clinical practice. Our data show that a kinesio taping and auricular acupressure decrease pain and drug intake in women with dysmenorrhoea. They are two techniques that are increasingly used by practitioners these days and can be performed safely with the appropriate training. This condition, and, in particular, the pain that is associated with it, has an important negative impact on the quality of life of women [2,5] which could be minimized with the use of the treatment approaches described in this study, as a complement to their pharmacological treatment.

Study Limitations

The main limitation of our study was the impossibility to blind the therapist that applied the techniques. Due to the nature of the treatment, they could clearly see which group the participant was allocated to.

Furthermore, we consider that it was important to analyze whether the drug intake and the type of medicine used for pain relief could influence these results. In order to assess this possible effect, a two-way multivariate ANOVA, considering as factors drug intake and type of drug, was carried out for each outcome measure. Although there were no significant results, neither for interaction nor for main effects, we cannot dismiss the possible influence. We do not have enough evidence to make a fair decision, since the number of participants that did not take any medicine was so small. In order to analyze the problem at that level, we consider that a bigger sample size would be needed.

5. Conclusions

Based on the results obtained in this pilot study, we can conclude that kinesio taping and auricular acupressure have a beneficial effect on pain relief in women with primary dysmenorrhoea. Although both groups showed similar improvements, the changes on the auricular-acupressure group seemed to last longer. The pain relief obtained by both treatment approaches suggests that these techniques could be used as complementary personalised therapies to the pharmacological treatment and not as a substitution. The participants of the kinesio taping and the auricular-acupressure group experienced a decrease in drug intake.

Supplementary Materials: The following are available online at https://www.mdpi.com/article/10.3390/jpm11080809/s1. Table S1: Descriptions of the interventions conducted following the Template for Intervention Description and Replication (TIDieR).

Author Contributions: Conceptualization, M.V.G.L.-A., E.M.-G. and J.M.-F.; methodology, E.M.-G., J.M.-F. and M.V.G.L.-A.; formal analysis, E.M.-G., M.V.G.L.-A. and J.M.-F.; investigation, E.M.-G. and M.V.G.L.-A.; writing—original draft preparation, M.V.G.L.-A., E.M.-G., E.M.G.-A. and J.R.-M.; writing—review and editing, E.M.-G., J.R.-M., M.V.G.L.-A., E.M.G.-A., J.M.-F. and J.R.-M. visualization, M.J.-P., E.M.-G., M.V.G.L.-A., E.M.G.-A., J.M.-F. and J.R.-M.; supervision E.M.-G., M.V.G.L.-A., E.M.G.-A., J.M.-F., M.J.-P. and J.R.-M. All authors have read and agreed to the published version of the manuscript.

Funding: This research received no external funding.

Institutional Review Board Statement: The study was conducted according to the guidelines of the Declaration of Helsinki, and approved by the Institutional Ethics Committee of the University of Extremadura (protocol code 58/2017 and date of approval: 7th of July 2017).

Informed Consent Statement: Informed consent was obtained from all subjects involved in the study.

Data Availability Statement: The data underlying this article cannot be shared publicly in order to maintain the privacy of individuals that participated in the study. The data will be shared upon reasonable request to the corresponding author.

Conflicts of Interest: The authors declare no conflict of interest.

References

1. Jaimeson, M.A. Disorders of menstruation in adolescent girls. *Pediatric Clin. N. Am.* **2015**, *62*, 943–961. [CrossRef]
2. Osayande, A.S.; Mehulic, S. Diagnosis and initial management of dysmenorrhea. *Am. Fam. Phys.* **2014**, *89*, 341–346.
3. Herrero-Gámiz, S.; Gómez, B.; Bajo, J.M. Síntomas de las ginecopatías. In *Fundamentos de Obstetricia (SEGO)*; Bajo, J.M., Melchor, J.C., Mercé, L.T., Eds.; 3M España: Madrid, Spain, 2007; pp. 111–118.
4. Latthe, P.; Latthe, M.; Say, L.; Gülmezoglu, M.; Khan, K.S. WHO systematic Review of prevalence of chronic pelvic pain: A neglected reproductive health morbidity. *BMC Public Health* **2006**, *6*, 177. [CrossRef]
5. Banikarim, C.; Chacko, M.R.; Kelder, S.H. Prevalence and impacto of dysmenorrhea on Hispanic female adolescents. *Arch. Pediatrics Adolesc. Med.* **2000**, *154*, 1226–1229. [CrossRef]
6. Peacock, A.; Alvi, N.S.; Mushtaq, T. Period problems: Disorders of menstruation in adolescents. *Arch. Dis. Child.* **2012**, *97*, 554–560. [CrossRef]
7. Ballina, J.; Carmona, L.; Laffon, A.; Grupo de estudio EPISER. Impacto del consumo de AINE en la población general española. Resultados del estudio EPISER. *Rev. Esp. Reumatol.* **2002**, *29*, 337–342.
8. López-Castellano, A.C.; Moreno-Royo, L.; Villagrasa-Sebastián, V. Uso racional del medicamento en el tratamiento del dolor. El farmacéutico en el tratamiento del dolor. In *Manual de Farmacología Guía para el uso Racional del Medicamento*; Elsevier: Madrid, Spain, 2005; pp. 258–262.
9. Aun, M.V.; Blanca, M.; Garro, L.S.; Ribeiro, M.R.; Kalil, J.; Motta, A.A.; Castells, M.; Giavina-Bianchi, P. Nonsteroidal anti-inflammatory drugs are mayor causes of drug-induced anaphylaxis. *J. Allergy Clin. Immunol. Pract.* **2014**, *2*, 414–420. [CrossRef]
10. Casado, M. El Rechazo al Tratamiento. Available online: http://www.ffomc.org/CursosCampus/Experto_Etica_Medica/U4_Rechazo%20al%20Tratamiento.pdf (accessed on 1 January 2021).
11. Margot, R.; Ortega, T. Anticonceptivos Hormonales: ¿Son Todos Iguales? Beneficios y Riesgos de su uso. Servicio de Obstetricia y Ginecología Hospital Universitario Virgen de las Nieves Granada. Available online: https://1library.co/document/q262wpez-servicio-obstetricia-ginecologia-hospital-universitario-granada-histerectomia-abdominal.html (accessed on 1 January 2021).

12. Vickers, A.J.; Vertosick, E.A.; Lewith, G.; MacPherson, H.; Foster, N.E.; Sherman, K.J.; Irnich, D.; Witt, C.M.; Linde, K.; Acupuncture Trialists' Collaboration. Acupuncture Trialists' Collaboration. Acupuncture for Chronic Pain: Update of an Individual Patient Data Meta-Analysis. *J. Pain* **2018**, *19*, 455–474. [CrossRef]
13. Jan, A.L.; Aldridge, E.S.; Rogers, I.R.; Visser, E.J.; Bulsara, M.K.; Niemtzow, R.C. Does Ear Acupuncture Have a Role for Pain Relief in the Emergency Setting? A Systematic Review and Meta-Analysis. *Med. Acupunct.* **2017**, *29*, 276–289. [CrossRef]
14. Yang, L.H.; Duan, P.B.; Hou, Q.M.; Du, S.Z.; Sun, J.F.; Mei, S.J.; Wang, X.Q. Efficacy of Auricular Acupressure for Chronic Low Back Pain: A Systematic Review and Meta-Analysis of Randomized Controlled Trials. *Evid. Based Complementary Altern. Med.* **2017**, *2017*, 6383649. [CrossRef]
15. Wu, P.L.; Lee, M.; Huang, T.T. Effectiveness of physical activity on patients with depression and Parkinson's disease: A systematic review. *PLoS ONE* **2017**, *12*, e0181515. [CrossRef]
16. Murakami, M.; Fox, L.; Dijkers, M.P. Ear Acupuncture for Immediate Pain Relief-A Systematic Review and Meta-Analysis of Randomized Controlled Trials. *Pain Med.* **2017**, *18*, 551–564. [CrossRef] [PubMed]
17. Lim, C.; Park, Y.; Bae, Y. The effect of the kinesio taping and spiral taping on menstrual pain and premenstrual syndrome. *J. Phys. Ther. Sci.* **2013**, *25*, 761–764. [CrossRef]
18. Tomás, M.I.; Palazón, A.; Martínez, D.R.; Toledo, J.V.; Asensio Mdel, R.; Gil, V.F. Effectiveness of medical taping concept in primary dysmenorrhoea: A two-armed randomized trial. *Sci. Rep.* **2015**, *5*, 16671. [CrossRef]
19. Wefers, C.; Pijnappel, H.F.J.; Stolwijk, N.M. Effect of CureTape on menstrual pain in women with primary dysmenorrhoea. [He effect van CureTape op pijn tijdens de menstruatie bij patiënten met primaire dysmenorrhoe]. *Ned. Tijdschr. Fysiother.* **2009**, *119*, 193–197.
20. Yum, K.S.; Kang, S.G.; Han, H.J. The effect of balance taping for prevention of menstrual pain in female middle school students. *J. Phys. Ther. Sci.* **2017**, *29*, 813–818. [CrossRef]
21. Yeh, M.L.; Hung, Y.L.; Chen, H.H.; Wang, Y.J. Auricular acupressure for pain relief in adolescents with dysmenorrhea: A placebo-controlled study. *J. Altern. Complement. Med.* **2013**, *19*, 313–318. [CrossRef]
22. Wu, R.D.; Zhang, H.D.; Lin, L.F. Observation on ear point taping and pressing therapy for treatment of primary dysmenorrhea. *Zhongguo Zhen Jiu* **2007**, *27*, 815–817. (In Chinese)
23. Cha, N.H.; Sok, S.R. Effects of Auricular Acupressure Therapy on Primary Dysmenorrhea for Female High School Students in South Korea. *J. Nurs. Scholarsh.* **2016**, *48*, 508–516. [CrossRef]
24. Rodriguez-Palencia, J. *Manual de Vendaje Neuromuscular: Aplicaciones Musculares*; Bubok: Madrid, Spain, 2013.
25. Kahanov, L. Kinesio taping, Part 1: An overview of its use in athletes. *Athl. Ther. Today* **2007**, *12*, 17–18. [CrossRef]
26. Kneeshaw, D. Shoulder taping in the clinical setting. *J. Bodyw. Mov. Ther.* **2002**, *6*, 2–8. [CrossRef]
27. Oleson, T. *Auriculoterapia. Sistemas Chino y Occidental de Acupuntura Auricular*, 3th ed.; Panamericana: Buenos Aires, Argentina, 2017.
28. Alimi, D.; Geissmann, A.; Gardeur, D. Auricular acupuncture stimulation measured on functional magnetic resonance imaging. *Med. Acupunct.* **2002**, *13*, 18–21.
29. Cho, Z.H.; Oleson, T.D.; Alimi, D.; Niemtzow, R.C. Acupuncture: The search for biologic evidence with functional magnetic resonance imaging and positron emission tomography techniques. *J. Altern. Complement. Med.* **2002**, *8*, 399–401. [CrossRef]
30. Andersch, B.; Milsom, I. An epidemiologic study of young women with dysmenorrhea. *Am. J. Obstet. Gynecol.* **1982**, *144*, 655–660. [CrossRef]
31. Huskisson, E.C. Measurement of pain. *Lancet* **1974**, *2*, 1127–1131. [CrossRef]
32. Hoffmann, T.C.; Glasziou, P.P.; Boutron, I.; Milne, R.; Perera, R.; Moher, D.; Altman, D.G.; Barbour, V.; Macdonald, H.; Johnston, M.; et al. Better reporting of interventions: Template for Intervention Description and Replication (TIDieR) checklist and guide. *BMJ* **2014**, *348*, g1687. [CrossRef]
33. Kannan, P.; Claydon, L.S. Some physiotherapy treatments may relieve menstrual pain in women with primary dysmenorrhea: A systematic review. *J. Physiother.* **2014**, *60*, 13–21. [CrossRef]
34. Xu, T.; Hui, L.; Juan, Y.L.; Min, S.G.; Hua, W.T. Effects of moxibustion or acupoint therapy for the treatment of primary dysmenorrhea: A meta-analysis. *Altern. Ther. Health Med.* **2014**, *20*, 33–42. [PubMed]
35. Akin, M.D.; Weingand, K.W.; Hengehold, D.A.; Goodale, M.B.; Hinkle, R.T.; Smith, R.P. Continuous low-level topical heat in the treatment of dysmenorrhea. *Obstet. Gynecol.* **2001**, *97*, 343–349. [CrossRef]
36. García Hurtado, B.; Chillón Martínez, R.; Rebollo Roldán, J.; Orta Pérez, M.A. Dismenorrea primaria y fisioterapia. *Fisioterapia* **2005**, *27*, 327–342. [CrossRef]
37. Ortiz, M.I.; Cortés-Márquez, S.K.; Romero-Quezada, L.C.; Murguía-Cánovas, G.; Jaramillo-Díaz, A.P. Effect of a physiotherapy program in women with primary dysmenorrhea. *Eur. J. Obstet. Gynecol. Reprod. Biol.* **2015**, *194*, 24–29. [CrossRef]
38. Abaraogu, U.O.; Igwe, S.E.; Tabansi-Ochiogu, C.S.; Duru, D.O. A Systematic Review and Meta-Analysis of the Efficacy of Manipulative Therapy in Women with Primary Dysmenorrhea. *Explore* **2017**, *13*, 386–392. [CrossRef]
39. Xu, Y.; Zhao, W.; Li, T.; Bu, H.; Zhao, Z.; Zhao, Y.; Song, S. Effects of acupoint-stimulation for the treatment of primary dysmenorrhoea compared with NSAIDs: A systematic review and meta-analysis of 19 RCTs. *BMC Complement. Altern. Med.* **2017**, *17*, 436. [CrossRef] [PubMed]

40. Asher, G.N.; Jonas, D.E.; Coeytaux, R.R.; Reilly, A.C.; Loh, Y.L.; Motsinger-Reif, A.A.; Winham, S.J. Auriculotherapy for Pain Management: A Systematic Review and Meta-Analysis of Randomized Controlled Trials. *J. Altern. Complement. Med.* **2010**, *16*, 1097–1108. [CrossRef]
41. Sun, L.; Liang, Y.; Li, X.; Liu, L.; Xu, X.; Ma, H.; Li, W.; Fei, S.; Gao, F. Efficacy of acupuncture combined with auricular point sticking on the content of serum prostaglandin F2α, and plasma arginine vasopressin in patients with menstrual headache. *Zhongguo Zhen Jiu* **2015**, *35*, 137–140.

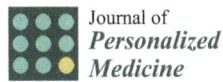

Article

Uncovering the Imprints of Chronic Disease on Patients' Lives and Self-Perceptions

Cheryl Lin [1], Rungting Tu [2], Brooke Bier [1] and Pikuei Tu [1,*]

[1] Policy and Organizational Management Program, Duke University, Durham, NC 27705, USA; c.lin@duke.edu (C.L.); brooke.bier@duke.edu (B.B.)
[2] College of Management, Shenzhen University, Shenzhen 518060, China; rungting@szu.edu.cn
* Correspondence: pikuei.tu@duke.edu

Abstract: Rheumatoid arthritis (RA) patients face psychological hardship due to physical discomfort, disabilities, and anxieties. Previous research indicated a bidirectional relationship and patient desire for emotional support from providers. This study examined lesser-understood RA experiences across the psychological and social contexts in relation to self-perception through the patients' expression of their struggles with these burdens. We conducted four semistructured focus groups and eleven interviews (total n = 31). A codebook was developed and refined through iterative transcript coding via NVivo-12. Four emerging themes were identified by inductive, thematic analysis: (1) the patients' healthy appearances were a myth, with subthemes revealing a conflict between an inclination to hide the disease and a desire for validation, while feeling embarrassed by symptom manifestations and disappointment at withdrawal from social interactions; (2) an identity crisis due to diminished functionality, autonomy, and sense of self; (3) RA constantly occupied the mind, as its unpredictability dictated daily schedules and altered plans; and (4) the disease's chronic nature influenced personal outlook to worry about or accept the uncertainty. Even with effective treatment, the invisibility of the disease, the fear and anticipation of flare-ups, and identity clashes caused emotional distress. The insights offer a different perspective on personalized medicine, complementing clinical treatments based on genetic or biomarker profile. For patient-centered holistic care, education is needed to prompt both patients and providers to discuss psychological issues for more customized, integrated interventions. The findings can help inform healthcare teams and families in recognizing and supporting these physical-psychological intertwined experiences, thereby ameliorating patients' wellbeing.

Keywords: patient-centered; personalized care; arthritis; autoimmune disease; sociopsychological factors; emotion; depression; self-identity; qualitative study; observational study

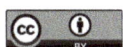

1. Introduction

Rheumatoid arthritis (RA) is a chronic, systematic inflammatory condition characterized by persistent and progressive joint and autoimmune dysfunction. It is estimated that up to 2% of the global population and about 1.5 million Americans suffer from RA; most are women with an age of onset between 40 and 60 years old [1,2]. The etiology of RA is relatively unknown. However, the resulting prolonged inflammation typically causes joint deformation, stiffness, excessive fatigue, as well as widespread and intense pain [3]. In addition, most patients face psychological hardship due to RA-imposed functional limitations and anxieties [4–6].

Numerous studies have described a bidirectional relationship between RA disease activities and poor mental functioning. The progression of RA often leads to feelings of helplessness, grief, and uncertainty [6–8]. This psychological distress further contributes to the intensification of pain and thus creates a vicious cycle of physical and emotional suffering [9–11]. RA patients have consistently reported a loss of enjoyable activities, a struggle to find and adhere to effective treatment, and difficulties in actively dealing with disease manifestations, implicating a 14–62% prevalence rate of depression in the RA community [6,12–15]. Moreover, illness-related shame and loneliness perpetuate social withdrawal, and the resulting lack of social support could lead to aggravated disease outcomes [16–18]. Recent studies have also discussed the impacts of the disease on self-esteem and outlook; patients express the loss of autonomy and low self-efficacy in maintaining a sense of independence due to physical disabilities [4,14,19].

These findings underscore the importance of a deeper understanding of the psychological nuances of RA's personal impacts. Previous research has explored such experiences to help plan treatments, but often focused on improving quality of life and coping strategies [14,15,20]. Other studies have deliberated how patient-centered care can complement clinical disease management for a more holistic approach [21,22]. Patient-centeredness encompasses a bio-psychosocial perspective to provide attentive, individualized care with emotional support and augmented communication for the patients' overall wellbeing [23,24]. While emerging personalized medicine emphasizes the individuals' distinctive genetic or biomarker profile to inform prevention and customize treatment [25,26], the patients' mental and contextual states are also critical in determining their response to medications and health outcomes.

Few existing studies have comprehensively explored the intricacies of these experiences faced by RA sufferers on a daily or long-term basis, or investigated personalized intervention techniques addressing such emotional and social struggles. It is imperative to hear and respect patients' voices and incorporate multidimensional therapies targeting biological and psychological pains concordantly [27–29]. Research in rheumatology and other medical disciplines have predominately evaluated the patients' conditions quantitatively [30,31]. This study utilized qualitative methods to uncover and synthesize lesser-understood psychological burdens, whether from or in combination with physical encumbrances. We captured the patients' narratives in their own words and examined the complex existence of RA in relation to the patients' self-perceptions and outlook in personal and social contexts. By identifying and analyzing novel domains of the impact of RA on lives and individual identities, these experiences and sentiments can be better recognized and legitimized. The findings also provide insights for more effective, personalized psychological interventions and support.

2. Methods

We conducted four focus groups ($n = 20$) and eleven individual interviews to elicit participants' descriptions of RA's presence in and influence on their lives (total $n = 31$ in 15 sessions). Eligibility criteria for participating in the study were age 18 years or older, clinically diagnosed with RA, and have received treatment for RA in the previous year. Focus-group participants were recruited and screened by a market research agency to ensure a diverse sample; two experienced moderators facilitated the four groups. Individual interviewees were recruited through flyers posted at local clinics, then screened and interviewed by the research team.

A semistructured discussion guide was constructed, incorporating inputs from the literature [6,30,32–35] and experts, and was used across all sessions. The discussions explored participants' history of diagnosis, hobbies, what a good day or bad day was like, awareness of and sentiments towards RA's impact or associated changes, sources and specifics of their emotional state, struggles with and strategies for managing the disease, and interactions with physicians and families. Participants were also asked to self-rate the extent to which their lives were impacted by RA on a scale of one to seven, one being "no impact" and seven being "extreme impact".

Group and individual interviews were recorded, transcribed, and de-identified. We uploaded text data into NVivo software version 12 for coding and analysis, utilizing an inductive, thematic approach [36]. A codebook was developed and refined through iterative coding by multiple researchers. Common experiences and sentiments emerging from the data were grouped together for potential theme categorization. Disagreements regarding coding and identification or naming of themes were discussed and resolved through consensus. Selective quotes were extracted to represent the essence of each theme in the participants' own words. The research protocol was approved by Duke University Institutional Review Board. Informed consents were obtained from individual participants before each session.

3. Results

3.1. Participant Characteristics

A total of 31 people were interviewed in groups or individually. Participants were heterogenous in terms of demographics (mean age 47.39, SD = 14.38; 77.42% female; 38.7% minorities; Table 1) and disease-related characteristics (mean disease duration: 11.76 years, SD = 8.71; mean RA impact: 4.29 on a scale of 1 to 7, SD = 1.19). The occurrences and intricacies of RA's impact were obtained via qualitative inquiries, described narratively and illustrated in a diagram below.

Table 1. Participant self-reported demographic and disease-related information.

Participant #	Gender	Race/Ethnicity	Employment Status	Household Income (USD)	Age (Years)	RA Impact *	Duration of Disease
1	Male	White	Disabled	<25 K	64	6	42 years
2	Female	Black	Unemployed	25–50 K	45	6	18 years
3	Male	White	Retired	25–50 K	67	4	4 years
4	Female	White	Retired	150–200 K	70	4	15 years
5	Female	Hispanic	Full Time	25–50 K	40	2	5 years
6	Female	Black	Full Time	50–75 K	50	3	4 years
7	Female	White	Full Time	25–50 K	47	3	19 years
8	Female	White	Part Time	100–150 K	60	4	20 years
9	Female	Hispanic	Full Time	50–75 K	38	4	10 years
10	Male	Black	Full Time	75–100 K	34	3	8 years
11	Female	Hispanic	Full Time	50–75 K	40	5	7 years
12	Male	White	Full Time	150–200 K	49	6	15 years
13	Female	White	Disabled	25–50 K	48	5	5 years
14	Male	White	Retired	100–150 K	52	5	5 years
15	Female	White	Retired	25–50 K	72	5	9 years
16	Female	White	Part Time	>200 K	41	4	10 years
17	Female	White	Part Time	75–100 K	46	6	16 years
18	Male	Black	Full Time	100–150 k	53	6	5 years
19	Female	White	Disabled	100–150 K	40	4	13 years
20	Female	White	Full Time	150–200 K	61	4	10 years
21	Female	Asian	Unemployed	100–150 K	65	3	35 years
22	Female	Asian	Full Time	25–50 K	58	4	10 years
23	Male	White	Student	150–200 K	22	4	10 years
24	Female	Hispanic	Student	25–50 K	23	4	7 years
25	Female	White	Full Time	50–75 K	28	6	13 years
26	Female	White	Full Time	50–75 K	37	4	2.5 years
27	Female	White	Unemployed	>200 K	62	2	10 years
28	Female	Asian	Unemployed	50–75 K	48	6	11 years
29	Female	Asian	Unemployed	<25 K	33	3	17 years
30	Female	White	Student	>200 K	18	4	7 years
31	Female	White	Unemployed	150–200 K	58	4	2 years

Participant number. * Participants were asked to rate how RA has impacted their life on a scale of 1–7, from "no impact" to "extreme impact".

3.2. Healthy Appearance as a Myth

3.2.1. Invisibility and Lack of Validation

A common struggle highlighted by participants was others' inability to comprehend that the participants were sick. Many endured physical impediments regularly but showed no discernible signs of disease. People often did not believe that the participants were experiencing pain or take the condition seriously, making it difficult for participants to feel supported and validated.

> *"It's one of those things you can't see it: I look fine, I look completely fine . . . . It's kind of like the silent suffering . . . because you don't look any different, you don't act any different, and I kind of learned to just deal with it."* (Participant #25)

> *"I've wondered a lot like is this all just in my head . . . and how much of this is real?"* (#24)

Relationships were strained by their friends' and family's incapacity to see the symptoms and consequently, to believe the participants or show sympathy. Friendships dissolved as people took offense when the participants had to cancel plans due to flare-ups or fatigue. This further loss of socialization brought participants to feel a sense of deprivation and resentment toward the disease.

> *"A lot of friends think you just don't want to hang out with them. I can plan and whatever I want to plan but, on the day, when it's time to do it, if I can't do it, I can't do it."* (#2)

> *"You have to cancel a lot on people, and that's really depressing."* (#8)

3.2.2. Preference to Hide RA from Others

Although several participants were frustrated by RA's invisibility, others reported purposefully hiding their symptoms or not mentioning they had the disease; some felt both sentiments simultaneously. Participants intended to minimize being perceived as ailing to achieve a desired sense of normalcy. They also attempted to disguise or counter (sometimes unsuccessfully) the anguish they experienced inside.

> *"(Acquaintances' response) is what I hate, they're like, 'Oh my God, I can't believe that you're so sick' . . . 'You look so healthy! How?' . . . I feel like sometimes they think differently of me so I don't like sharing it with people."* (#24)

> *"Every semester, I've had a moment where an advisor is like, 'hey, do you maybe not wanna do this semester?' And I'm like, 'No, I wanna do it!' . . . maybe more of a fear than a hope is being able to hold a full-time job and just live a normal life in that respect."* (#30)

> *"Some days my husband comes home and I'm with full makeup and full jewelry everything—I'm looking great—and he's like 'what's going on here? You feel really bad today, don't you?' and I'm like 'yep.'"* (#2)

3.2.3. Embarrassment from Physical Symptoms

Adding to their predicament of preferring to hide the disease yet desiring to be understood, participants also described discomfiture with apparent physical symptoms. More prominent disease manifestations were indicative of sickness. Such visible signs could cause embarrassment and disappointment.

> *"Your knees will look swollen, or your hands. And it was kind of embarrassing to go into dating because you tried to hide your twisted fingers."* (#9)

> *"I want to go walking but I can't. It's like excruciating pain. It's embarrassing sometimes, because I want to do things but can't move."* (#6)

3.3. Identity Crisis

Participants, moreover, indicated their dismayed realization that they were no longer the same person after diagnosis. Unable to perform daily tasks or forced to relinquish what they formerly enjoyed, many struggled to maintain their self-identity and described having difficulty recognizing themselves. The common misconception that RA only occurs at old age added to the confusion for both participants and others.

> *"I couldn't hold the book, I couldn't do anything. I just felt so helpless, useless and that's not my mode. I'm a very independent person, I don't like to ask anyone for help, and so having to do that was really problematic. It was even problematic—and I'm just going to be blunt—to go to the bathroom."* (#27)

"It was hard to think of myself as chronically ill." (#26)

"I am way too young to be ending up with RA because I thought of it as an older person's disorder." (#18)

The perpetual exertion of managing or suppressing symptoms took a toll both mentally and physiologically. Many participants experienced self-doubt, frequent mood-swings, and long-term changes to their personalities or worldview.

"I feel like I'm not as happy-go-lucky as I would like to be because it nags at you, distracts your mind." (#31)

"I was losing my mind. This is not like me." (#7)

"I was a very social person. I don't go out anymore...except for going to the doctors. I stopped any social engagement ... it affects EVERY part of life. I was living in a black-and-white world (with no color)." (#21)

RA also impacted fulfillment of responsibilities, which participants found upsetting and frustrating. They felt that their functionality as a parent, spouse, or employee was inadequate, and their performance of their roles within the household, office, or society seemed unsatisfactory. Some were confounded by the reversed role from caregiver to care-receiver.

"The days I can't are the days my kids want to do everything, like 'mom I want to do this, ride bikes,' and I'm like 'talk to your dad.' ... that for me, is hurtful." (#5)

"I couldn't have kids. And that's really sad when you come from a Latino family, and the family is the nucleus of everything." (#9)

"I left a really good job. I just couldn't handle the pressure and the stress with the RA symptoms." (#20)

3.4. Occupying the Mindset

RA became the determinant of all activities and plans. Many participants reported constantly thinking about RA, and that the fluctuating severity of symptoms dictated continuously how their day went. Even on a "good day" with minimal symptoms, the continuous dread or anticipation of pain or incapacity remained a burden.

"I think about it every morning when I put my feet on the floor. Like when I get up, I know what kind of day it's going to be based on how I get up out of bed." (#12)

"I get nervous, I know I will have pain even before I can feel it." (#22)

Participants also discussed the malevolent effects of RA on maintaining a sense of consistency in their lives and on their schedule. They regularly had to arrange for an alternative, bothersome plan. Many also shared nuisances due to the unpredictability of each day, whether simply getting out of bed, running errands, going to work, or taking a trip.

"I would get up and leave for work earlier so that I could go and sleep in my car for an extra hour before going into the office. Even the driving, I would get fatigued ... some days are just absolutely horrible." (#15)

"I might have a day when I'm feeling pretty good ... but then there's a day when I don't ... so then I get very frustrated because there are things I want to do or plan to do." (#17)

"It's really difficult to make plans living like that. I just committed myself to a 3-day trip with several friends and I'm wondering am I going to be able to go? And if I go, am I going to end up in the hotel the whole time?" (#13)

3.5. Chronic Nature of the Disease

The chronic nature of RA led to fear and despair, especially in the early stages of diagnosis. Participants expressed annoyance with the unknown of the disease and worried about their future, even with effective treatment or minor symptoms.

"It started in my forties, and so does that mean that when I'm in my sixties, is it going to be really bad? And how long can it be maintained at a reasonable level? What happens when something isn't working and it hurts? And how bad can it be?" (#14)

"The whole frustrating part is I have no idea what to expect moving forward." (#26)

As participants reluctantly adapted to an altered life, many found ways to improve their conditions by modifying their exercise routines, diets, or perspectives through positive thinking. Some had reached a neutral sense of acceptance or became at peace with RA. Through their experience battling the disease, participants described a sense of personal growth, gaining control and confidence in being able to persevere.

"I know I would have to take the medication for life, there is no cure. What can I do? It happens to me and I will just face it." (#29)

"I'm the kind of person that says other people have it worse. So I find someone who has it worse than me and I say I can do it, I can survive." (#27)

We further synthesized the themes and findings in Figure 1.

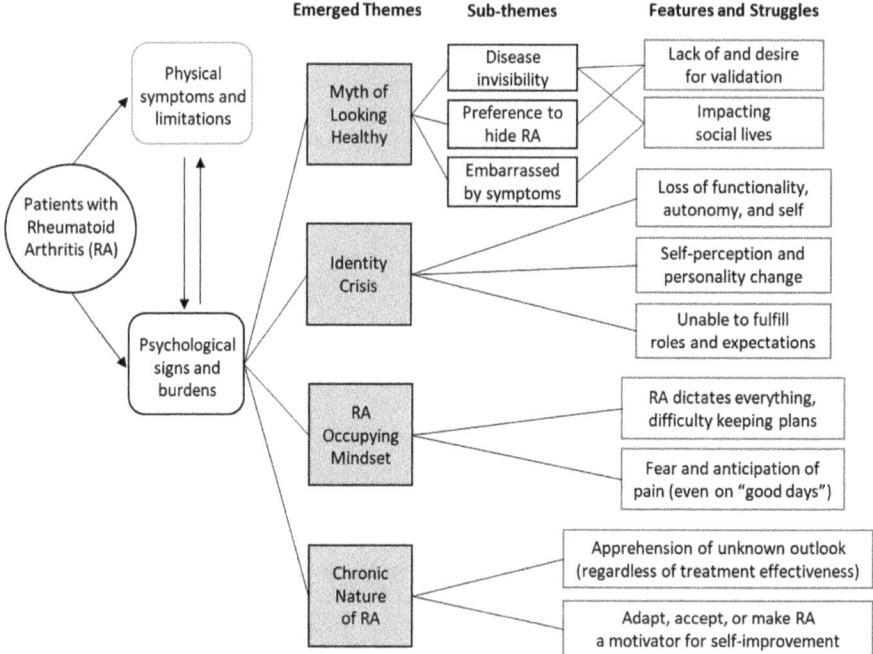

Figure 1. Identified themes and struggles from RA patient interviews.

4. Discussion

We identified four interconnected themes illustrating the imprints of RA on participants' lives and identities through in-depth focus groups and interviews. Their narrated experiences conveyed vivid accounts of the common mental and physical dilemmas patients regularly face. Participants expressed an overarching sense of frustration, apprehension, and lack of control in both managing RA symptoms and dealing with related social and psychological consequences. However, many were able to eventually come to terms with the illness and adapt, albeit reluctantly, to their new normal.

Earlier studies examined patients' preference for hiding symptoms and a desire for validation separately [4,37]. We uncovered the RA patients' concurrent intentions to conceal the disease and its manifestations while still seeking recognition to escape the disease's isolating effects. The suppression of knowledge about their illness might have made the disease feel even more confining and their experience invalidated. Other diseases have also been described as invisible, including fibromyalgia [38], chronic fatigue [39], and inflammatory bowel disease [40]. Our participants' qualitative reflections shed light on the seemingly contradictory inclinations encountered by RA and other patient populations.

These clashing sentiments are analogous to previous findings of RA's social impact, wherein patients described "illness-related shame" in being perceived as sickly and incapable [18]. Although the literature did not indicate whether this stigmatization was actualized or self-promulgated, our findings suggest a combination of both. Some participants were teased or treated differently by friends and family, but others tended to place guilt on themselves for not living up to expected roles. This self-disappointment was especially hurtful in a family context; such experiences were similar to that of mothers pervaded with guilt due to limited involvement in or forced exclusion from enjoyable family moments [41,42].

Moreover, our participants echoed an identity crisis pertaining to losing independence or self-esteem and feeling useless, which may contribute to personality change or depression. Participants were perceived differently by others, and came to (not) recognize themselves internally. These observations build upon existing understandings of RA-related identity conflict, where patients describe poor body-self unity in a physical sense [34,43]. Some felt uncomfortable in their own skin due to pain and bodily changes [5]. Others saw themselves as increasingly disabled and ineffective, propagating low self-confidence [7,8]. These findings highlight the far-reaching effect of RA on self-perception and altering identity. Both providers and support systems need to address these emotional hardships of RA patients, as psychological distress could lead to worsened disease and related mental health outcomes [16,44]. This is where patient-centered, integrative care involving a multidisciplinary consultation could be most beneficial [21,23].

Adding to the literature of disease-associated anxiety [6,16], our results underlined how RA remained prominent in the participants' minds. The ever-presence of the disease amended all plans and routines, and thereby minimized any sense of consistency. The participants further disclosed sentiments ranging from anxiety and concern about their future to neutrality and acceptance of the disease being part of their lives with the unending need for maintenance. However, even with effective treatment or absence of pain, the chronic nature of RA was nevertheless frustrating and worrisome for both new and seasoned patients. Many participants not only feared and actively avoided potentially distressing circumstances, but lived in a perpetual state of anticipation of symptom manifestation and a terror of possible disability. Personalized medicine needs to account for these non-somatic factors that could influence how patients take or react to medication, disease progression, and health outcomes.

Previous research has connected behavior modifications to the disease's conditions with positive results, such as decreased intensity of depression, reduced feelings of guilt and hopelessness, and improved physical functions [8,14,42]. Although no action may entirely remove the afflictions patients face, we also found encouraging evidence of patients turning illness impediments into motivation for self-improvement in other areas of their lives. Future exploration of this transformative change of mindset could offer valuable lessons for personalized therapies.

Analysis of patient perspectives from their own narratives is critical for supporting this population and understanding their reality. Yet the clinical practices necessary to recognize and validate these psychological symptoms and forced alterations remain sparse [20,45,46]. Instead, treatment strategies have primarily focused on the pharmacologic and physical aspects. Healthcare professionals tend not to probe for cognitive and emotional problems beyond the more frequent diagnoses of anxiety and depression [12,14]. Patients have indicated a desire for discussing social and emotional issues with their care team but less than a quarter of them receive such support [47]. Studies concur that this exclusion of psychological signs or inquiries is not a reflection of poor healthcare quality, but rather demonstrates the need for a greater understanding of the far-reaching impact of patients' struggles and multifaceted approaches to communication and treatment techniques [4,12,48]. The results of our qualitative investigation provided deeper insights into the complexity of psychological burdens in the RA population and informed education for both patients and providers for more holistic care. Future research into personalized medicine could explore the feasibility and effect of incorporating mental support in designing and evaluating treatment programs.

Numerous techniques have been proposed to better meet the psychological needs of RA patients, including encouraging patient involvement in medical decisions [15] and creating long-term goals [28], asking open-ended questions about the psychological impacts to allow for emotional venting [12,49], cognitive behavioral therapy [50], and the use of support groups [15,51]. These recommendations can help patients better address disease uncertainty and feelings of invalidation and uselessness. However, the effectiveness of these strategies on lesser-understood struggles has not been directly studied [47,48]. In addition, research is needed to determine if and how such therapies are actively sought by patients, or if physicians and nurses must encourage psychological counseling options as a complement to medications. Educational programs should also target the public so that families and communities can adequately offer support.

The current study has several limitations. First, the sample size was small. Different from quantitative studies, it is customary for qualitative studies to have a few dozen participants. A large majority of the participants were women, despite attention being paid to specifically recruit males as well, reflective of the doubly high incidence of RA in females (male−female ratio of RA prevalence is about 1:3) [2]. Future studies could incorporate more male perspectives, as existing findings are inconsistent as to whether men experience fewer, or perhaps differently expressed, psychological symptoms [28,34,48]. The heterogeneity of our participants in their demographic and disease-related characteristics ensured that the diverse perspectives of RA patients were represented. The subjective nature of qualitative coding could have introduced biases in the selection of themes and quotes. Other key ideas may have been overlooked due to confirmation or experimenter bias. Efforts were taken to reduce biases through consultation of the literature in developing the codebook and the utilization of multiple coders. Lastly, the volunteer-based sampling, though practical and common for similar observational studies, may have excluded patients who had different opinions or experiences but were unwilling or unable to participate.

5. Conclusions

There is a lack of qualitative research in rheumatic diseases and healthcare in general [30,52], signaling a gap in the literature. Future research should incorporate more in-depth examinations into patients' needs as well as investigate illness-induced cognitive and emotional processes that influence health outcomes. Our study provides a novel, comprehensive perspective of RA patients' experiences beyond somatic functionality and across a variety of contexts. Highlighting and connecting the sociopsychological burdens resulting from physical limitations adds to the knowledge of the impact of a chronic disease. These insights demonstrate the persistent need and the patients' desire for more personalized care that includes psychological support. This need has also been recognized in treatment guidelines but the demand has not been met, leaving care provision incomplete for many patients. In addition to providing pharmaceutical therapies, healthcare professionals must acknowledge and address these struggles when discussing and planning treatment strategies to both validate and ameliorate patients' experiences.

Author Contributions: Conceptualization C.L., R.T. and P.T.; data acquisition C.L. and P.T.; data analysis and interpretation C.L., R.T., B.B. and P.T.; manuscript drafting C.L. and B.B.; critical revisions C.L., R.T., B.B. and P.T. All authors have read and agreed to the published version of the manuscript.

Funding: This research was partially supported by Duke University Bass Connections.

Institutional Review Board Statement: The study was conducted according to the guidelines of the Declaration of Helsinki and approved by Duke University Institutional Review Board.

Informed Consent Statement: Informed consent was obtained from all participants involved in the study.

Data Availability Statement: The portion of the de-identified transcript directly pertaining to this paper is available from the corresponding author for one year from the date of publication upon reasonable request with a methodically sound proposal.

Acknowledgments: The authors would like to thank their research team's assistance in the data collection process and The Link Group's support in facilitating the focus groups and interviews. The authors are grateful for the study participants candidly sharing their experiences.

Conflicts of Interest: The authors declare no conflict of interest.

References

1. Almutairi, K.; Nossent, J.; Preen, D.; Keen, H.; Inderjeeth, C. The Global Prevalence of Rheumatoid Arthritis: A Meta-Analysis Based on a Systematic Review. *Rheumatol. Int.* **2021**, *41*, 863–877. [CrossRef]
2. Myasoedova, E.; Crowson, C.S.; Kremers, H.M.; Therneau, T.M.; Gabriel, S.E. Is the Incidence of Rheumatoid Arthritis Rising?: Results from Olmsted County, Minnesota, 1955–2007. *Arthritis Rheum.* **2010**, *62*, 1576–1582. [CrossRef]
3. Rheumatoid Arthritis-Symptoms and Causes. Available online: https://www.mayoclinic.org/diseases-conditions/rheumatoid-arthritis/symptoms-causes/syc-20353648 (accessed on 14 April 2021).
4. Bala, S.-V.; Samuelson, K.; Hagell, P.; Fridlund, B.; Forslind, K.; Svensson, B.; Thomé, B. Living with Persistent Rheumatoid Arthritis: A BARFOT Study. *J. Clin. Nurs.* **2017**, *26*, 2646–2656. [CrossRef]
5. Ryan, S. Psychological Effects of Living with Rheumatoid Arthritis. *Nurs. Stand.* **2014**, *29*, 52–59. [CrossRef]
6. Ziarko, M.; Siemiątkowska, K.; Sieński, M.; Samborski, W.; Samborska, J.; Mojs, E. Mental Health and Rheumatoid Arthritis: Toward Understanding the Emotional Status of People with Chronic Disease. *Bio. Med. Res. Int.* **2019**, *2019*, 1–8. [CrossRef] [PubMed]
7. Bacconnier, L.; Rincheval, N.; Flipo, R.-M.; Goupille, P.; Daures, J.-P.; Boulenger, J.-P.; Combe, B. Psychological Distress over Time in Early Rheumatoid Arthritis: Results from a Longitudinal Study in an Early Arthritis Cohort. *Rheumatology* **2015**, *54*, 520–527. [CrossRef] [PubMed]
8. Nagyova, I.; Stewart, R.E.; Macejova, Z.; van Dijk, J.P.; van den Heuvel, W.J.A. The Impact of Pain on Psychological Well-Being in Rheumatoid Arthritis: The Mediating Effects of Self-Esteem and Adjustment to Disease. *Patient Educ. Couns.* **2005**, *58*, 55–62. [CrossRef] [PubMed]
9. van Middendorp, H. Emotion Regulation Predicts Change of Perceived Health in Patients with Rheumatoid Arthritis. *Ann. Rheum. Dis.* **2005**, *64*, 1071–1074. [CrossRef]
10. Walker, J.G.; Jackson, H.J.; Littlejohn, G.O. Models of Adjustment to Chronic Illness: Using the Example of Rheumatoid Arthritis. *Clin. Psychol. Rev.* **2004**, *24*, 461–488. [CrossRef]
11. Ziarko, M.; Mojs, E.; Piasecki, B.; Samborski, W. The Mediating Role of Dysfunctional Coping in the Relationship between Beliefs about the Disease and the Level of Depression in Patients with Rheumatoid Arthritis. *Sci. World J.* **2014**, *2014*, 1–6. [CrossRef]
12. Leon, L.; Redondo, M.; Fernández-Nebro, A.; Gómez, S.; Loza, E.; Montoro, M.; Garcia-Vicuña, R.; Galindo, M. Expert Recommendations on the Psychological Needs of Patients with Rheumatoid Arthritis. *Rheumatol. Int.* **2018**, *38*, 2167–2182. [CrossRef]
13. Mahat, G. Perceived Stressors and Coping Strategies among Individuals with Rheumatoid Arthritis. *J. Adv. Nurs.* **1997**, *25*, 1144–1150. [CrossRef] [PubMed]
14. Moyano, S.; Scolnik, M.; Vergara, F.; Garcia, M.V.; Sabelli, M.R.; Rosa, J.E.; Catoggio, L.J.; Soriano, E.R. Evaluation of Learned Helplessness, Perceived Self-Efficacy, and Functional Capacity in Patients With Fibromyalgia and Rheumatoid Arthritis. *JCR J. Clin. Rheumatol.* **2019**, *25*, 65–68. [CrossRef]
15. Poh, L.W.; He, H.-G.; Lee, C.S.C.; Cheung, P.P.; Chan, W.-C.S. An Integrative Review of Experiences of Patients with Rheumatoid Arthritis. *Int. Nurs. Rev.* **2015**, *62*, 231–247. [CrossRef]
16. Benka, J.; Nagyova, I.; Rosenberger, J.; Macejova, Z.; Lazurova, I.; van der Klink, J.L.L.; Groothoff, J.W.; van Dijk, J.P. Social Participation in Early and Established Rheumatoid Arthritis Patients. *Disabil. Rehabil.* **2016**, *38*, 1172–1179. [CrossRef] [PubMed]
17. Kool, M.B.; Geenen, R. Loneliness in Patients with Rheumatic Diseases: The Significance of Invalidation and Lack of Social Support. *J. Psychol.* **2012**, *146*, 229–241. [CrossRef] [PubMed]
18. Trindade, I.A.; Duarte, J.; Ferreira, C.; Coutinho, M.; Pinto-Gouveia, J. The Impact of Illness-Related Shame on Psychological Health and Social Relationships: Testing a Mediational Model in Students with Chronic Illness. *Clin. Psychol. Psychother.* **2018**, *25*, 408–414. [CrossRef]
19. Vergara, F.; Rosa, J.; Orozco, C.; Bertiller, E.; Gallardo, M.; Bravo, M.; Catay, E.; Collado, V.; Gómez, G.; Sabelli, M.; et al. Evaluation of Learned Helplessness, Self-Efficacy and Disease Activity, Functional Capacity and Pain in Argentinian Patients with Rheumatoid Arthritis. *Scand. J. Rheumatol.* **2017**, *46*, 17–21. [CrossRef]

20. Anyfanti, P.; Gavriilaki, E.; Pyrpasopoulou, A.; Triantafyllou, G.; Triantafyllou, A.; Chatzimichailidou, S.; Gkaliagkousi, E.; Aslanidis, S.; Douma, S. Depression, Anxiety, and Quality of Life in a Large Cohort of Patients with Rheumatic Diseases: Common, yet Undertreated. *Clin. Rheumatol.* **2016**, *35*, 733–739. [CrossRef]
21. de Belvis, A.G.; Pellegrino, R.; Castagna, C.; Morsella, A.; Pastorino, R.; Boccia, S. Success Factors and Barriers in Combining Personalized Medicine and Patient Centered Care in Breast Cancer. Results from a Systematic Review and Proposal of Conceptual Framework. *J. Pers. Med.* **2021**, *11*, 654. [CrossRef]
22. Cramp, F. The Role of Non-Pharmacological Interventions in the Management of Rheumatoid-Arthritis-Related Fatigue. *Rheumatology* **2019**, *58*, v22–v28. [CrossRef]
23. Scholl, I.; Zill, J.M.; Härter, M.; Dirmaier, J. An Integrative Model of Patient-Centeredness-a Systematic Review and Concept Analysis. *PLoS ONE* **2014**, *9*, e107828. [CrossRef]
24. Castro, E.M.; Van Regenmortel, T.; Vanhaecht, K.; Sermeus, W.; Van Hecke, A. Patient Empowerment, Patient Participation and Patient-Centeredness in Hospital Care: A Concept Analysis Based on a Literature Review. *Patient Educ. Couns.* **2016**, *99*, 1923–1939. [CrossRef] [PubMed]
25. Collins, F. Personalized Medicine. Available online: https://www.genome.gov/genetics-glossary/Personalized-Medicine (accessed on 3 August 2021).
26. Pastorino, R.; Loreti, C.; Giovannini, S.; Ricciardi, W.; Padua, L.; Boccia, S. Challenges of Prevention for a Sustainable Personalized Medicine. *J. Pers. Med.* **2021**, *11*, 311. [CrossRef]
27. Romeyke, T.; Noehammer, E.; Stummer, H. Patient-Reported Outcomes Following Inpatient Multimodal Treatment Approach in Chronic Pain-Related Rheumatic Diseases. *Glob. Adv. Health Med.* **2020**, *9*, 1–12. [CrossRef]
28. Strand, V.; Wright, G.C.; Bergman, M.J.; Tambiah, J.; Taylor, P.C. Patient Expectations and Perceptions of Goal-Setting Strategies for Disease Management in Rheumatoid Arthritis. *J. Rheumatol.* **2015**, *42*, 2046–2054. [CrossRef]
29. Kvrgic, Z.; Asiedu, G.B.; Crowson, C.S.; Ridgeway, J.L.; Davis, J.M. "Like No One Is Listening to Me": A Qualitative Study of Patient-Provider Discordance Between Global Assessments of Disease Activity in Rheumatoid Arthritis. *Arthritis Care Res.* **2018**, *70*, 1439–1447. [CrossRef]
30. Kelly, A.; Tymms, K.; Fallon, K.; Sumpton, D.; Tugwell, P.; Tunnicliffe, D.; Tong, A. Qualitative Research in Rheumatology: An Overview of Methods and Contributions to Practice and Policy. *J. Rheumatol.* **2021**, *48*, 6–15. [CrossRef]
31. Bartkeviciute, B.; Lesauskaite, V.; Riklikiene, O. Individualized Health Care for Older Diabetes Patients from the Perspective of Health Professionals and Service Consumers. *J. Pers. Med.* **2021**, *11*, 608. [CrossRef]
32. Bay, L.T.; Ellingsen, T.; Giraldi, A.; Graugaard, C.; Nielsen, D.S. "To Be Lonely in Your Own Loneliness": The Interplay between Self-Perceived Loneliness and Rheumatoid Arthritis in Everyday Life: A Qualitative Study. *Musculoskelet. Care* **2020**, *18*, 450–458. [CrossRef]
33. Shaw, Y.; Bradley, M.; Zhang, C.; Dominique, A.; Michaud, K.; McDonald, D.; Simon, T.A. Development of Resilience Among Rheumatoid Arthritis Patients: A Qualitative Study. *Arthritis Care Res.* **2020**, *72*, 1257–1265. [CrossRef]
34. Lempp, H.; Scott, D.; Kingsley, G. The Personal Impact of Rheumatoid Arthritis on Patients' Identity: A Qualitative Study. *Chronic Illn.* **2006**, *2*, 109–120. [CrossRef]
35. Primdahl, J.; Hegelund, A.; Lorenzen, A.G.; Loeppenthin, K.; Dures, E.; Appel Esbensen, B. The Experience of People with Rheumatoid Arthritis Living with Fatigue: A Qualitative Metasynthesis. *BMJ Open* **2019**, *9*, e024338. [CrossRef]
36. Braun, V.; Clarke, V. Using Thematic Analysis in Psychology. *Qual. Res. Psychol.* **2006**, *3*, 77–101. [CrossRef]
37. McInnis, O.A.; McQuaid, R.J.; Bombay, A.; Matheson, K.; Anisman, H. Finding Benefit in Stressful Uncertain Circumstances: Relations to Social Support and Stigma among Women with Unexplained Illnesses. *Stress* **2015**, *18*, 169–177. [CrossRef] [PubMed]
38. Galvez-Sánchez, C.M.; Duschek, S.; Reyes del Paso, G.A. Psychological Impact of Fibromyalgia: Current Perspectives. *Psychol. Res. Behav. Manag.* **2019**, *12*, 117–127. [CrossRef]
39. Pilkington, K.; Ridge, D.T.; Igwesi-Chidobe, C.N.; Chew-Graham, C.A.; Little, P.; Babatunde, O.; Corp, N.; McDermott, C.; Cheshire, A. A Relational Analysis of an Invisible Illness: A Meta-Ethnography of People with Chronic Fatigue Syndrome/Myalgic Encephalomyelitis (CFS/ME) and Their Support Needs. *Soc. Sci. Med.* **2020**, *265*, 113369. [CrossRef] [PubMed]
40. Carter, B.; Rouncefield-Swales, A.; Bray, L.; Blake, L.; Allen, S.; Probert, C.; Crook, K.; Qualter, P. "I Don't Like to Make a Big Thing out of It": A Qualitative Interview-Based Study Exploring Factors Affecting Whether Young People Tell or Do Not Tell Their Friends about Their IBD. *Int. J. Chronic Dis.* **2020**, *2020*, 1–11. [CrossRef]
41. Flurey, C.A.; Hewlett, S.; Rodham, K.; White, A.; Noddings, R.; Kirwan, J.R. "You Obviously Just Have to Put on a Brave Face": A Qualitative Study of the Experiences and Coping Styles of Men With Rheumatoid Arthritis. *Arthritis Care Res.* **2017**, *69*, 330–337. [CrossRef]
42. Feddersen, H.; Mechlenborg Kristiansen, T.; Tanggaard Andersen, P.; Hørslev-Petersen, K.; Primdahl, J. Juggling Identities of Rheumatoid Arthritis, Motherhood and Paid Work–a Grounded Theory Study. *Disabil. Rehabil.* **2019**, *41*, 1536–1544. [CrossRef]
43. Bode, C.; van der Heij, A.; Taal, E.; van de Laar, M.A.F.J. Body-Self Unity and Self-Esteem in Patients with Rheumatic Diseases. *Psychol. Health Med.* **2010**, *15*, 672–684. [CrossRef]
44. ten Klooster, P.M.; Christenhusz, L.C.A.; Taal, E.; Eggelmeijer, F.; van Woerkom, J.-M.; Rasker, J.J. Feelings of Guilt and Shame in Patients with Rheumatoid Arthritis. *Clin. Rheumatol.* **2014**, *33*, 903–910. [CrossRef]
45. Hoving, J.L.; van Zwieten, M.C.B.; van der Meer, M.; Sluiter, J.K.; Frings-Dresen, M.H.W. Work Participation and Arthritis: A Systematic Overview of Challenges, Adaptations and Opportunities for Interventions. *Rheumatology* **2013**, *52*, 1254–1264. [CrossRef]

46. Kojima, M.; Kojima, T.; Ishiguro, N.; Oguchi, T.; Oba, M.; Tsuchiya, H.; Sugiura, F.; Furukawa, T.A.; Suzuki, S.; Tokudome, S. Psychosocial Factors, Disease Status, and Quality of Life in Patients with Rheumatoid Arthritis. *J. Psychosom. Res.* **2009**, *67*, 425–431. [CrossRef]
47. Dures, E.; Almeida, C.; Caesley, J.; Peterson, A.; Ambler, N.; Morris, M.; Pollock, J.; Hewlett, S. Patient Preferences for Psychological Support in Inflammatory Arthritis: A Multicentre Survey. *Ann. Rheum. Dis.* **2016**, *75*, 142–147. [CrossRef]
48. Kristiansen, T.M.; Primdahl, J.; Antoft, R.; Hørslev-Petersen, K. Everyday Life with Rheumatoid Arthritis and Implications for Patient Education and Clinical Practice: A Focus Group Study. *Musculoskelet. Care* **2012**, *10*, 29–38. [CrossRef]
49. Kelly, A.; Tymms, K.; Tunnicliffe, D.J.; Sumpton, D.; Perera, C.; Fallon, K.; Craig, J.C.; Abhayaratna, W.; Tong, A. Patients' Attitudes and Experiences of Disease-Modifying Antirheumatic Drugs in Rheumatoid Arthritis and Spondyloarthritis: A Qualitative Synthesis. *Arthritis Care Res.* **2018**, *70*, 525–532. [CrossRef]
50. Gettings, L. Psychological Well-Being in Rheumatoid Arthritis: A Review of the Literature. *Musculoskelet. Care* **2010**, *8*, 99–106. [CrossRef]
51. des Bordes, J.K.A.; Foreman, J.; Westrich-Robertson, T.; Lopez-Olivo, M.A.; Peterson, S.K.; Hofstetter, C.; Lyddiatt, A.; Willcockson, I.; Leong, A.; Suarez-Almazor, M.E. Interactions and Perceptions of Patients with Rheumatoid Arthritis Participating in an Online Support Group. *Clin. Rheumatol.* **2020**, *39*, 1775–1782. [CrossRef]
52. Chafe, R. The Value of Qualitative Description in Health Services and Policy Research. *Healthc. Policy* **2017**, *12*, 12–18. [CrossRef]

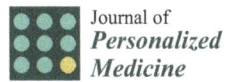

Review

Moving towards Integrated and Personalized Care in Parkinson's Disease: A Framework Proposal for Training Parkinson Nurses

Marlena van Munster [1,*], Johanne Stümpel [2,3], Franziska Thieken [1], David J. Pedrosa [1], Angelo Antonini [4], Diane Côté [5], Margherita Fabbri [6], Joaquim J. Ferreira [7,8,9], Evžen Růžička [10], David Grimes [11] and Tiago A. Mestre [11]

1. Department of Neurology, University Hospital Marburg, 35033 Marburg, Germany; thieken@staff.uni-marburg.de (F.T.); david.pedrosa@staff.uni-marburg.de (D.J.P.)
2. Cologne Center for Ethics, Rights, Economics, and Social Sciences of Health (CERES), University of Cologne, 50931 Cologne, Germany; Johanne.Stuempel@uk-koeln.de
3. Research Unit Ethics, University Hospital Cologne, 50931 Cologne, Germany
4. Parkinson and Movement Disorders Unit, University of Padua, 35122 Padua, Italy; angelo.antonini@unipd.it
5. The Ottawa Hospital Research Institute, Ottawa, ON K1Y 4E9, Canada; dianedenis0719@gmail.com
6. Department of Neurosciences, Clinical Investigation Center CIC 1436, Parkinson Toulouse Expert Center, NS-Park/FCRIN Network and NeuroToul COEN Center, TOULOUSE University Hospital, INSERM, University of Toulouse 3, 31062 Toulouse, France; margheritafabbrimd@gmail.com
7. Laboratory of Clinical Pharmacology and Therapeutics, Faculdade de Medicina, Universidade de Lisboa, 1649-028 Lisboa, Portugal; jferreira@medicina.ulisboa.pt
8. Instituto de Medicina Molecular João Lobo Antunes, Faculdade de Medicina, Universidade de Lisboa, 1649-028 Lisboa, Portugal
9. CNS—Campus Neurológico Sénior Torres Vedras, 2560-280 Torres Vedras, Portugal
10. Department of Neurology and Center of Clinical Neuroscience, First Faculty of Medicine, Charles University, General University Hospital in Prague, CZ-121 08 Prague, Czech Republic; evzen.ruzicka@lf1.cuni.cz
11. Parkinson Disease and Movement Disorders Centre, Division of Neurology, Department of Medicine, The Ottawa Hospital Research Institute, University of Ottawa Brain and Mind Research Institute, Ottawa, ON K1Y 4E9, Canada; dagrimes@toh.on.ca (D.G.); tmestre@toh.ca (T.A.M.)
* Correspondence: munster@med.uni-marburg.de

Abstract: Delivering healthcare to people living with Parkinson's disease (PD) may be challenging in face of differentiated care needs during a PD journey and a growing complexity. In this regard, integrative care models may foster flexible solutions on patients' care needs whereas Parkinson Nurses (PN) may be pivotal facilitators. However, at present hardly any training opportunities tailored to the care priorities of PD-patients are to be found for nurses. Following a conceptual approach, this article aims at setting a framework for training PN by reviewing existing literature on care priorities for PD. As a result, six prerequisites were formulated concerning a framework for training PN. The proposed training framework consist of three modules covering topics of PD: (i) comprehensive care, (ii) self-management support and (iii) health coaching. A fourth module on telemedicine may be added if applicable. The framework streamlines important theoretical concepts of professional PD management and may enable the development of novel, personalized care approaches.

Keywords: Parkinson's disease; nursing training; integrated care; Parkinson nurse; personalized care; multidisciplinary care

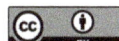

1. Introduction

Parkinson's disease (PD) is a progressive non-curable neurodegenerative disorder with an age of onset usually over 60 and presenting with complex motor and non-motor features such as cognitive impairment, mood and sleep disorders, autonomic dysfunction, and pain. In Europe, 1.2 million people are living with PD [1] with an increasing incidence in the elderly, so that the number of affected patients worldwide is expected to double by 2030 [2]. PD ranges among the top ten most resource intensive brain disorders in Europe [1] so that the need for PD services is expected to build up and consequently the burden on healthcare systems. This reality warrants the development and implementation of a care delivery model that conforms with society resources to guarantee its sustainability, while promoting better public policies, and reducing the overwhelming societal impact of PD [3]. The complexity of PD implies specific requirements for the design and delivery of care. Nevertheless, to date personalized care delivery models are rare [4]. While it has been shown that integrated and multidisciplinary care delivery models following a personalized care approach have positive implications for persons living with PD (PwPs), care partner and care providers, their implementation is difficult due to several reasons [3–5]. A key aspect for personalizing care services, is the availability of specialized staff [3]. Among these healthcare professionals, Parkinson Nurses (PN) can accomplish important tasks in the care process, such as providing mental health support, monitoring symptom progression and promoting patient navigation through the local healthcare system [3,6,7]. There has not been a consensus on defining the PN, but following Parkinsons UK, a PN can " ... provide expert care because they only work with people with the condition." They describe the major role of a PN in providing care as whilst " ... helping people to manage their medication" [8], the provided care by a PN will result in less side effects. Generally, PN help patients to manage their illness through making, for example by giving information and support to people with Parkinson's.

However, there are various definitions and descriptions not only of the role in the care team but there are also multiple approaches on the training of PNs as highlighted in Table 1.

Table 1. Existing Training Opportunities for Parkinson Nurses in different Countries.

Country	Role	Formal Education	Reference
United Kingdom	Being responsible for overall management within primary or secondary care teams Resource of Information and advice for PwPs Catalyst for improving public awareness	Provided via national universities Prerequisite: • Being a registered Nurse (registered no longer than three years) • Being registered at the Nursing and Midwifery Council (NMC) • Proving high level of experience working with and managing PD or other neurodegenerative disease Topics covered during education: • Strengthen experience through active involvement in clinical care • Education about principles of primary and secondary care • Responsibilities in care for PwPs • Aspects of multidisciplinary care coordination	[8,9]
Germany	Providing information and advice to patients and care givers on medication, symptoms and treatment options	Provided via German Parkinson Society (DPG), German Parkinson Association, (dPV), Parkinson Competence Network (KNP), Association of Parkinson Nurses and Assistants (VPNA) Prerequisite: • Completed 3-year regular nursing training + at least 2 years of working experience in the field Topics covered during education: • Specialist knowledge on special treatment procedures (e.g., medication pump or Deep Brain Stimulation) • Psychological counseling • Activating therapies • Handling of specific medications for PwPs	[7,10]

Table 1. Cont.

Country	Role	Formal Education	Reference
United States [1]	Role of APN (generally) • Care of patients • Education • Research • Consultation • Leadership They have: • Expert knowledge • Decision-making skills • Clinical competencies APNs are trained to work autonomously in specific care areas.	Advanced Practice Nurse (APN) → post-graduate education in nursing Two Types of APN roles have been recognized in the United States. • Nurse Practitioner (NP) • Clinical Nurse Specialist (CNP) Provided via national universities & national council Prerequisite: • Bachelor's degree in nursing + passed national council licensure Examination • For advanced nursing: master's degree in Nursing + specialty education Topics covered during education: • Advanced health assessment • Diagnosis • Disease management • Health promotion • Health prevention • Evaluation • Research	[11,12]
Canada [1]	Role of APN (generally) • Care of patients • Education • Research • Consultation • Leadership Role of NP • Legal authority to provide diagnosis and/or interpret diagnosis tests • Prescription of medication • Perform interventions • In Alberta, British Columbia and Ontario: Admission and discharge of patients from the hospital • NPs work in primary and community care setting • Responsible for health promotion, disease prevention, the diagnosis and management of acute illness and the management of the chronically ill Role of CNP: • Multi-faceted • Variable • Deployment in clinical care, education and research • Involvement in organizational leadership and professional development • Providing evidence-based practice and efforts on program development	Two types of APN roles have been recognized in Canada. • Nurse Practitioner (NP) • Clinical Nurse Specialist (CNP) Provided via national universities & national council NP → Registered nurses; completed NP education program; Bachelor- or Master's degree CNP → Master or Doctoral degree in nursing Topics covered during education for APNs: • Leadership • Accessibility of care • Safety of delivering care • Plan, coordinate, implement and evaluate programs to meet patients' needs • Promotion of community health	[13–16]

[1] In the United States and Canada, a variety of different forms of nurse education exist, and the nomenclature also holds a wide range of designations in both countries. The role and education of APNs (Advanced Practice Nurses) will be discussed here as an example. An explicit training as an advanced practice nurse for Parkinson's disease is not currently available in the United States and Canada.

Even though specialized training for PN on the delivery of personalized care services has been recommended [17], no framework has been proposed yet and existing curricular do not explicitly in cooperate it. By reviewing the specific requirements for the design and delivery of care in PD, we aim to propose a training framework for PN to facilitate the personalization and integration of care delivery.

2. Materials and Methods

We adopted a conceptual research approach to synthesize different perspectives on the theme of PD care and role of nurses. [18]. We entertained various conceptual streams from health care design, care delivery and medical prerequisites of PD. We considered the following questions to be essential to PN training: What are the care priorities for people living with PD (PwPs)? What type of PD-specific skills should a PN be equipped with in order to meet these needs?

The conceptualization of a training framework, may thus be seen a synthesis from various theoretical concepts which address care priorities for PD. We followed the structure of a line of reasoning to model this novel concept [19]. In this approach different hypothesis are formulated which then are integrated into a proposed model [19]. Following Lynham's Growth Cycle of Applied Theory-Building, the conceptualization of the training framework was informed by research, theory and practice [20]. A scoping literature review was conducted in order to identify relevant literature on care for PD. We chose The methodological approach of a scoping review, as it has been recommended to be particularly useful for categorizing the existing scientific literature in a defined research area in terms of its type, characteristics, and scope [21].The literature review was conducted in March 2020, (with an update in April 2021) by searching MEDLINE and Web of Knowledge (Figure 1), using the terms Parkinson's disease, concept and care. The search was not restricted in terms of the publication year. Studies were included if they described or theorized care models or concepts, relevant to PD and were either published in English or German. If a paper referred to another theory which was not focusing on PD but still relevant for the research aim (developing a PN training framework), the paper and theory reported also included. Opinion papers, literature reviews not proposing a new care model or studies testing short term interventions (i.e., physical therapy) were excluded. Publications focusing on palliative care were excluded, because this was seen as a different topic, where PwPs and care partners develop unique needs and concepts become relevant, which distinguish from other PD care literature. The search strategies, as well as a detailed list of in- and exclusion criteria can be accessed in the Supplementary Material (Table S1).

As a first step, publications retrieved from the literature review were grouped into 3 categories: intervention, practical care concept or theoretical concepts. Next, practical care concepts, guidelines and interventions were reviewed to identify care priorities for PD. Consecutively, a code was invented, whenever a new guiding care principle was mentioned following the approach of an undirected content analysis [22]. Thirdly, the identified care priorities informed the formulation of two hypothesis regarding a PN training framework. Fourth, the content of theoretical concepts was analyzed according to the previously identified care priorities. Finally, the content was used to construct a line of reasoning and to propose a framework for training PN. The literature research and coding, following the guidelines of PRISMA-ScR [23], was independently performed by two researchers (M.vM; J.S.). Discrepancies in coding and grouping were solved via discussion with a third researcher (F.T.). The final framework was commented by a range of PD experts for the iCARE-PD consortium (http://icare-pd.ca/, 1 June 2021), including PN, neurologists and scientists.

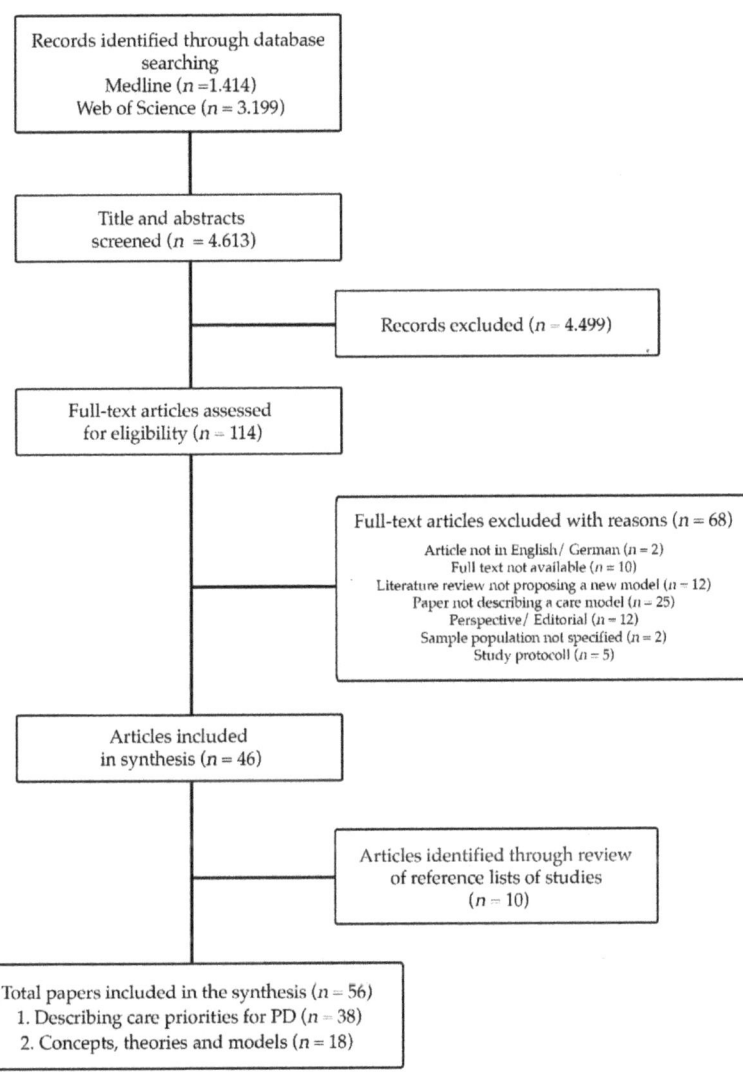

Figure 1. PRISMA flow diagram for the conducted scoping review.

3. Results

Fifty-six publications were included for final synthesis. (Figure 1).

The analysis included nine interventions implementing and evaluating a care model for PD, two guidelines for organizing PD care, 29 publications describing an implemented care model and 18 conceptual papers. Few publications described the same practical care model [24–27] whereas two reported the same care concept [28,29]. Consequently, 35 publications informed the definition of care priorities for PD care and 18 models informed the conceptualization of a PN training framework. Based on the implemented care models and recommendations, nine priorities for the organization and delivery of PD care were identified. The priorities and the frequency with which they were mentioned are summarized in Table 2.

Table 2. Care Priorities for Parkinson's Disease in Practical Care Concepts.

Care Priority	Citation (Frequency)	Reference
Multidisciplinary care	24	[19,24–27,30–51]
Patient-centeredness	17	[24–27,32,36,39–45,47,48,52–56]
Integrated care	16	[3,24–27,31,32,36,38,40,42,44–46,48,51,52,56,57]
Home-based care	13	[36,37,40–42,44,51,53,56–60]
Self-management	11	[24–27,36,39,40,44,45,55,57,61,62]
Community-centered care	9	[24–27,30,41,45,52,53,59,60,63]
Patient-/care partner education	7	[36,39,40,42,44,51,55]
Telemedicine	7	[30,42,44,56–59]
Professional education	1	[55]

The conceptual models covered the same care priorities as the practical care concepts. In addition to these priorities, the priority *personalized care* was observable in the conceptual models. The priorities and the frequency with which they were mentioned are summarized in Table 3. A content summary of the included models can be found in the Supplementary Material (Table S2).

Table 3. Care Priorities for Parkinson's Disease in Conceptual Models.

Care Priority	Citation (Frequency)	Reference
Patient-centeredness	9	[64–72]
Integrated care	8	[66,68,69,73–77]
Multidisciplinary care	6	[64,66,68,74,76,78]
Community-centered care	6	[67–69,71,77,78]
Home-based care	5	[28,29,65,68,73,79]
Personalized care	4	[70,75,78,80]
Self-management	4	[65,70,73,77]
Patient-/care partner education	2	[75,80]
Telemedicine	1	[28,29]
Professional education	1	[65]

Based on the identified care priorities for PD patients and their conceptualization in various care models, we present two hypotheses on the training requirements for PN, followed by relevant question(s) related to each hypothesis and their implication to the development of a PN training framework.

Hypothesis 1 (H1). *Parkinson Nurses should be trained to deliver comprehensive care for people living with parkinson's Disease and their care partner.*

Given the heterogeneous and progressive nature of PD, treatments require a high degree of personalization, as this enables the adjustment of the multiple existing management options to the clinical presentation, the individual symptoms and their progression, and the care needs of PwPs [81]. Based on the analyzed concepts of PD care, two models described personalized care management as important aspect [70,75] whereas two other models included the provision of tailored information [69,80].

What is personalized care? Personalizing care means adapting the care process to the patients' needs and preferences [78] (813) (p.813). Van Halteren et al. described five essential aspects of personalized care: providing information, proactively monitoring early detection signs and symptoms and the care process, coordinating care and navigating the patient in the healthcare system [78].

Implications for a PN curriculum: In reference to the conceptualization of a training framework, a PN ought to be competent to identify care needs and preferences for each individual. Additionally, they must be able to decide their implications for the care plan.

Personalizing care approaches means, that patients' perspective plays a central role in decision-making processes and leads to another frequently mentioned care priority: patient-centered care. Two models incorporated patient-centeredness as a pivotal aspect for care delivery [66,70] and three models highlighted the patients perspective as central component [65,68,71].

What is patient-centered care? Implementing a patient-centered perspective means '[...] ensuring that patient values guide all clinical decisions.' ([69], p. 360). Good communication is needed in order to identify these values [64,67]. PN must be able to meet patients and care partner with respect and empathy [64,67,69,72]. Providing emotional support and creating a trustful relationship has been mentioned as important element for implementing patient-centered care across all three identified concepts [67,69].

Implications for a PN curriculum: In reference to the conceptualization of a training framework, a PN ought to be trained in communicating with PwPs and care partner to enhance patient-centeredness.

What is integrated care? Integrated care is a form of multidisciplinary care. A multidisciplinary care approach can be described as an approach '[...] with contributions by experts from multiple complementary disciplines.' [49] (p.167). Bringing together these professions is what Goodwin described as professional integration [74]. Other concepts referred to this by highlighting the importance of incorporating physicians' perspectives in the care process; coordinating care across professions and implementing a clinical information system [64,68,77].

While there is a wide range of definitions, integrated care can be described as a care approach that aims '[...] bringing together key aspects in the design and delivery of care systems that are fragmented' [74] (p 1) (p.1). Three conceptual models described components that an integrated care approach should consider [66,74,76]. The Rainbow defines four primary domains of integration: clinical, professional, organizational, and systems integration, whereby functional and normative enablers play a role [76]. The Development Model of Integrated Care (DMIC) presents a nine-cluster model for organizational development in four phases with an emphasis on actual co-operation and commitment [66]. The DMIC also focuses on conditions for achieving effective collaboration, such as patient engagement, clarity of roles and responsibilities within the care delivery team [66]. Goodwin's work [74] distinguishes not only in the form in which integrated care should be designed (horizontal, vertical, sectoral, people-centered and whole-system), but also by how it is classified (by type, level, process, breadth and degree/intensity) [74].

An important aspect that was identifiable across the three integrated care concepts is care organization [66,74,76]. For PD, the inclusion of multiple healthcare professionals and the coordination of their care actions is of utmost importance [3]. Delivering integrated care has been described as central aspect for meeting PwPs complex care needs, reducing the burden of care partner and improving health care professional satisfaction [4].

Two of the conceptual models in integrated care services as important aspect for care delivery [73,75] and three models referred indirectly to the integration of care by mentioning a continuous collaboration of care providers, the organization of care and the selection of combined helping methods as important aspects of care organization [68,77].

Implications for a PN curriculum: PN fulfill important roles as clinical care integrators, navigators, support person and supervisor [4,75,82]. PNs, as part of the professional care team, should be able to design and implement a flexible routine network of service provider to support PwPs and their care partner in inpatient and outpatient settings.

What is home-based and community-centered care? Home-based care '[...] *refers to clinical practices that provide physician- or nurse practitioner led, longitudinal interdisciplinary care [...]*' at home ([79], p. 1). According to the Quality of Care Framework for Home-Based Medical Care [79], the essential elements are: assessment, care-coordination, patient and care partner education, provider competency, safety, provider competency and shared decision-making [79]. Additionally, factors such as patient and care partner experience, financial aspects and quality of life should be considered [79]. According to the model, patient-centered care can be promoted through the use of quality indicators that assess patients' access to care services, as well as their satisfaction with the expertise of care providers [79]. From the reviewed conceptual models, two referred indirectly to the organization of home-based care by mentioning the support of autonomy as important aspect for organizing patient-centered care [55,56]. Three models highlighted the need to assess available community resources [58,68], one model referred to the importance of assessing the personal lifestyle [59], one model defined quality criteria for the implementation of home-based telemedicine [19,20] and five models mentioned the navigation of the patient towards these resources and the reduction of barriers as important aspect for the organization of care and the selection of combined support methods as important aspects of care organization [59,60,62,68,69].

Delivering community-centered care means bringing '[. . .] care directly to the patients in the local community setting [. . .].' ([30], p. 1). Consequently, knowledge about the community and available resources is required. Based on the literature review, no model exclusively focusing on community-centered care was identified, however several concepts included available community resources as important quality aspects of care [67,77] as further detailed above.

Delivering care at home and within the community is important for PwPs and their care partners in order to enable access to care [3,73,83]. Additionally, home-based care for PwPs is becoming increasingly important from a demographic (e.g., aging, immobile population) and social (e.g., patients having a pronounced desire to continue living in their own homes) point of view [68].

Implications for a PN curriculum: Based on the concepts of home-based and community-centered care, we propose that the quality of care provided by PN may be influenced by level of coordination skills of different stakeholders in the healthcare system and knowledge about local healthcare resources. Thus, PN should be trained to map available community resources and navigate PwPs towards them.

Hypothesis 2 (H2). *Parkinson Nurses should be trained to deliver self-management support to persons with Parkinson's Disease and their care partner.*

Self-management support (SMS) and patient-education are critical elements of effective PD management [4,84], and key component of integrated care. SMS is a top priority for PwPs when asked about their care requirements [85]. SMS and patient-education help to reduce disease progression, complications and costs [4,84,85].

What is patient and care partner education? Based on Graham's concept, patient and care partner education are a form of knowledge translation [80]. The ability of lifelong learning is an important aspect of healthy aging and may be jeopardized by PD [70]. Implementing learning processes and empowering patients and care partner through education characterize integrated care concepts that were included in the analysis [66,69,75,77]. According to the Knowledge Translation Framework, patient education should be based on identified problems and adapted knowledge based on these problems. Patients and care partner should be motivated to use the delivered knowledge. Additionally, the identification of barriers and the use of knowledge should be evaluated continuously [80].

What is self-management support? Self-management support '[. . .] aims to empower patients with the skills and confidence necessary to manage their clinical disease.' ([73], p. 25). Activities include patient education, monitoring changes in symptoms and abilities, goal setting, and problem-solving [73]. Based on Orem's Self Deficit Theory, self-management support is needed, when the client's self-care demand exceeds the available self-care agency [68]. From the literature review, four conceptual models were identified that included self-management support as important aspect of care [65,70,73,77]. The Glasgow model (or 5-A's approach) describes five important actions that should be taken by the health-care professional when delivering SMS to the patient, namely: assessing, agreeing, advising, arranging and assisting. Another model, which is often referred to by SMS interventions for PwPs is the Chronic Care Model [77]. The model does not exclusively focus on SMS, but describes SMS as one of six dimensions, which should be addressed to improve care for patients with a chronic disease. According to the model, all dimensions affect each other, which is why all dimensions should be considered when aiming to improve care. The Chronic Disease Self-Management Model [77] is another model, which does not explicitly address PwPs but informed SMS approaches for PD [86]. Similar to the Glasgow model, it focuses on the relationship between the healthcare professional and the patient, however, a stronger focus is placed on the motivational aspect. According to the model, a good SMS-program pays attention to emotional and role management in addition to medical management and incorporates techniques to improve the patients' confidence.

Implications for a PN curriculum: PN play an important role in delivering SMS to PwPs [4,87,88], as good SMS relies on support from educated health professionals [88]. PN have a have a close patient contact and thus, are ideal professionals for delivering SMS [88]. In order to advise and assist PwPs properly, an understanding of the disease and its complexity is required, making it an essential part of a PN training framework. Considering the Knowledge Translation Framework, we propose that a PN training should include aspects of motivational interviewing in order to facilitate knowledge use by PwPs and their care partners [89].

Finally, one of the identified theoretical concepts considered telemedicine [28,29]. Telemedical applications can improve PwPs access to care, enhance quality of life and reduce the burden of care partner [90]. However, their purpose can vary greatly [28], which is why we propose to add a fourth module to the PN training framework when applicable, specifically focusing on the available technology.

Proposing a Framework for Training Parkinson Nurses to Deliver a Personalized Care Approach

In the previous section, we have formulated two hypotheses: (1) PN should be trained to deliver comprehensive care for PwPs and their care partner and (2) PD Nurses should be trained to deliver self-management support to PwPs and their care partner. Based on the review of conceptual models, we identified the following requirements to a framework for training PN:

(1) PN ought to be competent to identify needs and preferences. Additionally, they must be able to decide their implications for the care plan.
(2) PN require training in communicating with PwPs and care partner.
(3) PNs, as part of the professional care team, should be able to design and implement a flexible routine network of service providers to support PwPs and their care partner in inpatient and outpatient settings.
(4) The quality of care provided by PN may be influenced by specific training in the coordination of different stakeholders in the health care system and knowledge about local healthcare resources. Thus, PN should be trained to map available community resources and navigate PwPs towards them.
(5) In order to advise and assist PwPs properly, an understanding of the disease and its complexity is indispensable, making it an essential part of a PN training. Considering the Knowledge Translation Framework, we propose that a PN training should include aspects of motivational interviewing in order to facilitate knowledge use [89].
(6) Education on telemedicine should be incorporated whenever possible and applicable.
(7) Based on these requirements, we propose that PN should be trained in three central aspects in order to deliver a personalized care approach: i. understanding PD, ii. health coaching and iii. delivering comprehensive care. These aspects form the framework of the PN training displayed in Table 4.

Understanding the disease is a fundamental prerequisite for delivering care and, consequently, a foundational knowledge and skills for PN training [6,17,82]. PN must be able to adapt care delivery to the care requirements of PwPs and care partner, which change across the course of the disease. After completing the first module, PN are equipped with skills, that are important for integrating, personalizing and centering care around the patient. Besides a sound medical knowledge, PN must be able to understand and conduct clinical assessments [91]. These assessments may help the PN to evaluate patient needs as a starting point for discussion about care plans. Additionally, aspects of patient education and self-management support come into play when the PN discusses tests results or care plans with the patients. Consequently, we propose training on clinical assessments. And obtaining clinical conversation skills as central goal for the second training module: health coaching. Optimal care of PD should promote general health and wellbeing and care priorities should be defined together with PwPs and care partner [3]. Also, PwPs and care partner require a reference person that can be embodied by the PN through the empathic assessment of their care needs and the nurse's role as a care coordinator [3]. After the completion of this second training module, PN will have acquired the skills to assess personal care requirements of PwPs. The understanding of PD and health coaching skills merge, in line with the care priorities of home-based and community centered care, into a third and last module: delivering comprehensive tailored care. PwPs and care partner have to be navigated throughout the local healthcare system; multiple professions have to be incorporated in the care process and PwPs and care partner need motivation to use these resources. Consequently, we propose that PN should be trained to identify relevant local resources for PwPs and care partner, understand their living situation and motivate them to utilize available resources. Finally, a fourth module regarding available technologies can be added if applicable. This module will be discussed in greater detail in the following section.

Table 4. Conceptual framework for training Parkinson-Nurses to deliver a personalized care approach.

Module	Topic	Components	Goals
1	Understanding Parkinson's disease	• Understanding Parkinson's disease—symptoms and care requirements • Parkinson's disease stages and care needs • Aspects of Parkinson's disease management	Acquire fundamental knowledge about PD and management principles of motor and non-motor symptoms
2	Being a health coach	• Clinical assessments for people living with Parkinson's disease and care partners and their implications for care requirements • Acquire understanding of what's important when managing Parkinson's disease in a day-to-day practice and at home • Aspects of clinical conversations (identifying care priorities etc.)	Acquire skills and knowledge to assess patient-outcomes and identify personal care requirements
3	Aspects of care delivery for people living with Parkinson's disease and care partner	• Acquiring an overview of local care resources and important contact points for people living with Parkinson's disease and care partner • Building a local care network • Conversation training to motivate patients and care partners • Delivering self-management support based on the 5-As • Learning about the role of care partners as support person	Acquire knowledge about available local care resources and methods to motivate patients and care partners to use them
4	Telemedicine	• Adapted to the specific technology • Identify role of technology in care model: online monitoring, self-management support, enhance communication	Acquire knowledge about the technology

4. Discussion

This paper proposes a framework for a novel PN training in the context of integrated care. There is a scientific consensus that PNs will take a significant and prominent role in integrated, patient-centered home-/and community-based care in the future [92]. The PN is widely considered to be an important primary point of contact for PwPs and care partner alike. PNs are also recognized to be very helpful in the role of a multidisciplinary care team coordinator [93]. When PNs are available to provide home-based care, it has been shown that patients' quality of life improves [54,94]. The importance of professional education can be identified in both theoretical and intervention-based models [55,65].

When it comes to educating PN, a variety of training pathways exist in the various countries. Also, the recognition of nurses as important care coordinators differs. As it has been stated elsewhere, funding mechanisms and the structure of healthcare systems play an important task for defining a nurse's role [95]. This is also reflected in different education programs. Therefore, it is necessary to address country specific requirements when implementing the framework. Also, the structure of healthcare systems affects the availability of resources, which is why a sound understanding of the overall context is essential for implementing the framework presented here. We emphasize that module 3 of the framework should be adjusted to the country-specific context. Further research may aim to further defining this module and adapting it to a country-specific context. For countries with extensive training opportunities and high resources, such as the United States [95], we suggest, that single modules of the proposed training framework could be implemented in the basic training of nurses as prerequisite for a later specialization in the field. This would enable nurse students to better understand PD and prepare them to be empowered nursing advocates for PwPs in inpatient and outpatient settings. For countries, where the profession of PN is less well developed, such as Germany [7,95] the framework may be fully implemented and also be utilized to build an agenda for future research on how the role of PN can be strengthened.

When implementing the framework into pratice, one might face challenges and barriers. In some countries, the PN has been an integral part of the multidisciplinary care team for a long time [96], while in others PN are not present in every care team [7,17]. Also, it is necessary to clarify funding issues for implementing the framework and hire staff, such as experienced PN, to deliver the framework. Additionally the lack in certification of such training could be another barrier [7]. However, the framework introduced here may represent an crucial step towards a universal consensus on certification.

Concerning the fourth module, the framework is deliberately kept open. Telemedicine represents an increasingly studied and apparently beneficial instrument for the provision of medical care to the chronically ill [29,97,98]. However, telemedicine must always be evaluated in the context of its application, i.e., the technical prerequisites for widespread use must also be accessible to the individual patients [99]. Therefore, telemedicine is not yet part of this framework, but we strongly encourage its future integration. Due to the emerging possibility of remote patient monitoring (i.e., smart glasses, smart beds or wearables [83,100]), we emphasize future research on up-to-date tech-based home-based care solutions and the future role a PN may hold in this scenario of increasingly tech-based medical and social care delivery. This demand would also meet the need of care approaches to not only being responsive to specific care situations, but to incorporate proactive elements, such as the utilization of telemedicine [92,93].

For the future, the model being proposed here should configure a practical care concept that addresses effectively the identified care priorities for PD. One important aspect is the validation of the role of the PN and its training across cultures and societal contexts. Further research may focus on evaluating the implementation of the framework into a practical care concept and the development of a toolkit, which allows a flexible and streamlined adaptation of the training curriculum into different settings. Also, the model may be extended by reviewing care priorities for palliatve care.

5. Limitations

This review holds potential limitations. The quality of evidence, which was included in the review was not assessed, since the purpose was to review existing concepts as widely as possible. Further, the curriculum has not been implemented or evaluated in practice, which is why no claims about its feasibility can be made. Rather, it should be understood as stimulating and inspiring source of information for developing future PN curricula. Finally, the framework does not include country-specific differences of PN, which may affect its applicability.

6. Conclusions

A training framework for PN introduced here marks a pivotal contribution to increase the quality of care delivery for PwPs and their care partner following a care priority adapted approach. This framework is intended as an invitation to other researchers and practitioners to aid supporting the role of PNs and to move towards a standardized training. A shift towards a proactive role of a PN amongst healthcare providers is necessary and should be encouraged by legislation.

Supplementary Materials: The following are available online at https://www.mdpi.com/article/10.3390/jpm11070623/s1, Table S1: Search Strategy and In- and Exclusion Criteria, Table S2: Overview of Theoretical Concepts.

Author Contributions: Conceptualization, M.v.M., J.S., F.T., D.C. and T.A.M.; methodology, M.v.M., J.S.; formal analysis, M.v.M. and J.S.; investigation, M.v.M. and J.S.; resources, M.v.M., J.S., F.T. and T.A.M.; writing—original draft preparation, M.v.M., J.S.; writing—review and editing, F.T., D.J.P. and T.A.M.; visualization, M.v.M.; supervision, T.A.M.; funding acquisition, T.A.M., D.C., D.J.P., A.A., M.F., J.J.F., D.G., E.R. contributed with professional expertise and provided critical revisions of the intellectual content. All authors have read and agreed to the published version of the manuscript.

Funding: This research was funded by the Canadian Institutes of Health Research/EU Joint Programme—Neurodegenerative Disease Research, grant number 01789-000/HESOCARE-329-073.

Conflicts of Interest: M.v.M. declares no C.o.I. J.S. declares no C.o.I. F.T. declares no C.o.I. D.P. declares no C.o.I. A.A. has received compensation for consultancy and speaker related activities from UCB, Boehringer Ingelheim, General Electric, Britannia, AbbVie, Kyowa Kirin, Zambon, Bial, Neuroderm, Theravance Biopharma, Roche, Medscape; he receives research support from Bial, Lundbeck, Roche, Angelini Pharmaceuticals, Horizon 2020—Grant 825785, Horizon2020 Grant 101016902, Ministry of Education University and Research (MIUR) Grant ARS01_01081, Cariparo Foundation. He serves as consultant for Boehringer–Ingelheim for legal cases on pathological gambling. D.C. declares no C.o.I. M.F. declares no C.o.I. J.J.F. has held consultancy functions with GlaxoSmithKline, Novartis, TEVA, Lundbeck, Solvay, Abbott, Abbvie, BIAL, Merck-Serono, Merz, Ipsen, Biogen, NeuroDerm, Zambon, Sunovion, Affiris, ONO; has received lecture fees from Biogen, BIAL, Sunovion, ONO, Zambon, Abbvie; has received grants from GlaxoSmithKline, Grunenthal, MSD, Allergan, Novartis, Fundação MSD (Portugal), Medtronic and Teva; has been employed by Faculdade de Medicina de Lisboa and CNS—Campus Neurológico. D.G. received honorarium for speaking and consulting from Sunovion, Paladin Labs Inc, Clinical trials funding from Canadian Institutes of Health Research, Genzyme Corporation/Sanofi Canada, Eli Lilly and Company and grants from Canadian Institutes of Health Research, Parkinson Canada, Brain Canada, Ontario Brain Institute, PSI Foundation, Parkinson Research Consortium, EU Joint Programme—Neurodegenerative Disease Research, uOBMRI E. R. has been employed by First Faculty of Medicine, Charles University and General University Hospital in Prague, Czechia; received research funding form Czech Health Research Council and Michael J Fox Foundation; has no other relationships that present a potential conflict of interest. T.M. has received personal compensation for serving as a Consultant for CHDI, Sunovion, Valeo Pharma, Roche, Biogen and nQ, received personal compensation serving on a Speakers Bureau for Abbvie, Valeo Pharma, and has received research support from the Canadian Institutes of Health Research, EU Joint Programme—Neurodegenerative Disease Research, the Ontario Research Fund, Michael J Fox Foundation, Parkinson Canada, uOBMRI/Parkinson Research Consortium, Parkinson Canada, Brain Canada, Ontario Brain Institute, and PSI Foundation.

References

1. Gustavsson, A.; Svensson, M.; Jacobi, F.; Allgulander, C.; Alonso, J.; Beghi, E.; Dodel, R.; Ekman, M.; Faravelli, C.; Fratiglioni, L.; et al. Cost of disorders of the brain in Europe 2010. *Eur. Neuropsychopharmacol.* **2011**, *21*, 718–779. [CrossRef]
2. Dorsey, E.R.; Constantinescu, R.; Thompson, J.P.; Biglan, K.M.; Holloway, R.G.; Kieburtz, K.; Marshall, F.J.; Ravina, B.M.; Schifitto, G.; Siderowf, A.; et al. Projected number of people with Parkinson disease in the most populous nations, 2005 through 2030. *Neurology* **2007**, *68*, 384–386. [CrossRef]
3. Radder, D.L.M.; de Vries, N.M.; Riksen, N.P.; Diamond, S.J.; Gross, D.; Gold, D.R.; Heesakkers, J.; Henderson, E.; Hommel, A.L.A.J.; Lennaerts, H.H.; et al. Multidisciplinary care for people with Parkinson's disease: The new kids on the block! *Expert Rev. Neurother.* **2019**, *19*, 145–157. [CrossRef]
4. Rajan, R.; Brennan, L.; Bloem, B.R.; Dahodwala, N.; Gardner, J.; Goldman, J.G.; Grimes, D.A.; Iansek, R.; Kovács, N.; McGinley, J.; et al. Integrated Care in Parkinson's Disease: A Systematic Review and Meta-Analysis. *Mov. Disord.* **2020**, *35*, 1509–1531. [CrossRef]
5. Van der Marck, M.A.; Munneke, M.; Mulleners, W.; Hoogerwaard, E.M.; Borm, G.F.; Overeem, S.; Bloem, B.R. Integrated multidisciplinary care in Parkinson's disease: A non-randomised, controlled trial (IMPACT). *Lancet Neurol.* **2013**, *12*, 947–956. [CrossRef]
6. MacMahon, D.G. Parkinson's disease nurse specialists: An important role in disease management. *Neurology* **1999**, *52.7* (Suppl. 3), S21–S25.
7. Prell, T.; Siebecker, F.; Lorrain, M.; Tönges, L.; Warnecke, T.; Klucken, J.; Wellach, I.; Buhmann, C.; Wolz, M.; Lorenzl, S.; et al. Specialized Staff for the Care of People with Parkinson's Disease in Germany: An Overview. *J. Clin. Med.* **2020**, *9*, 2581. [CrossRef] [PubMed]
8. Parkinson's, U.K. *A Competency Frame-Work for Nurses Working in Parkinson's Disease Management*, 3rd ed.; Parkinson's U.K.: London, UK, 2016.
9. Morgan, E.; Moran, M. The Parkinson's disease nurse specialist. In *Parkinson's Disease in the Older Patient*, 2nd ed.; Palyfer, J., Hindle, J.V., Lees, A., Eds.; CRC Press: London, UK, 2008; pp. 314–323, ISBN 9781315365428.
10. Mai, T. Stand und Entwicklung der Rolle als Parkinson Nurse in Deutschland—Eine Online-Befragung. *Pflege* **2018**, *31*, 181–189. [CrossRef] [PubMed]
11. Schober, M.; Lehwaldt, D.; Rogers, M.; Steinke, M.; Turale, S.; Pulcini, J.; Roussel, J.; Stewart, D. *Guidelines on Advanced Practice Nursing*; International Council of Nurses: Geneva, Switzerland, 2020; ISBN 9789295099715.
12. Bryant-Lukosius, D.; Spichiger, E.; Martin, J.; Stoll, H.; Kellerhals, S.D.; Fliedner, M.; Roussel, J.; de Geest, S. Framework for evaluating the impact of advanced practice nursing roles. *J. Nurs. Scholarsh.* **2016**, *48*, 201–209. [CrossRef] [PubMed]
13. DiCenso, A.; Martin-Misener, R.; Bryant-Lukosius, D.; Bourgeault, I.; Kilpatrick, K.; Donald, F.; Kaasalainen, S.; Harbman, P.; Carter, N.; Kioke, S.; et al. Advanced practice nursing in Canada: Overview of a decision support synthesis. *Nurs. Leadersh.* **2010**, *23*, 15–34. [CrossRef]
14. Carter, F.D.; Harbman, P.; Kilpatrick, K.; Martin-Misener, R.; Sherifali, D.; Tranmer, J.; Valaitis, R. Report on Advanced Practice Nursing (APN) in Canada. In Proceedings of the Global Summit, Ottawa, ON, Canada, 28–29 July 2014. Available online: https://fhs.mcmaster.ca/ccapnr/documents/CanadianReportGlobalAPNSummit2014June12FINAL.pdf (accessed on 14 May 2021).
15. Bryant-Lukosius, D.; Carter, N.; Kilpatrick, K.; Martin-Misener, R.; Donald, F.; Kaasalainen, S.; Harbman, P.; Bourgeault, I.; DiCenso, A. The clinical nurse specialist role in Canada. *Nurs. Leadersh.* **2010**, *23*, 140–166. [CrossRef]
16. Canadian Nurses Association. *Advanced Practice Nursing. A Pan-Canadian Framework*; Canadian Nurses Association: Ottawa, ON, Canada, 2019.
17. Lennaerts, H.; Groot, M.; Rood, B.; Gilissen, K.; Tulp, H.; van Wensen, E.; Munneke, M.; van Laar, T.; Bloem, B.R. A Guideline for Parkinson's Disease Nurse Specialists, with Recommendations for Clinical Practice. *J. Parkinsons. Dis.* **2017**, *7*, 749–754. [CrossRef]
18. Fawcett, S.E.; Waller, M.A.; Miller, J.W.; Schwieterman, M.A.; Hazen, B.T.; Overstreet, R.E. A Trail Guide to Publishing Success: Tips on Writing Influential Conceptual, Qualitative, and Survey Research. *J. Bus Logist.* **2014**, *35*, 1–16. [CrossRef]
19. Jaakkola, E. Designing conceptual articles: Four approaches. *AMS Rev* **2020**, *10*, 18–26. [CrossRef]
20. Lynham, S.A. The General Method of Theory-Building Research in Applied Disciplines. *Adv. Dev. Hum. Resour.* **2002**, *4*, 221–241. [CrossRef]
21. Khalil, H.; Peters, M.; Godfrey, C.M.; McInerney, P.; Soares, C.B.; Parker, D. An Evidence-Based Approach to Scoping Reviews. *Worldviews Evid. Based Nurs.* **2016**, *13*, 118–123. [CrossRef]
22. Hsieh, H.-F.; Shannon, S.E. Three approaches to qualitative content analysis. *Qual. Health Res.* **2005**, *15*, 1277–1288. [CrossRef]
23. Tricco, A.C.; Lillie, E.; Zarin, W.; O'Brien, K.K.; Colquhoun, H.; Levac, D.; Moher, D.; Peters, M.D.J.; Horsley, T.; Weeks, L.; et al. PRISMA Extension for Scoping Reviews (PRISMA-ScR): Checklist and Explanation. *Ann. Intern. Med.* **2018**, *169*, 467–473. [CrossRef]
24. Bloem, B.R.; Rompen, L.; De Vries, N.M.; Klink, A.; Munneke, M.; Jeurissen, P. ParkinsonNet: A Low-Cost Health Care Innovation with A Systems Approach from The Netherlands. *Health Aff.* **2017**, *36*, 1987–1996. [CrossRef]
25. Nijkrake, M.J.; Keus, S.H.J.; Overeem, S.; Oostendorp, R.A.B.; Vlieland, T.P.V.; Mulleners, W.; Hoogerwaard, E.M.; Bloem, B.R.; Munneke, M. The ParkinsonNet concept: Development, implementation and initial experience. *Mov. Disord.* **2010**, *25*, 823–829. [CrossRef]

26. Tosserams, A.; de Vries, N.M.; Bloem, B.R.; Nonnekes, J. Multidisciplinary Care to Optimize Functional Mobility in Parkinson Disease. *Clin. Geriatr. Med.* **2020**, *36*, 159–172. [CrossRef] [PubMed]
27. Van der Eijk, M.; Bloem, B.R.; Nijhuis, F.A.P.; Koetsenruijter, J.; Vrijhoef, H.J.M.; Munneke, M.; Wensing, M.; Faber, M.J. Multidisciplinary Collaboration in Professional Networks for PD A Mixed-Method Analysis. *J. Parkinsons. Dis.* **2015**, *5*, 937–945. [CrossRef] [PubMed]
28. Larson, D.N.; Schneider, R.B.; Simuni, T. A New Era: The Growth of Video-Based Visits for Remote Management of Persons with Parkinson's Disease. *J. Parkinsons. Dis.* **2021**. [CrossRef] [PubMed]
29. Dorsey, E.R.; Okun, M.S.; Bloem, B.R. Care, Convenience, Comfort, Confidentiality, and Contagion: The 5 C's that Will Shape the Future of Telemedicine. *J. Parkinsons. Dis.* **2020**, *10*, 893–897. [CrossRef] [PubMed]
30. Aye, Y.M.; Liew, S.; Neo, S.X.; Li, W.; Ng, H.-L.; Chua, S.-T.; Zhou, W.-T.; Au, W.-L.; Tan, E.-K.; Tay, K.-Y.; et al. Patient-Centric Care for Parkinson's Disease: From Hospital to the Community. *Front. Neurol.* **2020**, *11*, 502. [CrossRef]
31. Cohen, E.V.; Hagestuen, R.; González-Ramos, G.; Cohen, H.W.; Bassich, C.; Book, E.; Bradley, K.P.; Carter, J.H.; Di Minno, M.; Gardner, J.; et al. Interprofessional education increases knowledge, promotes team building, and changes practice in the care of Parkinson's disease. *Parkinsonism Relat. Disord.* **2016**, *22*, 21–27. [CrossRef]
32. Eggers, C.; Dano, R.; Schill, J.; Fink, G.R.; Timmermann, L.; Voltz, R.; Golla, H.; Lorenzl, S. Access to End-of Life Parkinson's Disease Patients Through Patient-Centered Integrated Healthcare. *Front. Neurol.* **2018**, *9*, 627. [CrossRef]
33. Fleisher, J.E.; Klostermann, E.C.; Hess, S.P.; Lee, J.; Myrick, E.; Chodosh, J. Interdisciplinary palliative care for people with advanced Parkinson's disease: A view from the home. *Ann. Palliat. Med.* **2020**, *9*, S80–S89. [CrossRef]
34. Fründt, O.; Mainka, T.; Schönwald, B.; Müller, M.; Dicusar, P.; Gerloff, C.; Buhmann, C. The Hamburg Parkinson day-clinic: A new treatment concept at the border of in- and outpatient care. *J. Neural. Transm.* **2018**, *125*, 1461–1472. [CrossRef]
35. Giladi, N.; Manor, Y.; Hilel, A.; Gurevich, T. Interdisciplinary teamwork for the treatment of people with Parkinson's disease and their families. *Curr. Neurol. Neurosci. Rep.* **2014**, *14*, 493. [CrossRef]
36. Grimes, D.; Fitzpatrick, M.; Gordon, J.; Miyasaki, J.; Fon, E.A.; Schlossmacher, M.; Suchowersky, O.; Rajput, A.; Lafontaine, A.L.; Mestre, T.; et al. Canadian guideline for Parkinson disease. *CMAJ* **2019**, *191*, E989–E1004. [CrossRef]
37. Hack, N.; Akbar, U.; Monari, E.H.; Eilers, A.; Thompson-Avila, A.; Hwynn, N.H.; Sriram, A.; Haq, I.; Hardwick, A.; Malaty, I.A.; et al. Person-Centered Care in the Home Setting for Parkinson's Disease: Operation House Call Quality of Care Pilot Study. *Parkinsons. Dis.* **2015**, *2015*, 639494. [CrossRef]
38. Iansek, R. Interdisciplinary rehabilitation in Parkinson's disease. *Adv. Neurol.* **1999**, *80*, 555–559. [PubMed]
39. Jones, B.; Hopkins, G.; Wherry, S.-A.; Lueck, C.J.; Das, C.P.; Dugdale, P. Evaluation of a Regional Australian Nurse-Led Parkinson's Service Using the Context, Input, Process, and Product Evaluation Model. *Clin. Nurse Spec.* **2016**, *30*, 264–270. [CrossRef] [PubMed]
40. Kessler, D.; Hatch, S.; Alexander, L.; Grimes, D.; Côté, D.; Liddy, C.; Mestre, T. The Integrated Parkinson's disease Care Network (IPCN): Qualitative evaluation of a new approach to care for Parkinson's disease. *Patient Educ. Couns.* **2021**, *104*, 136–142. [CrossRef]
41. Keus, S.H.J.; Nijkrake, M.J.; Borm, G.F.; Kwakkel, G.; Roos, R.A.C.; Berendse, H.W.; Adang, E.M.; Overeem, S.; Bloem, B.R.; Munneke, M. The ParkinsonNet trial: Design and baseline characteristics. *Mov. Disord.* **2010**, *25*, 830–837. [CrossRef]
42. Loewenbrück, K.F.; Stein, D.B.; Amelung, V.E.; Bitterlich, R.; Brumme, M.; Falkenburger, B.; Fehre, A.; Feige, T.; Frank, A.; Gißke, C.; et al. Parkinson Network Eastern Saxony (PANOS): Reaching Consensus for a Regional Intersectoral Integrated Care Concept for Patients with Parkinson's Disease in the Region of Eastern Saxony, Germany. *J. Clin. Med.* **2020**, *9*, 2906. [CrossRef]
43. Monticone, M.; Ambrosini, E.; Laurini, A.; Rocca, B.; Foti, C. In-patient multidisciplinary rehabilitation for Parkinson's disease: A randomized controlled trial. *Mov. Disord.* **2015**, *30*, 1050–1058. [CrossRef]
44. Radder, D.L.M.; Nonnekes, J.; van Nimwegen, M.; Eggers, C.; Abbruzzese, G.; Alves, G.; Browner, N.; Chaudhuri, K.R.; Ebersbach, G.; Ferreira, J.J.; et al. Recommendations for the Organization of Multidisciplinary Clinical Care Teams in Parkinson's Disease. *J. Parkinsons. Dis.* **2020**, *10*, 1087–1098. [CrossRef]
45. Rompen, L.; De Vries, N.M.; Munneke, M.; Neff, C.; Sachs, T.; Cedrone, S.; Cheves, J.; Bloem, B.R. Introduction of Network-Based Healthcare at Kaiser Permanente. *J. Parkinsons. Dis.* **2020**, *10*, 207–212. [CrossRef]
46. Shrubsole, K. Implementation of an integrated multidisciplinary Movement Disorders Clinic: Applying a knowledge translation framework to improve multidisciplinary care. *Disabil. Rehabil.* **2019**, 1–13. [CrossRef] [PubMed]
47. Taylor, J.; Anderson, W.S.; Brandt, J.; Mari, Z.; Pontone, G.M. Neuropsychiatric Complications of Parkinson Disease Treatments: Importance of Multidisciplinary Care. *Am. J. Geriatr. Psychiatry* **2016**, *24*, 1171–1180. [CrossRef]
48. Tönges, L.; Ehret, R.; Lorrain, M.; Riederer, P.; Müngersdorf, M. Epidemiology of Parkinson's Disease and Current Concepts of Outpatient Care in Germany. *Fortschr. Neurol. Psychiatr.* **2017**, *85*, 329–335. [CrossRef] [PubMed]
49. Van der Marck, M.A.; Bloem, B.R. How to organize multispecialty care for patients with Parkinson's disease. *Parkinsonism Relat. Disord.* **2014**, *20*, S167–S173. [CrossRef]
50. Vaughan, C.P.; Prizer, L.P.; Vandenberg, A.E.; Goldstein, F.C.; Trotti, L.M.; Hermida, A.P.; Factor, S.A. A Comprehensive Approach to Care in Parkinson's Disease Adds Quality to the Current Gold Standard. *Mov. Disord. Clin. Pract.* **2017**, *4*, 743–749. [CrossRef]
51. Vickers, L.F.; O'Neill, C.M. An interdisciplinary home healthcare program for patients with Parkinson's disease. *Rehabil. Nurs.* **1998**, *23*, 286–289. [CrossRef]

52. Albanese, A.; Di Fonzo, A.; Fetoni, V.; Franzini, A.; Gennuso, M.; Molini, G.; Pacchetti, C.; Priori, A.; Riboldazzi, G.; Volonté, M.A.; et al. Design and Operation of the Lombardy Parkinson's Disease Network. *Front. Neurol.* **2020**, *11*, 573. [CrossRef] [PubMed]
53. Connor, K.I.; Cheng, E.M.; Barry, F.; Siebens, H.C.; Lee, M.L.; Ganz, D.A.; Mittman, B.S.; Connor, M.K.; Edwards, L.K.; McGowan, M.G.; et al. Randomized trial of care management to improve Parkinson disease care quality. *Neurology* **2019**, *92*, e1831–e1842. [CrossRef] [PubMed]
54. Fleisher, J.; Barbosa, W.; Sweeney, M.M.; Oyler, S.E.; Lemen, A.C.; Fazl, A.; Ko, M.; Meisel, T.; Friede, N.; Dacpano, G.; et al. Interdisciplinary Home Visits for Individuals with Advanced Parkinson's Disease and Related Disorders. *J. Am. Geriatr. Soc.* **2018**, *66*, 1226–1232. [CrossRef]
55. Marr, J.A.; Reid, B. Implementing managed care and case management: The neuroscience experience. *J. Neurosci. Nurs.* **1992**, *24*, 281–285. [CrossRef] [PubMed]
56. Pretzer-Aboff, I.; Prettyman, A. Implementation of an Integrative Holistic Healthcare Model for People Living with Parkinson's Disease. *Gerontologist* **2015**, *55* (Suppl. 1), S146–S153. [CrossRef]
57. Mestre, T.A.; Kessler, D.; Côté, D.; Liddy, C.; Thavorn, K.; Taljaard, M.; Grimes, D. Pilot Evaluation of a Pragmatic Network for Integrated Care and Self-Management in Parkinson's Disease. *Mov. Disord.* **2021**, *36*, 398–406. [CrossRef]
58. Achey, M.A.; Beck, C.A.; Beran, D.B.; Boyd, C.M.; Schmidt, P.N.; Willis, A.W.; Riggare, S.S.; Simone, R.B.; Biglan, K.M.; Dorsey, E.R. Virtual house calls for Parkinson disease (Connect.Parkinson): Study protocol for a randomized, controlled trial. *Trials* **2014**, *15*, 465. [CrossRef]
59. Dorsey, E.R.; Achey, M.A.; Beck, C.A.; Beran, D.B.; Biglan, K.M.; Boyd, C.M.; Schmidt, P.N.; Simone, R.; Willis, A.W.; Galifianakis, N.B.; et al. National Randomized Controlled Trial of Virtual House Calls for People with Parkinson's Disease: Interest and Barriers. *Telemed. J. E Health* **2016**, *22*, 590–598. [CrossRef] [PubMed]
60. Jorm, L.R.; Walter, S.R.; Lujic, S.; Byles, J.E.; Kendig, H.L. Home and community care services: A major opportunity for preventive health care. *BMC Geriatr.* **2010**, *10*, 26. [CrossRef]
61. Hellqvist, C.; Dizdar, N.; Hagell, P.; Berterö, C.; Sund-Levander, M. Improving self-management for persons with Parkinson's disease through education focusing on management of daily life: Patients' and relatives' experience of the Swedish National Parkinson School. *J. Clin. Nurs.* **2018**, *27*, 3719–3728. [CrossRef]
62. Hellqvist, C. Promoting Self-Care in Nursing Encounters with Persons Affected by Long-Term Conditions-A Proposed Model to Guide Clinical Care. *Int. J. Environ. Res. Public Health* **2021**, *18*, 2223. [CrossRef]
63. Schröder, S.; Martus, P.; Odin, P.; Schaefer, M. Impact of community pharmaceutical care on patient health and quality of drug treatment in Parkinson's disease. *Int. J. Clin. Pharm.* **2012**, *34*, 746–756. [CrossRef] [PubMed]
64. Coulter, A.; Cleary, P.D. Patients' experiences with hospital care in five countries. *Health Aff.* **2001**, *20*, 244–252. [CrossRef] [PubMed]
65. Sjödahl Hammarlund, C.; Westergren, A.; Åström, I.; Edberg, A.-K.; Hagell, P. The Impact of Living with Parkinson's Disease: Balancing within a Web of Needs and Demands. *Parkinsons. Dis.* **2018**, *2018*, 4598651. [CrossRef] [PubMed]
66. Minkman, M.M.N. Developing integrated care. Towards a development model for integrated care. *Int. J. Integr. Care* **2012**, *12*, e197. [CrossRef]
67. Murray, C.J.L.; Evans, D.B. *Health Systems Performance Assessment: Debates, Methods and Empiricism*; World Health Organization: Geneva, Switzerland, 2003; ISBN 9789241562454.
68. Hartweg, D. *Dorothea Orem: Self-Care Deficit Theory: Notes on Nursing Theories Volume 4*; SAGE Publications: Thousand Oaks, CA, USA, 1991; ISBN 0803942990.
69. Van der Eijk, M.; Faber, M.J.; Al Shamma, S.; Munneke, M.; Bloem, B.R. Moving towards patient-centered healthcare for patients with Parkinson's disease. *Parkinsonism Relat. Disord.* **2011**, *17*, 360–364. [CrossRef]
70. Fereshtehnejad, S.-M.; Lökk, J. Active aging for individuals with Parkinson's disease: Definitions, literature review, and models. *Parkinsons. Dis.* **2014**, *2014*, 739718. [CrossRef] [PubMed]
71. Glasgow, R.E.; Davis, C.L.; Funnell, M.M.; Beck, A. Implementing Practical Interventions to Support Chronic Illness Self-Management. *JT Comm. J. Qual. Saf.* **2003**, *29*, 563–574. [CrossRef]
72. Freeman, G.K.; Olesen, F.; Hjortdahl, P. Continuity of care: An essential element of modern general practice? *Fam. Pract.* **2003**, *20*, 623–627. [CrossRef]
73. Fabbri, M.; Caldas, A.C.; Ramos, J.B.; Sanchez-Ferro, Á.; Antonini, A.; Růžička, E.; Lynch, T.; Rascol, O.; Grimes, D.; Eggers, C.; et al. Moving towards home-based community-centred integrated care in Parkinson's disease. *Parkinsonism Relat. Disord.* **2020**, *78*, 21–26. [CrossRef]
74. Goodwin, N. Understanding Integrated Care. *Int. J. Integr. Care* **2016**, *16*, 6. [CrossRef] [PubMed]
75. Tenison, E.; Smink, A.; Redwood, S.; Darweesh, S.; Cottle, H.; van Halteren, A.; van den Haak, P.; Hamlin, R.; Ypinga, J.; Bloem, B.R.; et al. Proactive and Integrated Management and Empowerment in Parkinson's Disease: Designing a New Model of Care. *Parkinsons. Dis.* **2020**, *2020*. [CrossRef]
76. Valentijn, P.P.; Schepman, S.M.; Opheij, W.; Bruijnzeels, M.A. Understanding integrated care: A comprehensive conceptual framework based on the integrative functions of primary care. *Int. J. Integr. Care* **2013**, *13*, e010. [CrossRef] [PubMed]
77. Wagner, E.H.; Austin, B.T.; Davis, C.; Hindmarsh, M.; Schaefer, J.; Bonomi, A. Improving chronic illness care: Translating evidence into action. *Health Aff.* **2001**, *20*, 64–78. [CrossRef] [PubMed]

78. Van Halteren, A.D.; Munneke, M.; Smit, E.; Thomas, S.; Bloem, B.R.; Darweesh, S.K.L. Personalized Care Management for Persons with Parkinson's Disease. *J. Parkinsons. Dis.* **2020**, *10*, S11–S20. [CrossRef] [PubMed]
79. Ritchie, C.S.; Leff, B.; Garrigues, S.K.; Perissinotto, C.; Sheehan, O.C.; Harrison, K.L. A Quality of Care Framework for Home-Based Medical Care. *J. Am. Med. Dir. Assoc.* **2018**, *19*, 818–823. [CrossRef] [PubMed]
80. Graham, I.D.; Logan, J.; Harrison, M.B.; Straus, S.E.; Tetroe, J.; Caswell, W.; Robinson, N. Lost in knowledge translation: Time for a map? *J. Contin. Educ. Health Prof.* **2006**, *26*, 13–24. [CrossRef]
81. Titova, N.; Chaudhuri, K.R. Personalized medicine in Parkinson's disease: Time to be precise. *Mov. Disord.* **2017**, *32*, 1147–1154. [CrossRef] [PubMed]
82. Gopalakrishna, A.; Alexander, S.A. Understanding Parkinson Disease: A Complex and Multifaceted Illness. *J. Neurosci. Nurs.* **2015**, *47*, 320–326. [CrossRef] [PubMed]
83. Ferreira, J.J.; Godinho, C.; Santos, A.T.; Domingos, J.; Abreu, D.; Lobo, R.; Gonçalves, N.; Barra, M.; Larsen, F.; Fagerbakke, Ø.; et al. Quantitative home-based assessment of Parkinson's symptoms: The SENSE-PARK feasibility and usability study. *BMC Neurol.* **2015**, *15*, 89. [CrossRef] [PubMed]
84. Kessler, D.; Liddy, C. Self-management support programs for persons with Parkinson's disease: An integrative review. *Patient Educ. Couns.* **2017**, *100*, 1787–1795. [CrossRef]
85. Kessler, D.; Hauteclocque, J.; Grimes, D.; Mestre, T.; Côté, D.; Liddy, C. Development of the Integrated Parkinson's Care Network (IPCN): Using co-design to plan collaborative care for people with Parkinson's disease. *Qual. Life Res.* **2019**, *28*, 1355–1364. [CrossRef]
86. Lawn, S.; Schoo, A. Supporting self-management of chronic health conditions: Common approaches. *Patient Educ. Couns.* **2010**, *80*, 205–211. [CrossRef]
87. Tennigkeit, J.; Feige, T.; Haak, M.; Hellqvist, C.; Seven, Ü.S.; Kalbe, E.; Schwarz, J.; Warnecke, T.; Tönges, L.; Eggers, C.; et al. Structured Care and Self-Management Education for Persons with Parkinson's Disease: Why the First Does Not Go without the Second-Systematic Review, Experiences and Implementation Concepts from Sweden and Germany. *J. Clin. Med.* **2020**, *9*, 2787. [CrossRef]
88. Chenoweth, L.; Gallagher, R.; Sheriff, J.N.; Donoghue, J.; Stein-Parbury, J. Factors supporting self-management in Parkinson's disease: Implications for nursing practice. *Int. J. Older People Nurs.* **2008**, *3*, 187–193. [CrossRef] [PubMed]
89. Rollnick, S.; Miller, W.R. What is Motivational Interviewing? *Behav. Cogn. Psychother.* **1995**, *23*, 325–334. [CrossRef]
90. Achey, M.; Aldred, J.L.; Aljehani, N.; Bloem, B.R.; Biglan, K.M.; Chan, P.; Cubo, E.; Dorsey, E.R.; Goetz, C.G.; Guttman, M.; et al. The past, present, and future of telemedicine for Parkinson's disease. *Mov. Disord.* **2014**, *29*, 871–883. [CrossRef] [PubMed]
91. Bhidayasiri, R.; Martinez-Martin, P. Clinical Assessments in Parkinson's Disease: Scales and Monitoring. *Int. Rev. Neurobiol.* **2017**, *132*, 129–182. [CrossRef] [PubMed]
92. Bloem, B.R.; Henderson, E.J.; Dorsey, E.R.; Okun, M.S.; Okubadejo, N.; Chan, P.; Andrejack, J.; Darweesh, S.K.L.; Munneke, M. Integrated and patient-centred management of Parkinson's disease: A network model for reshaping chronic neurological care. *Lancet Neurol.* **2020**, *19*, 623–634. [CrossRef]
93. Bloem, B.R.; Okun, M.S.; Klein, C. Parkinson's disease. *Lancet* **2021**. [CrossRef]
94. Beck, C.A.; Beran, D.B.; Biglan, K.M.; Boyd, C.M.; Dorsey, E.R.; Schmidt, P.N.; Simone, R.; Willis, A.W.; Galifianakis, N.B.; Katz, M.; et al. National randomized controlled trial of virtual house calls for Parkinson disease. *Neurology* **2017**, *89*, 1152–1161. [CrossRef]
95. Bianchi, M.; Bagnasco, A.; Bressan, V.; Barisone, M.; Timmins, F.; Rossi, S.; Pellegrini, R.; Aleo, G.; Sasso, L. A review of the role of nurse leadership in promoting and sustaining evidence-based practice. *J. Nurs. Manag.* **2018**, *26*, 918–932. [CrossRef]
96. Reynolds, H.; Wilson-Barnett, J.; Richardson, G. Evaluation of the role of the Parkinson's disease nurse specialist. *Int. J. Nurs. Stud.* **2000**, *37*, 337–349. [CrossRef]
97. Ben-Pazi, H.; Browne, P.; Chan, P.; Cubo, E.; Guttman, M.; Hassan, A.; Hatcher-Martin, J.; Mari, Z.; Moukheiber, E.; Okubadejo, N.U.; et al. The Promise of Telemedicine for Movement Disorders: An Interdisciplinary Approach. *Curr. Neurol. Neurosci. Rep.* **2018**, *18*, 26. [CrossRef]
98. Dorsey, E.R.; Venkataraman, V.; Grana, M.J.; Bull, M.T.; George, B.P.; Boyd, C.M.; Beck, C.A.; Rajan, B.; Seidmann, A.; Biglan, K.M. Randomized controlled clinical trial of "virtual house calls" for Parkinson disease. *JAMA Neurol.* **2013**, *70*, 565–570. [CrossRef] [PubMed]
99. Chirra, M.; Marsili, L.; Wattley, L.; Sokol, L.L.; Keeling, E.; Maule, S.; Sobrero, G.; Artusi, C.A.; Romagnolo, A.; Zibetti, M.; et al. Telemedicine in Neurological Disorders: Opportunities and Challenges. *Telemed. J. E Health* **2019**, *25*, 541–550. [CrossRef] [PubMed]
100. Monje, M.H.G.; Foffani, G.; Obeso, J.; Sánchez-Ferro, Á. New Sensor and Wearable Technologies to Aid in the Diagnosis and Treatment Monitoring of Parkinson's Disease. *Annu. Rev. Biomed. Eng.* **2019**, *21*, 111–143. [CrossRef] [PubMed]

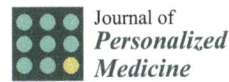

Article

Individualized Health Care for Older Diabetes Patients from the Perspective of Health Professionals and Service Consumers

Birute Bartkeviciute *, Vita Lesauskaite and Olga Riklikiene

Faculty of Nursing, Lithuanian University of Health Sciences, LT 44307 Kaunas, Lithuania; vita.lesauskaite@lsmuni.lt (V.L.); olga.riklikiene@lsmuni.lt (O.R.)
* Correspondence: birute.bartkeviciute@lsmuni.lt

Abstract: Background: Individualized nursing care as a form of person-centered care delivery is a well-known approach in the health care context and is accepted as best practice by organizations and professionals, yet its implementation in everyday practice creates serious challenges. The aim was to assess and compare the perceptions of health professionals and older diabetes patients on their individual care in regard to the patient's clinical situation, personal life situation, and decisional control. Methods: The quantitative study with a cross-sectional survey design was conducted from March 2019 until January 2021. The Individualized Care Scale was applied for the data collection. Health professionals (nurses and physicians, $n = 70$) and older diabetes patients ($n = 145$) participated in the study. The average duration of diabetes was 15.8 years (SD = 10.0) and type 2 diabetes was the most common (89.0%). The current glucose-lowering therapy for 51.0% of the patients was oral medications, 37.9% used injected insulin, and 11.1% were treated by combined therapy. Results: The highest-rated aspects of individualized care on both dimensions of the scale from the health professionals' perspective related to the clinical situation, and the scores for provision were significantly higher than those for support. The highest means of patients' ratings on the support dimension related to the clinical situation and the decisions over care sub-scale; for the care provision dimension, the highest individuality in care was assigned to the decisions over care sub-scale. The lowest ratings of individualized care, both in the health professionals' and patients' samples, related to the personal life situation sub-scale. Conclusions: Health professionals are more positive in regard to individualized care support and provisions for older diabetes patients than the patients themselves. Patient characteristics, such as the type of glucose-lowering therapy, education, and nutritional status, make a difference in patients' understanding and experience of individuality in care.

Keywords: individual care; nurses; older diabetes patients; physicians; support

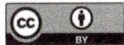

1. Introduction

Patient-centered care is a well-known and widely used approach in the health care context, as well as in education, management, and scientific investigations. The WHO global strategy on people-centered and integrated health services (2015) highlighted the importance of placing people and communities at the center of health services, which makes health services more comprehensive and responsive, more integrated, accessible, coordinated, safe, more focused on health needs and preferences, and more humane and holistic. Patient-centered care is understood as health services throughout the course of life that respond to the consumers' values and preferences, and are 'organized around the health needs and expectations of people rather than diseases' [1], p. 7.

A particular advantage of patient centralization in care, as mentioned by the WHO strategy, is an improved ability to respond to health care crises. Now, health care systems and societies, still guided by the global pandemic, have never been more clearly aware of the importance of patient-centered care for individuals' positive health outcomes and high-quality and continuity of care. As it was stated in the WHO document, a well-organized health system that is 'able to adapt to the needs of the people it serves is not only better positioned to respond to emerging threats, but is also more resilient to tackling the myriad of chronic diseases which plague our populations' [1], p. 5.

Several studies and reviews addressed care individuality, a form of person-centered care delivery, for chronic disease patients. The evidence was created on preferences for decision-making among chronic neurodegenerative disease (Parkinson's) patients [2] and the benefits of nurse-led patient education for adults with heart failure [3,4]. Nurse-led case management was tested on adults with cancer [5] and other chronic illnesses [6]. The effectiveness of community-based case management among adults who abuse substances [7] and nurse-led primary health care coordination were investigated for patients with complex needs [8]. The results of these studies indicated multidisciplinary teamwork, the delivery of personalized, integrated, and coordinated care, patient education, and self-management skill improvement as suitable strategies in solving complex patients' health and social care needs in the primary health care of chronic illnesses, including diabetes mellitus.

The number of new diabetes cases has been increasing globally, with a projected increase to 26.6 million cases of incidence, 570.9 million cases of prevalence, and 1.59 million deaths in 2025 without effective interventions [9]. There were 109,162 diabetes mellitus cases (0.8% were children) in Lithuania in 2018, that is, 1 in every 28 men and 1 in every 23 women. Complications of the illness were prevalent in 80.5% of patients with type 1, and in 46.1% of type 2 diabetes patients; 528 patients die annually from this disease or its complications. In 2019, the number of patients with diabetes increased to 110,136 (396.3/1000 pop.); 6421 (2.3/1000 pop.) had type 1 diabetes and 104,659 (37.46/1000) were ill with type 2 diabetes [10].

Health care service for patients with diabetes, besides the physical, psychological, and social consequences, brings remarkable financial expenses, creating an economical burden for national health care systems. In 2011, estimates of global health care expenditures due to diabetes were USD 376 billion, and for the whole European region, it was USD 105 billion (10% of total health care expenditures; USD 2046 per person), with expectations for it to increase to USD 490 billion by 2030 [11]. A study conducted by Domeikiene et al. (2014) calculated the direct health care costs needed for patients with type 2 diabetes mellitus (non-complicated and complicated cases) in Lithuania. The results revealed that costs, adjusted for the average annual cost per person with diabetes, increased gradually with the number of complications from USD 814.73 (95% CI, 697.22–932.24) in patients without complications to USD 1926.64 (95% CI, 1275.66–2577.61) in patients with three or more complications [12].

There is evidence that patient-centered care positively relates to reduced pain and discomfort, faster physical and emotional recovery, improved outcomes and quality of life [5,13], enhanced respect for persons and autonomy [2], increased adherence to the care plan [14], reduced hospital readmissions [3,13], and decreased health care utilization [15]. Similar patient health and care issues are intrinsic to older diabetes patients.

Various care strategies were suggested to improve the care and quality of life for patients with diabetes. In nursing, traditional nursing theoretical frameworks with patient education strategies were utilized for improving the care and self-care behaviors of people with diabetes [16–19]. To improve care for diabetes patients, an order of the Health Ministry on the requirements for the provision of nursing services for patients with diabetes mellitus was issued in Lithuania. The order states the right for diabetes nurses to provide primary and continuous consultations, and perform foot and leg ulcer care for patients independently or with a team [20]. Patient education becomes an important part of diabetes nurse service, as it encourages behavior changes in people with diabetes, which, in turn, may improve their chances for diabetes control. The clinical trial on continual diabetes education confirmed that values and achievement of the type 2 diabetes mellitus control improved after face-to-face individualized education sessions for patients [21]. During individual and group education, general information is provided, trying to correspond to the basic needs of the patients, enabling them to be active participants and creating a possibility to learn from the experiences of others. However, diabetes patients, particularly those of older age, are not always prepared to take an active role when discussing their care with health care professionals as they are lacking skills [22] or are not familiar with what their exact role in that discussion should be.

Even if the approach of patient-centered care is familiar to health care organizations and health professionals, the implementation of such care commonly creates challenges. The obstacles are related to the differences in the comprehension of the phenomenon, a necessary physical change of health facilities, a serious cultural shift of the paradigm in traditional care practices (e.g., a paternalistic approach vs a consumer-oriented approach to care), organizational initiatives, leadership capacities, and health care professionals' knowledge and skills [23,24]. To tackle the situation, it is important to analyze the providers' perspectives on the support and provision for individual care for patients. In addition, the consumers' feedback of their experiences in patient-centered care may be of great benefit for the improvement of the work at health care organizations [25].

To our knowledge, there is a lack of studies that explore older diabetes patients' perspectives on individualized care and compare the experiences of patients with those of health professionals (nurses and physicians). For the Republic of Lithuania and similar post-soviet states that began to transform the national health care system in the early 1990s by adopting the Western countries' principles of health service provision and modern nursing developments, the individualized approach to the care of older patients with chronic disease is a new practical reality where more evidence is needed. The results of this study highlight the need for more active involvement of older diabetes patients in care planning and provisions by communicating their preferences and making individual decisions. We also expect that increasing the data on Lithuanian nurses' perspectives on individualized care for diabetes patients will facilitate change by fostering the development of the independent role and expanding the competence of diabetes nurses in other countries where such specialty has not been introduced yet.

The aim of this study was to assess and compare the perceptions of health professionals and older diabetes patients on their individual care in regard to their patient clinical situation, personal life situation, and decisional control.

2. Materials and Methods

2.1. Design and Setting

A quantitative study with a cross-sectional survey design was conducted. The study was performed from March 2019 until January 2021.

The study was conducted at the primary health care institutions ($n = 10$) of the Kaunas region (i.e., the second largest city of Lithuania), where diabetes care for patients is provided by primary care physicians, physician endocrinologists, diabetes nurses, and general practice nurses. All institutions are funded by the national compulsory health insurance fund. Before the pandemic, questionnaires were distributed by the investigator when she met nurse managers at the study field, introduced the study, and asked for help in distributing and collecting the questionnaires to health professionals and patients. Patients, in most cases, picked up the questionnaire with a stamped envelope during their regular check-up, completed it at home, and returned it during the next visit or by mail. At the time of the pandemic and quarantine, health professionals were addressed through their work emails and were sent an e-questionnaire. The patients were not surveyed by e-mail.

2.2. Instruments

For this study, 2 versions of the Individualized Care Scale (ICS) [26–29] were applied for the data collection. The Nurse Version (ICS–Nurse) was filled in by the nurses and physicians who take care of older diabetes patients, and the Patient Version (ICS–Patient) of the instrument was delivered to older patients with either type 1 or type 2 diabetes mellitus.

The Individualized Care Scale–Nurse Version (ICS–Nurse) is a bipartite questionnaire designed to explore nurses' views about individualized care in two dimensions (A-ICS–

Nurse and B-ICS–Nurse) [29]. The current version of the scale includes 17 (A) and 17 (B) items, for a total of 34. The A-ICS–Nurse is a 17-item 5-point Likert-type scale (1 = strongly disagree, 2 = disagree to some extent, 3 = neither agree nor disagree, 4 = agree to some extent, 5 = strongly agree) designed to explore nurses' views on how they support patient individuality through nursing activities in general. For example, the nurse is asked to rate the items 'I talk with patients about their fears and anxieties' or 'I help patients take part in decisions concerning their care'. The B-ICS–Nurse is also a 17-item 5-point Likert-type scale exploring the extent to which nurses perceive that the care they provide is individualized (e.g., 'I took into account their needs that require care and attention') [30,31]. Both scales consist of 3 sub-scales: (1) clinical situation (Clin A and B), (2) personal life situation (Pers A and B), and (3) decisional control over care (Dec A and B).

The Individualized Care Scale–Patient Version (ICS–Patient) is a 34-item self-reporting measure that was developed for the purposes of exploring patients' views on how patient individuality was supported through specific nursing activities (A-ICS–Patient) and the extent to which patients perceived their care as individualized (B-ICS–Patient) [27].

Both dimensions consist of 3 sub-scales eliciting information on the following: (1) patient characteristics in the clinical situation caused by hospitalization (or, for this study, a visit to an outpatient clinic) (Clin A and B), (2) the patient's personal life situation (Pers A and B), and (3) decisional control over care (Dec A and B). Both dimensions, that is, A and B-ICS–Patient, share the same structure in terms of their content. The questions are differently worded in that some A-ICS–Patient items ask the patients how nurses' activities have facilitated their individual existence in care, whereas some B-ICS–Patient items present the question as to how individual or individualized the care for the patients has been. The following response categories were used: 1 = fully disagree, 2 = disagree to some extent, 3 = neither disagree nor agree, 4 = agree to some extent, and 5 = fully agree. Higher scores indicated higher individuality in care from the patient perspective.

The ICS–Nurse and ICS–Patient versions have been previously translated and validated in various European countries with nurses of different specialties (e.g., general surgery, orthopedic surgery, maternity ward, geriatric, rehabilitation) and patients (e.g., patients from surgical, internal medicine, oncological, and gynecological wards) [28–33]. For this study, the Individualized Care Scale (ICS) was forward-translated into the Lithuanian language and back-translated into English following the methodological considerations for double translation and reconciliation [34].

To assess the psychometric properties, Cronbach's alpha was calculated for internal consistency for both scales (ICS-A and ICS-B) and 6 sub-scales of both instruments, for nurses and patients. In this study, 1 item from the sub-scales A and B (No. 17) that related to the patient's preference of washing time in a day was excluded from the Lithuanian version of the Individualized Care Scale (ICS) in the Nurse and Patient Versions, as it was not relevant for the primary health care service profile.

The 2 scales and 6 sub-scales of the Individualized Care Scale–Nurse Version (ICS–Nurse) had Cronbach's alpha (α) values ranging from 0.79 to 0.92; the Cronbach's alpha (α) for the Individualized Care Scale–Patient Version (ICS–Patient) ranged from 0.77 to 0.96, indicating appropriate (from satisfactory to excellent) internal consistency of the instrument for both samples (Table 1). When compared with the Dutch validation study, we observed that the internal consistency of the Lithuanian version of the ICS was weaker [33].

Table 1. Reliability statistics for the Lithuanian version of the Individualized Care Scale–Nurse Version (ICS–Nurse) and Patient Version (ICS–Patient).

Individualized Care Scale	Cronbach's Alpha	
	ICS–Nurse	ICS–Patient
A-ICS	0.90	0.96
A-ICS–Clinical	0.84	0.94
A-ICS–Personal	0.84	0.85
A-ICS–Decision	0.80	0.92
B_ICS	0.92	0.96
B-ICS–Clinical	0.85	0.94
B-ICS–Personal	0.79	0.77
B-ICS–Decision	0.84	0.90
Total	0.95	0.91

The Individualized Care Scale–Nurse Version (ICS–Nurse) was used for health care professionals that provide care for older diabetes patients. Even if the ICS is primarily aimed at nurses' support and provision of individualized care, we used this scale for physicians as well. By not separating physician and nurse contributions to individualized care, we argue that nurses and physicians work as a team while providing care for older patients with diabetes. Thus, the team is responsible for finding the means to assure that their care plan implements each patient's preferences and enables him/her to actively participate in their care by making decisions about their own care. Moreover, the scale items appear to be generic (not specific to only nursing activities) and ask patients to respond about general features of an individual approach to care. It is also expected that the study results will help to detect the weakest points of patient-centered care implementation for the specific population of our study, that is, older diabetes patients, and will serve as a basis for further joint educational initiatives for both physicians and nurses.

The following background data about the nurses' and physicians' characteristics were requested from the participants: age, gender, education, occupation/job title (nurse/physician), and years of professional experience. In addition, the patients were asked to provide their age, gender, education level, height and weight, type of diabetes, most recent HbA1c, and duration of illness.

2.3. Participants

Nurses and physicians (n = 126, response rate—96.9%), as well as older patients with diabetes (n = 145, response rate—72.5%), participated in the anonymous survey. The enrollment criteria for the study for nurses and physicians was the provision of care for older diabetes patients for more than one year. Every nurse and physician from the institutions involved in the study that suited the inclusion criteria were invited to participate in the study.

Among the health care professionals (N = 70), the majority were nurses (81.4%, 57) and the others were physicians (28.6%, 13). Regarding gender, all the respondents were female. The mean age of the respondents (nurses and physicians) was 48.57 ± 9.33 years (range of 24–65, median of 49.5 y.). More than half of the health care professionals (65.7%, 46) had completed higher education (university or college), and the others (34.3%, 24) had received a vocational education (nursing school with a diploma). The average duration of professional experience was 24.37 ± 10.96 years (range of 1–43); 34.3% worked in their professional practice for fewer than 20 years, and the others (65.7%, 46) for 20 years or more.

Patients were consecutively enrolled based on the following criteria: age of 65+, with a confirmed diagnosis of type 1 or type 2 diabetes mellitus, with more than 1 year of the disease's duration, having Lithuanian language reading and writing skills, and being able to comprehend the questions. Each older diabetes patient that visited a primary health care center or outpatient unit of the hospital during the study period (23 months in total) was invited to participate in the study. Those who declined to answer the questionnaire explained being busy at the time, not being interested in the study, or having vision or Lithuanian language problems. The characteristics of the patient sample are presented in Table 2.

Table 2. Characteristics of the patient sample (N = 145).

Variables	
Age (mean ± SD; median)	71.9 ± 6.2; 70.0
(Range)	65–92
Disease duration (mean ± SD)	15.7 ± 10.0
(Range)	1–46
	% (N)
Gender	
Female	59.3 (86)
Male	40.7 (59)
Age (in years)	
65–70	51.7 (75)
≥71	48.3 (70)
Education level	
Degree (university or college)	18.6 (27)
Less than degree	81.4 (118)
Place of residence	
Urban	71.7 (104)
Rural	28.3 (41)
Type of current glucose-lowering therapy	
Tablets	51.0 (74)
Insulin injections	37.9 (55)
Combined therapy (oral antidiabetics and injectable medications)	11.1 (16)
Type of diabetes mellitus	
Type 1	11.1 (16)
Type 2	88.9 (129)
Years of diabetes diagnosis	
1–10	37.9 (55)
11–20	37.9 (55)
≥21	24.2 (35)
Glucose profile (HbA1c) in %, (N = 143)	
Less than 7	44.1 (63)
7–9	43.4 (62)
>9	12.6 (18)
Body mass index, (N = 142)	
<30	47.9 (68)
≥30	52.1 (74)

2.4. Ethical Considerations

Permission to conduct the study was obtained from the Kaunas Regional Biomedical Research Ethics Committee on 13 March 2019, No. BE-2-29.

2.5. Statistical Data Analysis

The data were analyzed using the Statistical Package for Social Sciences (IBM SPSS Statistics) version 25.0. To assess the psychometric properties of the scale, Cronbach's alpha was calculated for the internal consistency of the individual items and the sub-scales; the internal consistency of $\alpha > 0.6$ was considered to be acceptable [35].

The results were presented in percentages for the qualitative variables and the means with standard deviation (SD) were calculated for the quantitative variables. For the ICS, the higher the mean scores, the better patient individuality was supported (ICS-A–Nurse) and the higher the perceptions were of the maintenance of individuality in care (ICS-B–Nurse).

The nonparametric Kolmogorov–Smirnov normality test was used to test the normal distribution of the data. As normality was absent, the nonparametric Mann–Whitney U test was used to compare the distributions of the quantitative variables for the independent groups. The Wilcoxon signed-ranks test was applied to compare the results from the 2 ICS dimensions. The significance of the differences was defined by a p-value of <0.05.

3. Results

At the sub-scale level, health professionals scored the perception of individual care provided to the patient (B-ICS–Clinical) (mean 4.17) and views on support to the patient (A-ICS–Clinical) (mean 4.13) at clinical situations as the highest. The lowest professionals' and patients' scores in both domains (support and provision) of individualized care were associated with the patient's personal life situation (Table 3). Accordingly, the highest means of patients' ratings of individualized care in the support dimension related to the clinical situation (mean of 3.55) and decisions related to care (mean of 5.54) sub-scales. For the care provision dimension, the highest individuality in care from the patients' perspective was related to the decisions over care domain (mean of 3.65). Moreover, the ratings of support for individualized care and such care provision were significantly higher for the health professionals than for the patients in each sub-scale of the ICS (Table 3).

Table 3. Health professionals' and patients' assessments of individualized care at the ICS dimension and sub-scale level.

Individualized Care Scale—ICS	Health Professionals Mean (SD)	Patients Mean (SD)	p
A-ICS (Total)	4.00 (0.54)	3.51 (0.92)	<0.001
A-ICS–Clinical	4.13 (0.55)	3.55 (1.00)	<0.001
A-ICS–Personal	3.82 (0.78)	3.40 (1.03)	0.008
A-ICS–Decision	3.99 (0.55)	3.54 (0.97)	0.003
B-ICS (Total)	4.08 (0.54)	3.58 (8.71)	<0.001
B-ICS–Clinical	4.17 (0.51)	3.60 (0.92)	<0.001
B-ICS–Personal	3.95 (0.60)	3.45 (0.95)	<0.001
B-ICS–Decision	4.06 (0.61)	3.65 (0.92)	0.003

At the ICS item level, significant differences between the health professionals' and patients' perspectives towards the support of individuality in care were determined for the majority of the items (Part A); the scores of the health professionals were higher than those of the patients (Table 4). In contrast, no differences were revealed in the answers about previous experiences of hospitalization and patients' participation in decision making.

Regarding the support scorings, the health professionals' and patients' perspectives on the provision of individual care for older patients also varied significantly; the professionals were more positive in their answers than the patients were (Table 5). The nurses and physicians thought similarly to the patients only in the cases of the patients' chance to take responsibility as far as possible and their knowledge preferences (what they want to know about illness/health condition).

A comparative analysis of ratings among health professionals revealed statistically significant differences between the two dimensions of the ICS, that is, the professionals' views on support to the patient through care activities and the professionals' perception of individual care provided to the patients. The differences were related to the personal life situation and the decisional control over care sub-scales; the health professionals' ratings of provision were significantly higher than those for support ($p = 0.046$ and $p = 0.037$, respectively, based on the Wilcoxon test).

Within the health professionals' sample, there were no differences in the scores (neither at the dimension nor at the sub-scale level) of individualized care between physicians and nurses. The sociodemographic characteristics in the total sample of health professionals did not make any differences for individualized care scores as well.

As all the physicians (N = 13) had a higher university education, we separately analyzed the nurses' (N = 57) ratings on the ICS sub-scales in relation to their education.

Nurses who take care of older diabetes patients and who have had vocational education scored support for individual care (Part A) with significantly higher scores than nurses with a college education (the means were 4.11 and 3.68, $p = 0.039$, respectively,). In addition, it was observed that the tendency for nurses with a university education rated provision (Part B) higher than nurses with a college education; the means were 4.16 and 3.66, $p = 0.052$, respectively.

Several factors made a difference in the perception of individual care in older patients with diabetes. The highest differences in diabetes patients' assessments of individualized care dimensions and sub-scales were observed in relation to the current type of glucose-lowering therapy. Patients with combined therapy rated each sub-scale of the provision dimension and particular sub-scales of the support dimension of individual care significantly higher than those with oral or injectable medications (Table 6).

Table 4. Health professionals' and patients' assessments of the support of patient individuality: item-level analysis.

Items of the Individualized Care Scale	Health Professionals (Mean (SD))	Patients (Mean (SD))	p
	Clinical situation		
A01—Feelings about illness/health condition	4.21 (0.83)	3.54 (1.16)	<0.001
A02—Needs that require care and attention	4.27 (0.74)	3.66 (1.11)	<0.001
A0—Chance to take responsibility as far as possible	4.16 (0.65)	3.62 (1.17)	0.002
A04—Identify changes in how they have felt	4.21 (0.56)	3.59 (1.14)	<0.001
A05—Talk with patients about fears and anxieties	4.03 (0.79)	3.39 (1.23)	<0.001
A06—Find out how their health conditions affect them	4.07 (0.68)	3.55 (1.15)	0.003
A07—What the illness/health condition means to them	3.96 (0.89)	3.54 (1.16)	0.018
	Personal life situation		
A08—What kinds of things they do in their everyday life	3.87 (0.91)	3.49 (1.16)	0.040
A09—Previous experience of hospitalization	3.63 (0.95)	3.39 (1.15)	0.252
A10—Everyday habits	3.86 (0.92)	3.41 (1.21)	0.011
A11—Family take part in their care	3.94 (0.88)	3.35 (1.14)	<0.001
	Decisional control over care		
A12—Instructions to patients	4.31 (0.64)	3.67 (1.18)	<0.001
A13—What they want to know about illness/health condition	4.21 (0.72)	3.66 (1.20)	0.003
A14—Patients' personal wishes with regards to their care	3.96 (0.75)	3.59 (1.07)	0.021
A15—Help patients take part in decisions	4.00 (0.68)	3.66 (1.06)	0.064
A16—Encourage patients to express their opinions	4.06 (0.83)	3.59 (1.10)	0.003

Table 5. Health professionals and patients' assessments of the provision of individualized care: item-level analysis.

Items of the Individualized Care Scale	Health Professionals (Mean (SD))	Patients (Mean (SD))	p
	Clinical situation		
B01—Feelings about illness/health condition	4.13 (0.65)	3.58 (1.02)	<0.001
B02—Needs that require care and attention	4.20 (0.62)	3.71 (1.03)	0.001
B03—Chance to take responsibility as far as possible	4.03 (0.65)	3.69 (1.07)	0.061
B04—Identify changes in how they have felt	4.27 (0.58)	3.64 (1.09)	<0.001
B05—Talk with patients about fears and anxieties	4.19 (0.64)	3.50 (1.14)	<0.001
B06—Find out how their health conditions affect them	4.26 (0.69)	3.52 (1.05)	<0.001
B07—What the illness/health condition means to them	4.19 (0.68)	3.68 (1.07)	0.001
	Personal life situation		
B08—What kinds of things they do in their everyday life	3.96 (0.75)	3.57 (1.04)	0.014
B09—Previous experience of hospitalization	3.77 (0.72)	3.43 (1.12)	0.045
B10—Everyday habits	3.99 (0.73)	3.47 (1.10)	0.001
B11—Family take part in their care	4.10 (0.78)	3.40 (1.18)	<0.001
	Decisional control over care		
B12—Instructions to patients	4.20 (0.75)	3.82 (1.05)	0.018
B13—What they want to know about illness/health condition	4.13 (0.74)	3.84 (1.03)	0.103
B14—Patients' personal wishes with regards to their care	4.10 (0.68)	3.66 (1.03)	0.002
B15—Help patients take part in decisions	4.09 (0.67)	3.63 (1.06)	0.002
B16—Encourage patients to express their opinions	4.10 (0.70)	3.67 (1.04)	0.003

In addition, patients with lower than a degree education level rated the support dimension (Part A) higher than those with a college or university education; the means were 3.60 and 3.12, $p = 0.032$, respectively.

Body mass index (BMI) was also a variable that resulted in variations in the patients' perceptions of support for individual care. Older diabetes patients with a BMI of <30 rated the support dimension significantly lower than patients with a BMI of ≥ 30; the means for Part A of the ICS were 3.34 and 3.68 respectively ($p = 0.032$).

Moreover, a tendency was observed in relation to the patients' ages and their opinions on individual care; patients of 71 years and over rated the support for their personal life situation (A-ICS–Personal) higher than those who were 70 years old or below ($p = 0.054$).

Table 6. Patients' assessments of individualized care at the ICS dimension and sub-scale levels in relation to the current type of glucose-lowering therapy.

Individualized Care Scale—ICS	Type of Therapy	Mean Rank	p *	Type of Therapy	Mean Rank	p *
A-ICS (Total)	1 3	43.07 56.75	0.057	2 3	33.92 43.16	0.115
A-ICS–Clin	1 3	43.33 55.53	0.089	2 3	34.19 42.22	0.170
A-ICS–Pers	1 3	42.77 58.13	0.032	2 3	33.89 43.25	0.108
A-ICS–Dec	1 3	42.92 57.44	0.043	2 3	33.55 44.41	0.063
B-ICS (Total)	1 3	42.20 60.75	0.010	2 3	32.98 43.16	0.048
B-ICS–Clin	1 3	42.43 59.69	0.016	2 3	33.39 44.97	0.022
B-ICS–Pers	1 3	42.59 58.97	0.022	2 3	32.99 46.34	0.034
B-ICS–Dec	1 3	42.42 59.75	0.016	2 3	33.21 45.59	0.022

* Mann–Whitney U test; 1—tablets ($n = 74$), 2—insulin injections ($n = 55$), 3—combined ($n = 16$).

4. Discussion

A patient-centered approach to care sees individuals as active recipients of health care provision. Patients are expected to collaborate with medical professionals, discuss their clinical and life situations, and make decisions related to their care plan. Health professionals (nurses and physicians) taking care of older diabetes patients in the Lithuanian primary health care organization had an opinion that they support patient individuality, in general, and provide care that takes into account the particular patient's situation. The highest scores from the professionals' perspective were for the support and provision of individual care in regard to the clinical situation of the patient. These results generally correspond to the comparative cross-cultural study on individualized nursing care in seven countries [31]. Very similar nurses' positive perceptions of individualized care, especially for the clinical situation and patients' decisional control over care, were also found by Finnish researchers [36].

Notably, patients in our study rated the support for individual care higher than patients from internal medicine and surgical units of teaching hospitals in Turkey, although the results of both studies correspond in regard to the patients' ratings of the personal life situation aspect of the support dimension, where the mean was the lowest [32]. Similar to a study on orthopedic and trauma patients [37], the personal life preferences of the patient were also at least discussed during care provision for the Lithuanian older diabetes patients from both patients' and health professionals' points of view.

In all cases, the ratings of support for individualized care and such care provision through care activities were significantly higher for the health professionals than for the patients. An international study among five European countries revealed similar differences in patients' and nurses' assessments of individualized nursing, where nurses, compared with patients, assessed that they supported patient individuality more often [30]. In Lithuania, the data about chronically ill patients' preferences and readiness for active participation in care and in decision-making, particularly, is scarce and creates difficulties for a valid interpretation of the current results. The arguments for a lower rating of individual care support and provision in the patient sample might be twofold: either they wish but lack actual possibilities to participate, discuss, and make decisions, or their understanding and knowledge about such possibilities is incomplete and they are not even motivated to be an active participant in their care. Such an interpretation is consistent with the findings of du Pon et al. (2019), in which patients with diabetes were found to have limited necessary skills to be adequately prepared for a consultation and achieve an active role [22]. In prior research on the preferences and participation in decision-making among patients with Parkinson's disease, the authors suggest that in some contexts or situations, patients prefer less autonomy in medical decision-making and choose shared decisions, or even find it acceptable to be excluded from decision-making as their illness worsens. Some patients preferred to make the final decision, some wanted the decision-making process to be evenly shared, while others preferred to delegate final decisions to the doctor [2]. Further research applying a rigorous quantitative and qualitative design to larger populations of diabetes patients is recommended. Future work should also address how different groups of patients understand and prefer individuality in care, and how this care is linked with other relevant factors.

The ratings of individual care for the ICS dimensions and sub-scales did not vary among health professionals in regard to their qualification, that is, being a nurse or physician. Although, education level made a difference in how nurses comprehend and practice their individual approach in the care of older diabetes patients, as the nurses with a vocational education were more positive and rated higher individual care proposed and provided for the older diabetes patients than the college degree nurses. These results are in contrast with those of Suhonen et al., (2009) who found that higher scores supporting the delivery of individualized care could have been expected from nurses with higher education [38]. Such results may be explained by the differences that were introduced in the nursing curriculum in the last decade, when nursing education was elevated from a diploma to a college or university-based system. As a condition for membership in the European Union (EU), nursing programs were harmonized with the EU requirements, which caused remarkable transitions of nursing education from a strongly biomedical, technical approach toward a more sensitive, patient-centered, holistic approach to care [39]. We propose that higher educated nurses are well equipped with the knowledge of modern nursing and have a clearer vision of what care should be in relation to safeguarding the patient's individuality. This is the reason they are more critical in assessing the current situation, which is lacking a full integration of the patient-centered approach in older diabetes patient care practice.

Our results revealed that patients with combined glucose-lowering therapy rated some aspects of support and all the aspects of the provision of individuality in their care higher than those patients who were treated by oral or injectable medications. We propose that a complex type of treatment requires the physicians and nurses to give more attention to an individual patient's case through collecting health information, assessing health status, instructing, and educating. In addition, the integration and monitoring of patient-reported outcomes facilitates holistic interdisciplinary care and takes into account patient-relevant endpoints [40]. Such a relatively prolonged communication and going into the situation creates for the patient an impression of greater consideration for his or her particular case. A similar interpretation might be true in regard to the body mass index, as diabetes patients with a BMI of ≥ 30 had more positive opinions about individual care support than those patients with a lower BMI.

Patients' perceptions of individualized nursing care are related to their education level. In our study, older diabetes patients with a lower than degree education level rated the support dimension (Part A) higher than those with a college or university education. Other researchers similarly reported that a lower educational level is associated with a perception of more individualized care in patients [36,41].

The findings of this study provide the initial evidence of the perception and provision of the individualized care approach to the care of older diabetes patients. For improvements in clinical practice and fostering the actual implementation of a patient-centered approach of care, complex means would be the most effective for unifying professional, organizational, and policy development. The research showed that older patients' perceptions of individuality in care were associated with the care environment, especially a patient-centered care climate [42]. In order to be responsible in personal care decisions and adhere to health recommendations (e.g., medications, nutrition, and physical activity), patients require adequate 'education and support they need to make decisions and participate in their own care' [1], p. 7. It might be assumed that continuous patient–provider communication, regular contact, and careful consideration of individual values, knowledge, habits, and behaviors motivate and empower older and chronically ill patients to change. Further continuing education of physicians and nurses, joining them in one class and with the same teaching content, would help to expand their unified understanding of patient-centered care components, principles, and practical implementation in caring for older diabetes patients.

This study was one of the first attempts to study individual patient care in our country. For further research, physicians' and nurses' work environment characteristics that can also affect the provision of individualized have to be considered [43]. There are more factors of the professional practice environment found that correlate with the nurses' perceptions about the support of individuality and their views on the individual care provided [44]. This means that for a real shift toward an individual approach to care, health care institutions need to expand their philosophy of service to support the new roles of care providers and consumers at an organizational level.

This study has several limitations. Firstly, the Individualized Care Scale–Nurse Version (ICS–Nurse) was initially developed and validated to assess nurses' points of view about individual care support and the provision of such care through nursing activities, particularly. The evidence for the validation of this scale among other health care professionals is lacking and should be separately addressed in further studies. Secondly, the construct of the scale (a bipartite structure with a rather similar wording of items for both dimensions) may influence the clear comprehension and accuracy of the responses when applying it to older persons with chronic illnesses. Specific considerations would be important during the selection of an appropriate data collection method (e.g., a structural face-to-face interview instead of a survey). Thirdly, the sample size of patients was small and has a limited representation of only the institutions involved in the study. The study is lacking generalizability across settings and countries; wider studies are recommended for the future, including older diabetes patients with experiences of inpatient settings as well. Finally, half of the data collection was conducted during the pandemic period when a rather large extent of routine health care services for chronically ill patients were suspended or provided by different means (e.g., phone calls). This fact should be taken into consideration when interpreting and comparing the results of this study with any other sources.

5. Conclusions

Health professionals have a more positive perception in regard to individualized care support and provision for older diabetes patients than the patients themselves. Individual personal life preferences of the patient are at least discussed during care provisions for the older diabetes patients from both health professionals' and patients' points of view. Patient characteristics, such as the type of glucose-lowering therapy, education, and body mass index, make a difference for older diabetes patients in their understanding and experience of individuality in care.

A change needs to be made to provide better individualized care for older diabetes patients, and the next steps would be to interview patients to see how the care can be improved and what will motivate patients to be more active in their care planning and implementation. Careful consideration of individual patients' values, knowledge, habits, and behaviors would assist and assure that their personal life situation is taken into account during care processes.

Author Contributions: Conceptualization, B.B., V.L. and O.R.; methodology, B.B. and O.R.; software, B.B.; formal analysis, B.B.; investigation, B.B.; data curation, B.B.; writing—original draft preparation, B.B.; writing—review and editing, V.L. and O.R.; visualization, B.B.; supervision, V.L. All authors have read and agreed to the published version of the manuscript.

Funding: This research received no external funding.

Institutional Review Board Statement: The study was conducted according to the guidelines of the Declaration of Helsinki, and approved by the Kaunas Regional Biomedical Research Ethics Committee on 13 March 2019, No. BE-2-29.

Informed Consent Statement: Informed consent was obtained from all subjects involved in the study.

Acknowledgments: The authors acknowledge Patti Hamilton, Texas Woman's University for her valuable critical comments on the manuscript and her help with English language editing.

Conflicts of Interest: The authors declare no conflict of interest.

References

1. WHO. WHO Global Strategy on People-Centred and Integrated Health Services. 2021. Available online: https://apps.who.int/iris/bitstream/handle/10665/155002/WHO_HIS_SDS_2015.6_eng.pdf?sequence=1 (accessed on 29 May 2021).
2. Zizzo, N.; Bell, E.; Lafontaine, A.; Racine, E. Examining chronic care patient preferences for involvement in health-care decision making: The case of Parkinson's disease patients in a patient-centred clinic. *Health Expect.* **2016**, *20*, 655–664. [CrossRef]
3. Rice, H.; Say, R.; Betihavas, V. The effect of nurse-led education on hospitalization, readmission, quality of life and cost in adults with heart failure. A systematic review. *Patient Educ. Couns.* **2018**, *101*, 363–374. [CrossRef] [PubMed]
4. Cui, X.; Zhou, X.; Ma, L.; Sun, T.; Bishop, L.; Gardiner, F.W.; Wang, L. A nurse-led structured education program improves self-management skills and reduces hospital readmissions in patients with chronic heart failure: A randomized and controlled trial in China. *Rural. Remote. Health* **2019**, *19*, 5270. [CrossRef]
5. Joo, J.; Liu, M. Effectiveness of Nurse-Led Case Management in Cancer Care: Systematic Review. *Clin. Nurs. Res.* **2018**, *28*, 968–991. [CrossRef] [PubMed]
6. Joo, J.; Liu, M. Case management effectiveness for managing chronic illnesses in Korea: A systematic review. *Int. Nurs. Rev.* **2018**, *66*, 30–42. [CrossRef]
7. Joo, J.Y.; Huber, D.L. Community-based case management effectiveness in populations that abuse substances: Effectiveness of community-based case management. *Int. Nurs. Rev.* **2015**, *62*, 536–546. [CrossRef] [PubMed]
8. Karam, M.; Chouinard, M.-C.; Poitras, M.-E.; Couturier, Y.; Vedel, I.; Grgurevic, N.; Hudon, C. Nursing care coordination for patients with complex needs in primary healthcare: A scoping review. *Int. J. Integr. Care* **2021**, *21*, 16. [CrossRef]
9. Lin, X.; Xu, Y.; Pan, X.; Xu, J.; Ding, Y.; Sun, X.; Song, X.; Ren, Y.; Shan, P.-F. Global, regional, and national burden and trend of diabetes in 195 countries and territories: An analysis from 1990 to 2025. *Sci. Rep.* **2020**, *10*, 1–11. [CrossRef]
10. Higienos Institutas Stat. Hi. Lt. Available online: https://stat.hi.lt/default.aspx?report_id=256 (accessed on 28 May 2021).
11. Giorda, C.B.; Manicardi, V.; Diago Cabezudo, J. The impact of diabetes mellitus on healthcare costs in Italy. *Expert. Rev. Pharm. Outcomes Res.* **2011**, *11*, 709–719. [CrossRef]
12. Domeikienė, A.; Vaivadaitė, J.; Ivanauskienė, R.; Padaiga, Ž. Direct cost of patients with type 2 diabetes mellitus healthcare and its complications in Lithuania. *Medicina* **2014**, *50*, 54–60. [CrossRef]
13. Jaén, C.R.; Ferrer, R.L.; Miller, W.L.; Palmer, R.F.; Wood, R.; Davila, M.; Stewart, E.E.; Crabtree, B.F.; Nutting, P.A.; Stange, K.C. Patient outcomes at 26 months in the patient-centered medical home National Demonstration Project. *Ann. Fam. Med.* **2010**, *8* (Suppl. 1), S57–S67. [CrossRef]
14. Beach, M.C.; Keruly, J.; Moore, R.D. Is the quality of the patient-provider relationship associated with better adherence and health outcomes for patients with HIV? *J. Gen. Intern. Med.* **2006**, *21*, 661–665. [CrossRef] [PubMed]
15. Bertakis, K.D.; Azari, R. Patient-centered care is associated with decreased health care utilization. *J. Am. Board Fam. Med.* **2011**, *24*, 229–239. [CrossRef]
16. Carroll, K. Bringing nursing care to patients living with diabetes mellitus. *Nurs. Sci. Q.* **2019**, *32*, 187–188. [CrossRef]
17. Araújo, E.S.S.; Silva, L.F.; Moreira, T.M.M.; Almeida, P.C.; Freitas, M.C.; Guedes, M.V.C. Nursing care to patients with diabetes based on King's Theory. *Rev. Bras. Enferm.* **2018**, *71*, 1092–1098. [CrossRef]
18. Karota, E.; Marlindawani Purba, J.; Simamora, R.H.; Lufthiani Siregar, C.T. Use of King's theory to improve diabetics self-care behavior. *Enferm. Clin.* **2020**, *30* (Suppl. 3), 95–99. [CrossRef] [PubMed]
19. Husband, A. Application of King's Theory of Nursing to the care of the adult with diabetes. *J. Adv. Nurs.* **1988**, *13*, 484–488. [CrossRef] [PubMed]
20. V-337 Dėl Lietuvos Respublikos Sveikatos Apsaugos Ministro 2008 m. Spalio 10 d. Įsakymo Nr. V-982. [Oder of the Minister of the Health of the Republic of Lithuania on 10th October, 2008, No. V-982). Available online: https://e-seimas.lrs.lt/portal/legalAct/lt/TAD/TAIS.396536?jfwid=-15kurkg48i (accessed on 28 May 2021).
21. De la Fuente Coria, M.C.; Cruz-Cobo, C.; Santi-Cano, M.J. Effectiveness of a primary care nurse delivered educational intervention for patients with type 2 diabetes mellitus in promoting metabolic control and compliance with long-term therapeutic targets: Randomised controlled trial. *Int. J. Nurs. Stud.* **2020**, *101*, 103417. [CrossRef] [PubMed]
22. du Pon, E.; Wildeboer, A.T.; van Dooren, A.A.; Bilo, H.J.G.; Kleefstra, N.; van Dulmen, S. Active participation of patients with type 2 diabetes in consultations with their primary care practice nurses—what helps and what hinders: A qualitative study. *BMC Health Serv. Res.* **2019**, *19*, 814. [CrossRef]

23. Fix, G.M.; VanDeusen Lukas, C.; Bolton, R.E.; Hill, J.N.; Mueller, N.; LaVela, S.L.; Bokhour, B.G. Patient-centred care is a way of doing things: How healthcare employees conceptualize patient-centred care. *Health Expect.* **2018**, *21*, 300–307. [CrossRef]
24. Gluyas, H. Patient-centred care: Improving healthcare outcomes. *Nurs. Stand.* **2015**, *30*, 50–57. [CrossRef]
25. Wong, E.; Mavondo, F.; Fisher, J. Patient feedback to improve quality of patient-centred care in public hospitals: A systematic review of the evidence. *BMC Health Serv. Res.* **2020**, *20*, 530. [CrossRef]
26. Suhonen, R. *Individualized Care from the Surgical Patient's Point of View. Developing and Testing a Model. Annales Universitatis Turkuensis D 523*; University of Turku: Turku, Finland, 2002.
27. Suhonen, R.; Leino-Kilpi, H.; Välimäki, M. Development and psychometric properties of the Individualized Care Scale. *J. Eval. Clin. Pract.* **2005**, *11*, 7–20. [CrossRef]
28. Suhonen, R.; Schmidt, L.A.; Radwin, L. Measuring individualized nursing care: Assessment of reliability and validity of three scales. *J. Adv. Nurs.* **2007**, *59*, 77–85. [CrossRef] [PubMed]
29. Suhonen, R.; Gustafsson, M.-L.; Katajisto, J.M.V.; Leino-Kilpi, H. Individualized Care Scale—Nurse version: A Finnish validation study. *J. Eval. Clin. Pract.* **2010**, *16*, 145–154. [CrossRef] [PubMed]
30. Suhonen, R.; Efstathiou, G.; Tsangari, H.; Jarosova, D.; Leino-Kilpi, H.; Patiraki, E.; Karlou, C.; Balogh, Z.; Papastavrou, E. Patients' and nurses' perceptions of individualized care: An international comparative study: Individualized care—An international study. *J. Clin. Nurs.* **2012**, *21*, 1155–1167. [CrossRef]
31. Suhonen, R.; Papastavrou, E.; Efstathiou, G.; Lemonidou, C.; Kalafati, M.; da Luz, M.D.A.; Idvall, E.; Berg, A.; Acaroglu, R.; Sendir, M.; et al. Nurses' perceptions of individualized care: An international comparison: Nurses' perceptions of individualized care. *J. Adv. Nurs.* **2011**, *67*, 1895–1907. [CrossRef] [PubMed]
32. Rasooli, A.; Zamanzadeh, V.; Rahmani, A.; Shahbazpoor, M. Patients' Point of View about Nurses' Support of Individualized Nursing Care in Training Hospitals Affiliated with Tabriz University of Medical Sciences. *J. Caring Sci.* **2013**, *2*, 203–209.
33. Theys, S.; Van Hecke, A.; Akkermans, R.; Heinen, M. The Dutch Individualised Care Scale for patients and nurses—A psychometric validation study. *Scandinavian J. Caring Sci.* **2021**, *35*, 308–318. [CrossRef]
34. Maneesriwongul, W.; Dixon, J.K. Instrument translation process: A methods review. *J. Adv. Nurs.* **2004**, *48*, 175–186. [CrossRef]
35. Bland, J.M.; Altman, D.G. Statistics notes: Cronbach's alpha. *BMJ* **1997**, *314*, 572. [CrossRef] [PubMed]
36. Land, L.; Suhonen, R. Orthopaedic and trauma patients' perceptions of individualized care. *Int Nurs Rev.* **2009**, *56*, 131–137. [CrossRef] [PubMed]
37. Suhonen, R.; Gustafsson, M.; Katajisto, J.; Välimäki, M.; Leino-Kilpi, H. Nurses' perceptions of individualized care. *J. Adv. Nurs.* **2010**, *66*, 1035–1046. [CrossRef]
38. Suhonen, R.; Välimäki, M.; Leino-Kilpi, H. The driving and restraining forces that promote and impede the implementation of individualised nursing care: A literature review. *Int. J. Nurs. Stud.* **2009**, *46*, 1637–1649. [CrossRef]
39. Riklikiene, O.; Vozgirdiene, I.; Karosas, L.M.; Lazenby, M. Spiritual care as perceived by Lithuanian student nurses and nurse educators: A national survey. *Nurse Educ. Today* **2016**, *36*, 207–213. [CrossRef]
40. Romeyke, T.; Noehammer, E.; Stummer, H. Patient-Reported Outcomes Following Inpatient Multimodal Treatment Approach in Chronic Pain-Related Rheumatic Diseases. *Glob. Adv. Health Med.* **2020**, *9*, 216495612094881. [CrossRef] [PubMed]
41. Köberich, S.; Feuchtinger, J.; Farin, E. Factors influencing hospitalized patients' perception of individualized nursing care: A cross-sectional study. *BMC Nurs.* **2016**, *15*, 14. [CrossRef]
42. Stolt, M.; Koskenvuori, J.; Edvardsson, D.; Katajisto, J.; Suhonen, R. Validation of the Finnish Person-Centered care Climate Questionnaire-Patient and testing the relationship with individualized care. *Int. J. Older People Nurs.* **2021**, *16*, e12356. [CrossRef]
43. Suhonen, R.; Charalambous, A.; Stolt, M.; Katajisto, J.; Puro, M. Caregivers' work satisfaction and individualized care in care settings for older people: Work satisfaction and individualized care. *J. Clin. Nurs.* **2013**, *22*, 479–490. [CrossRef]
44. Charalambous, A.; Katajisto, J.; Välimäki, M.; Leino-Kilpi, H.; Suhonen, R. Individualized care and the professional practice environment: Nurses' perceptions: Individualized care and practice environment. *Int. Nurs. Rev.* **2010**, *57*, 500–507. [CrossRef] [PubMed]

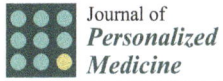

Article

Validation of the Patient-Centred Care Competency Scale Instrument for Finnish Nurses

Riitta Suhonen [1,2,3,*], Katja Lahtinen [1,4], Minna Stolt [1], Miko Pasanen [1] and Terhi Lemetti [1,5]

1. Department of Nursing Science, University of Turku, 20014 Turku, Finland; katlahz@utu.fi (K.L.); minna.stolt@utu.fi (M.S.); misapas@utu.fi (M.P.); terhi.lemetti@hus.fi (T.L.)
2. Turku University Hospital, 20014 Turku, Finland
3. City of Turku Welfare Division, 20014 Turku, Finland
4. City of Helsinki, Department of Social and Health Care, 00099 Helsinki, Finland
5. University Hospital, 00029 Helsinki, Finland
* Correspondence: riisuh@utu.fi; Tel.: +358-50-435-0662

Abstract: Patient-centredness in care is a core healthcare value and an effective healthcare delivery design requiring specific nurse competences. The aim of this study was to assess (1) the reliability, validity, and sensitivity of the Finnish version of the Patient-centred Care Competency (PCC) scale and (2) Finnish nurses' self-assessed level of patient-centred care competency. The PCC was translated to Finnish (PCC-Fin) before data collection and analyses: descriptive statistics; Cronbach's alpha coefficients; item analysis; exploratory and confirmatory factor analyses; inter-scale correlational analysis; and sensitivity. Cronbach's alpha coefficients were acceptable, high for the total scale, and satisfactory for the four sub-scales. Item analysis supported the internal homogeneity of the items-to-total and inter-items within the sub-scales. Explorative factor analysis suggested a three-factor solution, but the confirmatory factor analysis confirmed the four-factor structure (Tucker–Lewis index (TLI) 0.92, goodness-of-fit index (GFI) 0.99, root mean square error of approximation (RMSEA) 0.065, standardized root mean square residual (SRMR) 0.045) with 61.2% explained variance. Analysis of the secondary data detected no differences in nurses' self-evaluations of contextual competence, so the inter-scale correlations were high. The PCC-Fin was found to be a reliable and valid instrument for the measurement of nurses' patient-centred care competence. Rasch model analysis would provide some further information about the item level functioning within the instrument.

Keywords: patient-centred care; competence; assessment; instrument; measurement; validity; reliability

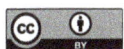

1. Introduction

Patient-centeredness in care has been reported to be a core health care value [1,2], and the optimal design for the delivery of healthcare [3,4] requiring specific competences from healthcare professionals [5,6]. Patient-centred care has also been found to be a healthcare core competency [7]. This core competency describes the professionals' ability to identify patient expectations, preferences, and values, facilitating joint decision making, and acting with individual patients to deliver safe, effective, and compassionate care [8]. Patient-centred care is, therefore, a care approach which considers individual patient's specific care needs [4,9,10] and is regarded as patients' preferred care delivery process [11,12]. Importantly, patient-centeredness in care has been used as an attribute and indicator of quality [2,13] and patient safety [6], especially in the interaction between the patient and care provider [14].

The concept of patient-centred care is multidimensional, and includes domains at the individual, human level and at organizational levels [2,4,15–17]. The concepts of patient-centred care and person-centred care have been used interchangeably in the literature, e.g., [18], and defined in many ways. However, regardless of the particular title, the concepts include very similar core elements, with elements specific to professional groups in healthcare. Scholl and colleagues [18] (p. 1), in their model of patient-centredness in professionals and healthcare, identified 15 dimensions: "essential characteristics of the clinician; the clinician-patient relationship; clinician-patient communication; the patient as a unique person; the biopsychosocial perspective; patient information; patient involvement in care; involvement of family and friends; patient empowerment; physical support; emotional support; the integration of medical and non-medical care; teamwork and teambuilding; access to care; and the coordination and continuity of care".

The difference between the concepts may be the intent of the focus on or viewpoint to ill-health issues or patient as a person, or the balance on these. However, the approach, typical in nursing is bringing the person to the centre of care, seeing the individual, trying to maintain their personhood, and valuing their personal experiences of life in relations with others in their social environment [19,20].

Competence has typically been defined in terms of "complex combinations of knowledge, skills, performance, attitudes and values" [20,21]. However, there seems to be no consensus about the meaning of these terms within the nursing profession [21–23]. Demonstrating this complexity further, both subjective (self-assessment) and objective (knowledge test and simulations) evaluations of competence have been used to assess competence. This complexity and lack of consensus is not surprising as assessing competence is many-sided, and rarely comprehensive [24].

Competence has been assessed and measured as a behavioural objective, within a psychological construct which includes decision-making and justifications for actions. In these assessments the self-assessing individuals justify their preferences and activities against defined, predetermined criteria. Measuring competence using self-assessment and standard instruments in this behavioural context has been criticized as reductionism, simplifying the assessed issues, dividing the complex processes of healthcare activities into single tasks, or sets of tasks, activities, and targets [24]. Helpfully, competence has also been divided into professional competence [25,26] and clinical competence, e.g., [27,28]. In a similarly helpful way, patient-centred care has also been separated into care competence needed by all professionals and specific competence, being context specific [29] and possibly varying between individual professionals [26]. As with general competence, the patient-centered care competence has been found to be multidimensional and can be conceptualised and operationalised in multiple ways [6].

Although the concept of patient-centred care has been used for many years and is considered widely to be fundamental for individualised healthcare [30,31], the competence requirements for such care provision remain largely undefined. Although empirical studies about patient-centred care competence are limited [6] these studies have pointed out the clear need for a special competence required for the provision of patient-centred care [5,6]. It follows that the assessment of patient-centred care competence forms the basis of support for the development and enhancement of patient-centred clinical care provision by nurses for patients [6]. The Patient-centred Care Competency (PCC) instrument was developed for measuring professional nurses' competence in the delivery of patient-centred care in hospitals [6]. Within the PCC instrument, patient-centred care competence is defined in terms of knowledge, skills, and attitudes [6] (p. 45) and applies components from the Quality and Safety Education for Nurses (QSEN) faculty study [32]. The QSEN study [32] included the following components of competence for nurses: patient-centred care, advance event management, contributions to patient safety culture, effective communication, optimisation of human and environmental factors, risk management, and teamwork. The results of this study and the work of Hwang [6], formulating the PCC instrument, suggests that assessment could be based around the use of core competencies for nursing professionals including patient-centred care, as defined in terms of earlier literature, e.g., [11,19,33–36]. Thus, the PCC instrument includes assessment of the knowledge, skills and attitudes required in terms of respecting patients' perspectives; promoting patient involvement in care processes; providing for patient comfort; and advocating for patients [6].

The aim of this current study was to assess (1) the reliability, validity, and sensitivity of the Finnish version of the PCC scale and (2) the self-assessed level of patient-centred care competency in two samples of Finnish nurses.

2. Materials and Methods

2.1. Design, Setting and Sampling

The assessment of the PCC uses the data from two earlier studies as secondary data where the PCC was used. These two studies employed cross-sectional survey designs and used the PCC instrument [6] (with permission from Hwang, also from Elsevier) as part of them. These separate datasets, labelled Dataset 1 and Dataset 2, were used to analyse the psychometric properties of the PCC, not fully reported previously.

Dataset 1 was collected electronically, between October 2016 and January 2017, from registered nurses working in one major university hospital in Southern Finland using self-administered questionnaires. Digitally delivered questionnaires were used in one organisation, with the assistance of the member of the organisation. Nurses were recruited with the help of nurse managers, who emailed the information letter and a link to the survey to potential participants. Inclusion criteria for participation were that respondents would: (1) be a registered nurse (RN) and (2) work in an acute hospital in-patient unit that cares for older patients. The researcher, together with the nurse managers, identified the units where older people form most of the patients cared for in the unit, including internal medicine units. In total 770 invitations were sent to a convenience sample of RNs working in 14 in-patient units, 223 nurses responded giving the response rate of 29%. The respondents' mean age was 38.9 (standard deviation (SD) 11.6, range 23–64) and most of the respondents were female (n = 206). The highest level of nurse education was registered nurse (college or baccalaureate, n = 210). A few of the respondents had a master's degree in nursing (n = 4) or had taken postgraduate classes in nursing (n = 9). The mean length of the work experience in the nurses' current employment was 7.6 years (SD 7.3, range 0.1–35).

Dataset 2 was collected in written form, between October 2017 and June 2018 from nurses working in a University hospital and in primary health care units in Southern Finland. Paper-pencil format was the only useful technique as many organisations participated and access to study sites was demanding due to many participating organisations. A cluster sampling approach was used to recruit nurses from one university hospital (hospital) and two major cities (primary health care) offering care for older people in Finland. Respondents were informed about the study verbally and in writing. If the respondents were interested in participating in the study, they completed the paper questionnaire by hand, sealed it in an envelope and sent it to the researcher by mail. A total of 1435 questionnaires were delivered to potential respondents from 41 units in the university hospital and 19 units in primary health care: health centres: (n = 13); long-term care units (n = 2); home care (n = 2); and city hospitals (n = 2).

A total of 443 completed questionnaires (response rate 30.9%) were returned by hospital nurses (n = 240) and primary health care nurses (n = 203). The respondents mean age was 43.2 (SD 11.2, range 22–67) and most of the respondents were female (n = 426). The highest level of nurse education was that of Registered Nurse (college or polytechnic, n = 385). However, some of respondents' highest level of nurse education was master of healthcare (polytechnic, n = 14), bachelor of healthcare (university, n = 19) or Master of healthcare (university, n = 14). The mean length of the work experience in their current unit was for nurses working in the university hospital, 8.6 years (SD 9.0, range 0.6–37.2) and for nurses working in primary health care, 6.2 (SD 6.3, range 0.8–32.0).

2.2. Instrument

The PCC scale [6] was used in both Finnish studies. The PCC was originally developed in Korea for the measurement of patient-centred competence of nurses in hospital settings. The competence was defined in terms of knowledge, skills and attitudes related to patient-centred care. The PCC consists of four sub-scales including Respecting patients' perspectives (6 items), Promoting patient involvement in care processes (5 items), Providing for patient comfort (3 items) and Advocating for patients (3 items). The instrument uses a five-point Likert scale (1 minimal, 2 below average, 3 average, 4 good, 5 excellent) which the respondents used to rate their competencies. (subjective, self-assessment).

The 41 PCC items were developed, based on earlier literature and the QSEN faculty framework of competence in patient-centred care [32]. The items were then analyzed by experts who reduced the preliminary 41 items, to 25 after using the Content Validity Index (CVI) and cut off criterion of 0.70, and psychometric testing [6]. The expert panel members were eight members of the board of directors (Korean Quality Improvement Nurses Society) and three nursing professors, and they assessed the relevance of the proposed 41 items. The first version of the PCC was pretested in the sample of two head nurses and two registered nurses to verify the comprehensibility and clarity of the items. The PCC was then tested with a sample of 577 hospital nurses. Explorative factor analysis supported a four-factor solution explaining 64.7% of the variance and suggesting the final 17 items for the PCC [6]. The overall Cronbach's alpha coefficients for the 17-item instrument was 0.92, and for the sub-scales, 0.80–0.85. Concurrent validity was assessed using the single item on patient-centred care performance using VAS (0–100), with Pearson's correlation coefficient of 0.60 ($p < 0.001$).

2.3. Translation of the Instrument

The PCC with 17 items created by Hwang [6] was used, and the English language items were used. A standard forward-back translation method [37] was used to translate the PCC from the English version to the Finnish version by an official translator, whose work was analysed by two researchers, mainly interested in ensuring nursing terminology was well matched. Secondly, the translated version was back-translated into English by another official translator. Thirdly, the back translated version was compared with the original English language instrument. Finally, all three instrument versions were analysed at the same time by two experienced researchers. The final Finnish version included some minor changes of terms (professional terminology and most suitable term from two suggested) and the deletion of some redundant words. As languages differ from each other, the semantic, cultural, conceptual equivalence, and linguistic terminology were ensured [37].

2.4. Data Analysis

Data were analysed statistically using the SPSS for Windows (IBM SPSS, Chicago, IL, USA) version 22.0/24.0 and lavaan (0.6–7) package from R (version 4.0.2) statistical software. Firstly, descriptive statistics were calculated which described the two samples and study variables at the total scale and sum-variable level for the four sub-scales. The sum-variables were formed based on the theoretical background of the original instrument, see [6]. Secondly, the internal consistency reliability was examined using the Cronbach's alpha coefficients and item analysis in both data sets (criterion ≥ 0.70) [38,39]. Item analysis included item-to-total correlations (criterion ≥ 0.30) and the percentage of the appropriate inter-item correlations (criterion $0.30 \leq r \leq 0.70$). Thirdly, an explorative factor analysis (EFA) was conducted in the sample of 233 respondents (Dataset I). The Kaiser–Meyer–Olkin measure of sampling adequacy was 0.895, (acceptable value > 0.5) [40] and Bartlett's test of sphericity (<0.001; where a p value less than 0.05 indicates that a factor analysis may be useful with the data) [41]. These two measures were used to assess the preconditions for factor analysis. An EFA, with principal axis factoring as the extraction method, and Promax with Kaiser Normalization for rotation method was computed. Fourthly, a confirmatory factor analysis (CFA) with maximum likelihood estimation was used to investigate the conceptualised four-dimensional structure (KMO = 0.92, Bartlett's test < 0.001). Several indices with criteria were used to examine the goodness-of-fit of the model with Dataset 2: goodness-of-fit index (GFI); adjusted goodness-of-fit index (AGFI); Tucker–Lewis index (TLI) and the comparative fit index (CFI) (criterion >0.90 threshold for all mentioned fit indices [42,43], root mean square error of approximation (RMSEA <0.08) [42], and standardized root mean square residual (SRMR <0.08) [42]. Fifthly, to examine whether the PCC sub-scales measure distinct dimensions, inter-scale correlations between the PCC sub-scales were analysed. Finally, analysis of the sensitivity of the PCC was assessed comparing the PCC total and sub-scale scores within the two different facilities (contrasting groups), university hospital care (n = 233) and primary health care (n = 201) in Dataset 2 (n = 434). The distributions were non-normal and therefore, the Mann–Whitney U-test was used.

2.5. Ethical Considerations

Permissions for data collection were obtained from the participating organisations according to their specific ethical procedures. The studies using Dataset 1 and Dataset 2 were approved by the Ethics Committee of the University (34/2016/6 June 2016 and 4/2016/15 February 2016 respectively). Permission to use the PCC instrument was granted by the developer Jee-In Hwang (email) and Elsevier (reprint of the items). The respondents gave their voluntary informed consent for the studies by completing the questionnaires sent to them and posting them to the researcher, after having all information about the study in an introductory letter. Respondents were informed that they could withdraw from the study at any time.

3. Results

3.1. Descriptive Statistics on the Patient-Centred Care Competency (PCC) and Sub-Scales

In total, patient-centred care competence in Dataset I was rated in the 'good', level 4.04 (SD 0.46) and was higher compared to Dataset 2 (3.90, SD 0.42). At the sub-scale level (dataset 2 in parenthesis), competence providing for patient comfort was evaluated the highest in both data sets 4.31, SD 0.56 (4.13, SD 0.55) at the 'good' level. Competence in respecting patients' perspectives 4.12 SD 0.49 (3.99, SD 0.42) and advocating for patients 4.03 SD 0.56 (3.84, SD 0.56) was also rated 'good'. Competence promoting patient involvement in care processes was assessed the lowest at 3.78 SD 0.56 (3.70, SD 0.49).

3.2. Psychometric Properties of the PCC

3.2.1. Internal Consistency Reliability

The internal consistency measured using Cronbach's alpha coefficients (Dataset 2 in parenthesis) was α = 0.93 (0.91) for the total scale and ranged from α = 0.78 (0.74) to α = 0.85 (0.83) for the sub-scales (Table 1). Item analysis (Dataset I) provided some evidence about the internal consistency of the items within the total scale and its four sub-scales. All items were closely tied to its construct as all item-to-total correlations reached an acceptable level (≥ 0.40). Correlations between the items in the given sub-scale (inter-item correlations) were acceptable in three sub-scales (PCC2–4), as was 87% of the inter-item correlations within the PCC total and the sub-scale PCC1 (Table 1).

Table 1. Descriptive statistics of the Patient-centred Care Competency (PCC) total and sub-scales, Cronbach's alpha and item analysis.

Scale	n of Items	n	Mean (SD)	α *	Item-to Total r Range (% Criteria) §	Average Inter-Item r (Range), % Criteria #
Dataset 1						
PCC total	17	223	4.04 (0.46)	0.93	0.518–0.704 (100)	0.437 (0.035–0.70) 87%
Respecting patients' perspectives	6	223	4.13 (0.49)	0.84	0.444–0.681 (100%)	0.472 (0.243–0.637) 87%
Promoting patient involvement in care processes	5	223	3.78 (0.56)	0.85	0.571–0.705 (100%)	0.531 (0.414–0.628) 100%
Providing for patient comfort	3	223	4.31 (0.56)	0.85	0.686–0.743 (100%)	0.655 (0.619–0.700) 100%
Advocating for patients	3	223	4.03 (0.56)	0.78	0.552–0.679 (100%)	0.537 (0.456–0.613) 100%
Dataset 2						Inter-item range (5) #
PCC total	17	434	3.90 (0.42)	0.91	0.51–0.64 (100%)	0.28–0.54 (92%)
Respecting patients' perspectives	6	434	3.99 (0.44)	0.82	0.52–0.67 (100%)	0.31–0.60 (100%)
Promoting patient involvement in care processes	5	434	3.70 (0.49)	0.77	0.50–0.58 (100%)	0.31–0.48 (100%)
Providing for patient comfort	3	433	4.13 (0.55)	0.83	0.60–0.74 (100%)	0.55–0.69 (100%)
Advocating for patients	3	431	3.84 (0.56)	0.74	0.52–0.61 (100%)	0.43–0.55 (100%)

* α Cronbach's alpha coefficient. § item to total correlation r > 0.3. # inter item correlation 0.30 < r < 0.70.

3.2.2. Construct Validity

Firstly, the exploratory factor analysis of Dataset I suggested a three-factor solution based on scree plot and eigen values (criterion eigen value ≥ 1). The Pattern matrix showed a clear structure for three sub-scales (Factors 3, 2 and 1) which explained 57.7% of the variance. However, the fourth sub-scale was not independent as the items loaded on the first sub-scale (Factor 1, item 15) and the third sub-scale (Factor 3, item 16 and item 17). A four-factor model was also examined, with a 61.2% explained variance, and an eigen value range of 8.04–0.87, and a last factor with an eigen value of less than 1.0. (Table 2).

Table 2. Exploratory factor analysis (EFA) Pattern matrix, Dataset I (n = 223), items of competence in the PCC.

Item	Respecting Patients' Perspectives	Communality	Factor 1	Factor 2	Factor 3
Item 1	Value seeing health-care situations through patients' eyes	0.587	−0.002	0.160	**0.604**
Item 2	Elicit patient values, preferences and needs as part of clinical interview, implementation of care plan, and evaluation of care	0.617	−0.167	0.421	**0.509**
Item 3	Integrate understanding of multiple dimensions of patient-centred care such as patient and family preferences	0.633	−0.102	0.320	**0.555**
Item 4	Communicate patient values, preferences and need to other health-care team members	0.603	−0.144	0.142	**0.686**
Item 5	Provide patient-centred care with sensitivity and respect for the diversity of human experience	0.640	0.210	−0.334	**0.902**
Item 6	Support patient-centred care for individuals and groups whose values differ from own	0.483	0.276	0.003	**0.389**
	Promoting Patient Involvement in Care Processes				
Item 7	Examine barriers to active involvement of patients in the care processes	0.593	−0.002	**0.430**	0.386
Item 8	Assess level of patient's decisional conflict and provide access to resources	0.611	0.060	**0.641**	0.159
Item 9	Describe strategies to empower patients or families in all aspects of care process	0.623	−0.156	**0.897**	−0.017

Table 2. Cont.

Item	Respecting Patients' Perspectives	Communality	Factor 1	Factor 2	Factor 3
Item 10	Engage patients or designated surrogates in active partnerships that promote health, safety and well-being, and self-care management	0.578	0.221	**0.775**	−0.195
Item 11	Respect patient preferences for degree of active engagement in care process	0.574	0.281	**0.310**	0.231
	Providing for Patient Comfort				
Item 12	Assess presence and extent of pain and suffering	0.631	**0.855**	−0.042	−0.061
Item 13	Assess levels of physical and emotional comfort	0.627	**0.914**	−0.157	−0.003
Item 14	Elicit expectations of patient and family for relief pain, discomfort and suffering	0.698	**0.709**	0.230	−0.062
	Advocate for Patients				
Item 15	Facilitate informed patient consent for care	0.659	**0.505**	0.165	0.201
Item 16	Communicate care provided and needed at each transition in care	0.608	**0.303**	0.108	0.424
Item 17	Participate in building consensus or resolving conflict in the context of patient care	0.533	**0.231**	0.191	0.398
	Eigen value		8.041	1.924	0.996
	% of explanation		44.8	9.3	3.6
	Cumulative % of explanation		44.8	54.057	57.7

Extraction Method: principal axis factoring; Rotation method: Promax with Kaiser normalization. Bold: representing original structure. Items reprinted from *Nursing Outlook* 55(1), Cronenwett et al. Quality and safety education for nurses 122–131, Table 1. Copyright (2007), with permission from Elsevier.

Secondly, a Confirmatory Factor Analysis was conducted using the Dataset 2 (n = 421 valid cases). The Chi-square test did not show a model fit (χ^2 = 283.70, df = 113, p < 0.01) possibly due to the large sample size. Other goodness-of-fit indices were as follows: CFI 0.93, TLI 0.92, GFI 0.99 and adjusted AGFI 0.99, all at an acceptable level (criterion >0.90). The RMSEA was 0.065 (criterion <0.08) and the SRMR of 0.045 (criterion <0.08) was also a good fit to the model. The Item loadings ranged were: PCC1 (0.584–0.729), PCC2 (0.612–0.681), PCC3 (0.726–0.824) and PCC4 (0.699–0.707), all of which were acceptable (criterion >0.40) (Figure 1).

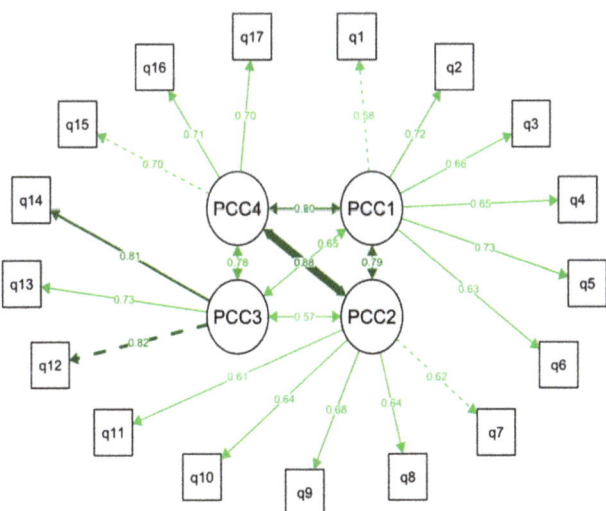

Figure 1. Construct validity of the Patient-centred Care (PCC) instrument based on confirmatory factor analysis (CFA) and inter-scale correlations PCC1–PCC4. q refers to items, numbers refer to factor loadings within each sub-scale. Model fit statistics: comparative fit index (CFI) 0.93, Tucker–Lewis index (TLI) 0.92, goodness-of-fit index (GFI) 0.99, adjusted goodness-of-fit index (AGFI) 0.99, root mean square error of approximation (RMSEA) 0.065, standardized root mean square residual (SRMR) 0.045.

The average variance extracted (AVE), the amount of variance captured by a construct in relation to the amount of variance due to measurement error) [44] was 0.44 (PCC1), 0.41 (PCC2), 0.49 (PCC3) and 0.47 (PCC4) implying that the discriminant validity may not be ideal but includes variance based on measurement bias. However, the factor loadings were as follows, PCC1 (0.584–0.729, composite reliability (CR) 0.82), PCC2 (0.612–0.681, CR 0.77), PCC3 (0.726–0.824, CR 0.83) and PCC4 (0.699–0.707, 0.82), some being lower than 0.70.

3.2.3. Inter Scale Correlations

The correlations between the PCC sub-scales ranged from 0.57 to 0.88 showing the scales are related to each other and to the latent variable, PSS (Figure 1).

3.3. Sensitivity to Context/Contrasting Groups

The competence assessments by nurses working in specialised hospital care and those working in primary health care were not statistically significantly different in the total scale or any of the sub-scales (total PCC, Mann–Whitney U =20,804, p = 0.659), PCC1 (U = 22,484, p = 0.628), PCC2 (U = 21,763, p = 0.519), PCC3 (U = 23,620, p = 0.745) or PCC4 (U = 20,110, p = 0.980).

4. Discussion

Two datasets (1 and 2) were used to validate the PCC instrument in the Finnish healthcare context. The psychometric properties computed suggest acceptable reliability, content and construct validity and sensitivity. The PCC was developed and tested in the hospital environment in Korea by Hwang [6] to measure patient-centred care competency, and the findings in this current study are similar to those of Hwang [6]. The purpose of the PCC instrument is clearly defined, has meaningful content in the Finnish context and has acceptable internal consistency, face validity and construct validity [45]. These results demonstrate that the instrument is a useful measure of patient-centred care competency. In the Finnish studies the nurses assessed their overall patient-centred care competency higher 4.04 (Dataset I), 3.90 (Dataset 2) compared to the Korean studies, 3.58 [6] and 3.61 [46] respectively. The sub-scale "providing for patient comfort" was assessed the highest and the sub-scale "promoting patient involvement" was assessed the lowest in all four studies, increasing the inter-rater reliability of the instrument.

This current study also shows that the instrument is suitable for use in different health care environments, for example, home care and long-term care units (Dataset 2) as the findings are comparable between Dataset I and Dataset 2. However, because the data from home care and long-term care units, Dataset 2, is limited, and the staffing profiles differ from those in hospital environments, more research is needed to be more certain of this.

The sub-scales contain items related to general patient relations, patient involvement, safety, and teamwork [6,46] which are shared goals of all health care workers, for example clinicians and practical nurses. Therefore, it can be argued that although the instrument was originally developed for use in nursing studies, it could be used, with minor adaptations, to measure the patient-centred care competency of other healthcare workers such as physiotherapists and public health nurses.

Translating instruments for nursing studies is necessary [47] for researchers to have access to the many valid and reliable instruments available [37]. The standard forward-back translation method [37] for the Finnish version of the PCC achieved equivalence [47] with the original English and also Korean version. The Likert-type response options of the PCC are sensitive, and the instrument is comprehensible to the healthcare respondents as it suits their demographic and educational backgrounds [48]. The PCC is easy to complete taking a short time only, making it a useful research tool [48]. However, more research is needed to further validate the instrument, for example in diverse healthcare environments and among different professionals working in health care.

Patient-centred care competence is a multidimensional concept which can be defined and measured from different perspectives and multiple ways. This study provides more information about the validation of one instrument, the PCC instrument [6], used for measuring nurses' patient-centred care competence. The results of this study suggest that the PCC instrument is a valid, reliable, and sensitive instrument that could be used to measure Finnish nurses' patient-centred care competence and may be adapted to measure the patient-centred competence of other health care workers. Cowan et al. [24] suggests that the self-assessed instrument oversimplifies a complex process, applying also to PCC. However, this instrument provides important information about nurses' own views of their patient-centred care competence. Combining this information with other measurements, for example, peer, co-workers' and patients' perspectives, can provide a more comprehensive understanding of patient-centred care competence in the workplace.

Methodological Considerations, Validity and Limitations

Some of the methodological considerations of the study, relate to data collection, sample size and instrumentation, and warrant further discussion. The data in this study were taken from two independent studies, using same instrument, the PCC [6]. Due to the secondary nature of the data, it was not possible to increase the sample size. However, the recommended sample size for a study like this, is at least five respondents per item in cross-sectional survey studies [38,39] which was realized in both studies. The PCC was translated to Finnish following the recommended forward-back translation process and semantic and linguistic equivalence were confirmed. As the PCC is a self-assessment instrument, the results may be affected by social desirability bias [49], as the participants may have evaluated their competence higher than in reality. This is to be expected as patient-centeredness in care, strongly rooted in the value-based healthcare, and often discussed in policy and strategic documents is a pillar of professional nurse education. There is no method available to evaluate competence in such value-laden activities, including the knowledge, skills, and attitudes objectively [21,24]. The PCC items self-assess knowledge, skills, and attitudes of the practicing nurse. The next step could be the development of a more objective assessment method. However, it might be very challenging objectively to measure all the aforementioned dimensions of competence. This may possibly lead to behavioural level assessment. It has been criticized that the competence of healthcare professionals is multidimensional, demanding several assessment methods.

Cronbach's alpha coefficients, indicating the level of internal consistency homogeneity of the total scale, in both datasets were (0.91–0.93). This high value suggests some scale items have similar meaning, requiring item deletion. However, the Cronbach's alpha coefficients are lower and more acceptable at the sub-scale level in both datasets (0.78–0.85 and 0.74–0.83). The correlation coefficients (also in the CFA) between the factors, especially between PCC4 and the other factors PCC1, PCC2 and PCC3, are high, suggesting there may be some overlap within the scales. The chi-square statistics did not show a model fit with a p value less than 0.05. However, this statistic is known to be sensitive to sample size [50] and is, therefore, insufficient in this study for the assessment of goodness-of-fit. The other goodness-of-fit indices were all acceptable.

The average variance extracted (AVE 0.41–0.49 within the sub-scales) implied that the discriminant validity may not be ideal and includes variance based on measurement bias. The factor loadings were mostly acceptable PCC1 (0.584–0.729), composite reliability CR 0.82), PCC2 (0.612–0.681, CR 0.77), PCC3 (0.726–0.824, CR 0.83) and PCC4 (0.699–0.707, 0.82). The criteria given (0.5 > AVE > 0.4) [44] if the composite reliability CR >0.6, is acceptable (here all CR > 0.7), but may suggest revision for the total scale, by deleting some possibly redundant items. The PCC scale could benefit from a Rasch analysis which would further analyse item-level reliability and provide information about how participants response patterns relate to the difficulty of the items. For the known-group validity testing, the findings regarding the total scale or its sub-scales indicate that competence was assessed in the hospital care context and in primary health care context in similar ways, even though there was a variety of service provision.

5. Conclusions

Patient-centred care has a central role in healthcare worldwide [30,31] and has been found to improve health literacy and patient engagement, be effective and cost-effective [31] and can be used as an important indicator of care quality [2,13] and patient safety [6]. In nursing, patient-centred care competence has been identified as a core competency for nurses [7,32] and is needed to guide the development of care. The PCC instrument measures nurses' patient-centred care competence in terms of knowledge, skills, and attitudes through self-assessment. In this current study, the PCC was validated in the Finnish healthcare system by registered nurses using self-assessment. The PCC has proven reliability, construct validity and sensitivity for the measurement of non-contextual, specific competence. Further research into the analysis of item-level discrimination with, for example, Rasch modelling, will identify any overlapping items and person fit in evaluations, including the identification of nurse-related characteristics. The results of this study showed there is some room for improvement in the promotion of patient involvement in their care.

Author Contributions: Conceptualization, R.S., T.L., K.L.; methodology, R.S., M.S., M.P.; formal analysis, M.P.; investigation, T.L., K.L.; data curation, T.L., K.L.; writing—original draft preparation, R.S., K.L., T.L.; writing—review and editing, R.S., M.S., T.L., K.L., M.P.; visualization, M.P.; supervision, R.S., M.S., T.L.; project administration, R.S., T.L.; funding acquisition, R.S. All authors have read and agreed to the published version of the manuscript.

Funding: This research was funded by The Turku University Hospital, special grant-in aid VTR, grant number 13238.

Institutional Review Board Statement: The study was conducted according to the guidelines of the Declaration of Helsinki and approved by the Ethics Committee of the University of Turku (34/2016/6 June 2016; dataset I) as well as the study with dataset 2 (4/2016/15 February 2016).

Informed Consent Statement: Informed consent was obtained from all subjects involved in the study as advised by returning of the anonymous questionnaires to the researchers.

Data Availability Statement: No new data were created or analyzed in this study. Data sharing is not applicable to this article.

Acknowledgments: We acknowledge Norman Rickard for the language edition. We would like to thank Statistician Pauli Puukka and Jouko Katajisto for their expertise in the earlier steps with the statistics, as this was the secondary analysis.

Conflicts of Interest: The authors declare no conflict of interest. The funders had no role in the design of the study; in the collection, analyses, or interpretation of data; in the writing of the manuscript; or in the decision to publish the results.

References

1. Hudon, C.; Fortin, M.; Haggerty, J.; Loignon, C.; Lambert, M.; Poitras, M.E. Measuring patients' perceptions of patient-centered care: A systematic review of tools for family medicine. *Ann. Fam. Med.* **2011**, *9*, 155–164. [CrossRef] [PubMed]
2. Pelletier, L.R.; Stichler, J.F. Patient-centered care and engagement: Nurse leaders' imperative for health reform. *J. Nurs. Adm.* **2014**, *44*, 473–480. [CrossRef] [PubMed]
3. Coyle, J.; Williams, B. Valuing people as individuals: Development of an instrument through a survey of person-centredness in secondary care. *J. Adv. Nurs.* **2001**, *36*, 450–459. [CrossRef] [PubMed]
4. Sidani, S.; Fox, M. Patient-centered care: Clarification of its specific elements to facilitate interprofessional care. *J. Interprof. Care.* **2014**, *28*, 134–141. [CrossRef] [PubMed]
5. Jakimowicz, S.; Perry, L. A concept analysis of patient-centred nursing in the intensive care unit. *J. Adv. Nurs.* **2015**, *71*, 1499–1517. [CrossRef] [PubMed]
6. Hwang, J.I. Development and testing of a patient-centered care competency scale for hospital nurses. *Int. J. Nurs. Pract.* **2015**, *21*, 43–51. [CrossRef]
7. Yaqoob Mohammed Al Jabri, F.; Kvist, T.; Azimirad, M.; Turunen, H. A systematic review of healthcare professionals' core competency instruments. *Nurs. Health Sci.* **2021**, *23*, 87–102. [CrossRef]
8. Delaney, L.J. Patient-centered care as an approach to improving health care in Australia. *Collegian* **2018**, *25*, 119–123. [CrossRef]
9. Mead, N.; Bower, P.; Hann, M. The impact of general practitioners' patient-centredness on patients' post-consultation satisfaction and enablement. *Soc. Sci. Med.* **2002**, *55*, 283–299. [CrossRef]

10. McCance, T.; McCormack, B.; Dewing, J. An exploration of person-centredness in practice. *Online J. Issues Nurs.* **2011**, *31*, 1. [CrossRef]
11. Edvardsson, D.; Fetherstonhaugh, D.; Nay, R.; Gibson, S. Development and initial testing of the Person-centered Care Assessment Tool (P-CAT). *Int. Psychogeriatr.* **2010**, *22*, 101–108. [CrossRef]
12. Coelho, T. A patient advocate's perspective on patient-centered comparative effectiveness research. *Health Aff.* **2010**, *29*, 1885–1890. [CrossRef] [PubMed]
13. Mead, N.; Bower, P. Patient-centredness: A conceptual framework and review of the empirical literature. *Soc. Sci. Med.* **2000**, *51*, 1087–1110. [CrossRef]
14. Lusk, J.M.; Fater, K. A concept analysis of patient-centered care. *Nurs. Forum* **2013**, *48*, 89–98. [CrossRef]
15. Edvardsson, D.; Koch, S.; Nay, R. Psychometric evaluation of the English language Person-centred Climate Questionnaire–staff version. *J. Nurs. Manag.* **2010**, *18*, 54–60. [CrossRef]
16. Huppelschoten, A.G.; Verkerk, E.W.; Appleby, J.; Groenewoud, H.; Adang, E.M.; Nelen, W.L.; Kremer, J.A. The monetary value of patient-centred care: Results from a discrete choice experiment in Dutch fertility care. *Hum. Reprod.* **2014**, *29*, 1712–1720. [CrossRef] [PubMed]
17. Scholl, I.; Zill, J.M.; Härter, M.; Dirmaier, J. An integrative model of patient-centeredness—A systematic review and concept analysis. *PLoS ONE* **2014**, *17*, e107828. [CrossRef] [PubMed]
18. Entwistle, V.A.; Watt, I.S. Treating Patients as Persons: A Capabilities Approach to Support Delivery of Person-Centered Care. *Am. J. Bioethics.* **2013**, *13*, 29–39. [CrossRef] [PubMed]
19. McCormack, B.; McCance, T.V. Development of a framework for person-centred nursing. *J. Adv. Nurs.* **2006**, *56*, 472–479. [CrossRef]
20. Edvardsson, D.; Winblad, B.; Sandman, P.O. Person-centered care for people with severe Alzheimer's disease: Current status and ways forward. *Lancet Neurol.* **2008**, *7*, 362–367. [CrossRef]
21. Cowan, D.T.; Norman, I.J.; Coopamah, V.P. Competence in nursing practice: A controversial concept: A focused review of literature. *Nurse Educ. Today* **2005**, *25*, 355–362. [CrossRef]
22. Milligan, F. Defining and assessing competence: The distraction of outcomes and the importance of educational process. *Nurse Educ. Today* **1998**, *18*, 273–280. [CrossRef]
23. Valloze, J. Competence: A concept analysis. *Teach. Learn. Nurs.* **2009**, *4*, 115–118. [CrossRef]
24. Cowan, D.T.; Wilson-Barnett, J.D.; Norman, I.J.; Murrells, T. Measuring nursing competence: Development of a self-assessment tool for general nurses across Europe. *Int. J. Nurs. Stud.* **2008**, *45*, 902–913. [CrossRef] [PubMed]
25. Randolph, P.K.; Hinton, J.E.; Hagler, D.; Mays, M.Z.; Kastenbaum, B.; Brooks, R.; DeFalco, N.; Weberg, D. Measuring competence: Collaboration for safety. *J. Contin. Educ. Nurs.* **2012**, *43*, 541–547. [CrossRef]
26. Flinkman, M.; Leino-Kilpi, H.; Numminen, O.; Jeon, Y.; Kuokkanen, L.; Meretoja, R. Nurse Competence Scale: A systematic and psychometric review. *J. Adv. Nurs.* **2017**, *73*, 1035–1050. [CrossRef] [PubMed]
27. Watson, R.; Stimpson, A.; Topping, A.; Porock, D. Clinical competence assessment in nursing: A systematic review of the literature. *J. Adv. Nurs.* **2002**, *39*, 421–431. [CrossRef]
28. Löfmark, A.; Mårtensson, G. Validation of the tool assessment of clinical education (AssCE): A study using Delphi method and clinical experts. *Nurse Educ. Today* **2017**, *50*, 82–86. [CrossRef]
29. Eraut, M. *Developing Professional Knowledge and Competence*; Falmer Press: London, UK, 1994.
30. World Health Organization. Framework on Integrated, People-Centred Health Services. 2016. Available online: https://apps.who.int/gb/ebwha/pdf_files/WHA69/A69_39_en.pdf?ua=1&ua=1 (accessed on 4 April 2021).
31. World Health Organization. What are Integrated People-Centred Health Services? 2021. Available online: https://www.who.int/servicedeliverysafety/areas/people-centred-care/ipchs-what/en/ (accessed on 4 April 2021).
32. Cronenwett, L.; Sherwood, G.; Barnsteiner, J.; Disch, J.; Johnson, J.; Mitchell, P.; Sullivan, D.T.; Warren, J. Quality and Safety Education for Nurses. *Nurs. Outlook* **2007**, *55*, 122–131. [CrossRef]
33. McCormack, B. A conceptual framework for person-centred practice with older people. *Int J. Nurs Pract.* **2003**, *9*, 202–209. [CrossRef]
34. Stewart, M.; Brown, J.B.; Donner, A.; McWhinney, I.R.; Oates, J.; Weston, W.W.; Jordan, J. The impact of patient-centered care on outcomes. *J. Fam. Pract.* **2000**, *49*, 796–804. [PubMed]
35. Edvardsson, D.; Innes, A. Measuring person-centered care: A critical comparative review of published tools. *Gerontologist* **2010**, *50*, 834–846. [CrossRef]
36. Rokstad, A.M.; Engedal, K.; Edvardsson, D.; Selbaek, G. Psychometric evaluation of the Norwegian version of the Person-Centred Care Assessment Tool. *Int. J. Nurs. Pract.* **2012**, *18*, 99–105. [CrossRef] [PubMed]
37. Sousa, V.D.; Rojjanasrirat, W. Translation, adaptation and validation of instruments or scales for use in cross-cultural health care research: A clear and user-friendly guideline. *J. Eval. Clin. Pract.* **2011**, *17*, 268–274. [CrossRef] [PubMed]
38. DeVon, H.A.; Block, M.E.; Moyle-Wright, P.; Ernst, D.M.; Hayden, S.J.; Lazzara, D.J.; Savoy, S.M.; Kostas-Polston, E. A psychometric toolbox for testing validity and reliability. *J. Nurs. Sch.* **2007**, *39*, 155–164. [CrossRef]
39. Rattray, J.; Jones, M.C. Essential elements of questionnaire design and development. *J. Clin. Nurs.* **2007**, *16*, 234–243. [CrossRef] [PubMed]
40. Kaiser, H.F.; Rice, J. Little Jiffy, Mark Iv. *Educ. Psychol. Meas.* **1974**, *34*, 111–117. [CrossRef]

41. Williams, B.; Onsman, A.; Brown, T. Exploratory factor analysis: A five-step guide for novices. *Australas. J. Paramed.* **2010**, *8*, 1–13. [CrossRef]
42. Browne, M.W.; Cudeck, R. Alternative ways of assessing model fit. In *Testing Structural Equation Models*; Bollen, K.A., Long, J.S., Eds.; Sage: Newbury Park, CA, USA, 1993; pp. 136–162.
43. Hu, L.; Bentler, P.M. Cutoff criteria for fit indexes in covariance structure analysis: Conventional criteria versus new alternatives. *Struct. Equ. Modeling* **1999**, *6*, 1–55. [CrossRef]
44. Fornell, C.; Larcker, D.F. Evaluating structural equation models with unobservable variables and measurement error. *J. Market. Res.* **1981**, *18*, 39–50. [CrossRef]
45. Kimberlin, C.L.; Winterstein, A.G. Validity and reliability of measurement instruments used in research. *Am. J. Health Syst. Pharm.* **2008**, *65*, 2276–2284. [CrossRef] [PubMed]
46. Hwang, J.; Kim, S.W.; Chin, H.J. Patient Participation in Patient Safety and Its Relationships with Nurses' Patient-Centered Care Competency, Teamwork, and Safety Climate. *Asian Nurs. Res.* **2019**, *13*, 130–136. [CrossRef]
47. Maneesriwongul, W.; Dixon, J.K. Instrument translation process: A methods review. *J. Adv. Nurs.* **2004**, *48*, 175–186. [CrossRef] [PubMed]
48. Frank-Stromborg, M.; Olsen, S.J. *Instruments for Clinical Health-Care Research*, 3rd ed.; Jones and Bartlett Publisher: London, UK, 2004.
49. Meisters, J.; Hoffmann, A.; Much, J. Controlling social desirability bias: An experimental investigation of the extended crosswise model. *PLoS ONE* **2020**, *7*, e0243367. [CrossRef]
50. Byrne, B.M. *Structural Equation Modeling with Amos: Basic Concepts, Applications, and Programming*; Routledge: New York, NY, USA, 2016.

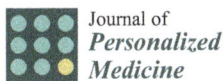

Article

Older Adults' Perceived Barriers to Participation in a Falls Prevention Strategy

Júlio Belo Fernandes [1,*], Sónia Belo Fernandes [2,*], Ana Silva Almeida [3], Diana Alves Vareta [3] and Carol A. Miller [4]

1 Department of Nursing, Escola Superior de Saúde Egas Moniz/PaMNEC—CiiEM, Almada, Rua António José Batista n°116, 3esq., 2910-397 Setúbal, Portugal
2 Department of Nursing, Projetar Enfermagem, 1600-577 Lisboa, Portugal
3 Department of Nursing, Centro Hospitalar de Setúbal, 2910-397 Setúbal, Portugal; anasilvalmeida@gmail.com (A.S.A.); diana_vareta@hotmail.com (D.A.V.)
4 Independent Care Manager at Care & Counseling, Brecksville, OH 44141, USA; cmiller4321@ameritech.net
* Correspondence: juliobelo01@gmail.com (J.B.F.); soniabelo@sapo.pt (S.B.F.); Tel.: +351-968392976 (J.B.F.)

Abstract: There is a need to increase older adults' access and adherence to falls prevention strategies. This study aims to explore older adults' perceived barriers to participation in a fall prevention strategy. A qualitative descriptive approach was used. Semi-structured interviews were conducted with 18 older adult users of a Day Care Unit from a Private Institution of Social Solidarity in the region of Lisbon and Tagus Valley in Portugal. The recruitment was made in September 2019. The interviews were recorded transcribed verbatim and analysed thematically using the method of constant comparisons. The barriers to participation in a fall prevention strategy are healthcare system gaps, social context, economic context, health status, psychological capability, and lack of knowledge to demystify myths and misconceptions about falls. There are different barriers to participate in a fall prevention strategy. It is urgent to eliminate or reduce the effect of these barriers to increase older adults' participation in fall prevention strategies.

Keywords: accidental falls; fall prevention; older adults; barriers; patient compliance

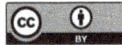

1. Introduction

Every year, one out of three older adults falls. It is estimated that each year, more than 640,000 people die as a result of falls [1]. Falls are the second leading cause of non-fatal and fatal injuries among older adults [2–4]. Older adults with a high risk of falls are in the high-risk group for fall injury [5] and fall-related death [6]. Fall related injury can range from minor trauma to severe injuries requiring hospitalization. The most common severe injuries include fractured bones and soft tissue injuries [7,8].

Preventing falls and fall-related injuries is challenging because of its multifactorial nature [9]. Several studies have identified more than 400 potential risk factors for falling [10]. Results from numerous researches have suggested that multidimensional falls prevention strategies can be effective in reducing the number of falls [11–13]. Furthermore, several guidelines have been developed to summarise the best evidence and guide healthcare professionals in their clinical practice [14,15]. Despite these facts, many fallers do not seek any type of help to prevent further falls [16], as well as many older adults, do not engage in fall prevention strategies even after referrals are made [17].

To improve access and adherence to falls prevention strategies, health care policy-makers and health administrators should contemplate older adults' perspectives when developing these strategies [18]. Little is known about the barriers to engage in a fall prevention strategy in the Portuguese population, therefore this research seeks to fill this evidence gap by exploring barriers to participation in a fall prevention strategy from the perspective of Portuguese older adults with a high risk of falling. By seeking this evidence we can provide insight into developing a more effective fall prevention strategy and take measures to minimise those obstacles and therefore increasing enrolment and participation.

2. Methods

2.1. Study Design

A qualitative descriptive study was conducted using semi-structured interviews, which enabled an in-depth exploration of older adults' perceived barriers to participation in a fall prevention strategy. To ensure quality in the research report we followed the con-solidated criteria for reporting qualitative research (COREQ) [19].

2.2. Setting

The study setting was a Day Care Unit from a Private Institution of Social Solidarity in the region of Lisbon and Vale do Tejo in Portugal that caters to a population of over 80,000 people.

2.3. Sampling and Recruitment

The study population consists of older adults who are users of the Day Care Unit. The sampling method selection was non-probabilistic by convenience. The inclusion criteria included: (1) have a high risk of falling; (2) have participated in a falls prevention strategy.

Researchers used the fall risk test developed by VeiligheidNL [20] to screen older adults. The test contains three simple questions: 'Did you fall during the past twelve months?', 'Do you experience problems with movement and balance?', and 'Are you afraid of falling?' When participants answer "yes" to the first question or two of the overall questions, they are considered at high risk of falling.

The recruitment was made in September 2019. Eligible participants were invited by telephone to participate in the interviews. All older adults available at the time of data collection that met the inclusion criteria were included in the study.

2.4. Participants

Of the 26 older adults who agreed to participate in the study, 8 were excluded based on not meeting the inclusion criteria. We conducted 18 interviews, the participants were mostly male (61.1%). The mean age of participants was 76.2 (range 69–83 years) and the standard deviation was 4.16215 years.

2.5. Data Collection

The interviews were conducted by the first author at the Day Care Unit facilities and lasted approximately 20 min. All interviews were audiotaped, transcribed verbatim into written data, anonymised, and analysed.

The semi-structured interview guide was developed based on data gathered from previous studies and with contributions from experts. Examples of questions used in the guide are: 'Were there any factors that limit you to participate in a falls prevention program?' 'Tell me about a particular example of a barrier to undertake a falls prevention program?' 'What do you think could difficult people to participate in a falls prevention program?' 'Do you have any suggestions for how services could improve its contributions for older adults to engage in a falls prevention program?'

2.6. Data Analyses

In the process of analysis, Braun, Clarke, Hayfield, and Terry's [21] procedures were followed. Researchers listened to the audio records to obtain an overall sense and then transcribed verbatim into written data. The data was separated into meaning units, based on similarity. Meaning unit codes were developed based on participants' own words. Initially, the transcribed verbatim was reviewed independently by two study team members and manually coded using inductive content analysis to identify common themes. To ensure credibility, the researchers discussed and compared the emergent themes and categories. Afterward, the other study team member reviewed the participant quotes and matched each quote to one of the identified themes.

2.7. Ethics and Procedures

Before conducting the study, a research protocol was analysed and approved by the Institutional Review Board. Prior to the interviews, all participants sign a written informed consent to record, anonymously report and publish the research data.

3. Results

Six themes emerged from the analysis of focus group data. These themes included several categories as showed in Table 1, and examples are provided in the following section.

Table 1. Barriers to undertaking a fall prevention strategy.

Themes	Categories	Participants (N = 18)
Healthcare system gaps	Access shortage	12
	Lack of personalised interventions	7
Social context	Stigma associated with fall	8
	Social awkwardness	7
Economic context	Financial capacity	12
Health status	Lack of physical fitness	7
	Impaired mobility	5
Psychological capability	Fear of falling and injuries	9
Lack of knowledge	Falls perceived as inevitable and not preventable	4
	Underestimation of risk	4

3.1. Healthcare System Gaps

3.1.1. Access Shortage

Participants highlighted a shortage of program offers. Hence, they were unable to engage in a fall prevention program.

> 'There are not many offers of these types of programs. While I was in the hospital, I participated in an exercise program to prevent falls, but after discharged I questioned everyone and nobody was able to refer me to a community-based program. There is a real shortage.' (P11)

3.1.2. Lack of Personalised Interventions

In addition to the offer shortage, participants reported that the ones they attended lack personalised interventions. They felt that to solve their problem, they should have been targets of tailored programs. Program participants had different problems, so they should receive interventions personalised to their different needs.

> 'There's no personalised intervention. There were around ten or twelve people in a room doing the same thing. My problem was not the same as the others, so how does the same intervention solve different problems.' (P3)

3.2. Social Context

3.2.1. Stigma Associated with Fall

Participants described stigma as a barrier to engage in a fall prevention strategy because they associate falls with the need to receive institutional care. They fear that by participating in a falls prevention strategy, their families might assume they lack the physical capacity to take care of themselves and therefore institutionalize them to nursing homes.

> 'It is unlikely for me to assume the need to undertake a fall prevention program because as soon as they feel that I lack capabilities to take care of me, they will search for a nursing home.' (P4)

3.2.2. Social Awkwardness

The group environment made participants state social awkwardness as they felt uncomfortable and unease in a group-based exercise program.

'At this age, it isn't normal for us to do training exercises in a gym. You look around and realise everybody feels uncomfortable. Life is full of awkward and uncomfortable situations. We can avoid them. You have a lot of say-so in how you feel as you grow older.' (P8)

3.3. Economic Context
Financial Capacity

Participants referred that their financial capacity is a major barrier to undertaking a falls prevention strategy. Even considering the offer of free programs, in some cases, the costs associated with travel in itself harm their family budget.

'Even if there was a greater offer of fall prevention programs, they are not free and you have to add travel costs. As you grow older, the money you spend on our health increases a lot.' (P10)

3.4. Health Status
3.4.1. Lack of Physical Fitness

Participants reported their experience of facing physical challenges. They consider that despite thinking that they were able to perform the physical component of the fall prevention program, they lacked physical fitness.

'It was a bit more than I could manage. I thought I was capable to perform the exercises without any problems, but the reality was different. I felt short of breath and tired. I went there once and gave up.' (P7)

3.4.2. Impaired Mobility

Besides their lack of physical fitness, participants also reported their inability to face physical challenges due to impaired mobility. This impairment has an impact not only on the ability to perform exercises but also on the ability to travel from home to the facilities where the training program takes place.

'There were several problems. First, my impaired mobility has a tremendous impact on my ability to travel to the clinic. Then I was unable to do more than half of the exercise because of my mobility.' (P2)

3.5. Psychological Capability
Fear of Falling and Injuries

Participants referred to the fear of falling and injuries as a barrier. They stated that after several falls, even if they did not sustain any injuries, they become afraid of falling and this leads them to feel more and more limited in terms of their autonomy and physical independence.

'Who wants to participate in any exercise program if they have to leave their house and risk falling again. It's a big problem because you fall, and fall again and then you became afraid. Fear sets in and you don't want to do any daily activities.' (P12)

3.6. Lack of Knowledge
3.6.1. Falls Perceived as Inevitable and Not Preventable

Participants referred that their lack of knowledge about falls led them to think that this was an issue that only affected frail older adults and that falls are accidental and, therefore, inevitable and not preventable.

'There is a belief that falls only happen to frail older adults. I thought they were an inevitable event associated with ageing. It wasn't just me who thought that. My sons also thought the same. Lack of knowledge leads to these common misconceptions.' (P12)

3.6.2. Underestimation of Risk

Participants reported that some older adults refused to admit that they are at risk of falling and thus underestimate the consequences of certain behaviours to increase the risk of fall.

'Sometimes people do not want to admit their weakness and they are careless, underestimate the consequences of their behaviours and then fall and sustain injuries.' (P1)

4. Discussion

Understanding the barriers to undertaking a falls prevention strategy may influence the guideline to change the process of selecting and more appropriately target the person at risk of falling.

It is well known from information gathered in other researches that before choosing the program interventions, decision-makers need to understand the target group, setting, and barriers to change [18].

This research found that access shortage and lack of personalised interventions are healthcare system gaps that could act as barriers for older adults to undertake a falls prevention strategy. Participants described difficulties with accessing any type of fall prevention programs due to access shortage. Older adults require opportunities within their environment to attend these types of programs. There must be a variety of offers so that the person can choose a program that best suits one's personhood [22].

It seems clear, that for the successful implementation of a fall prevention strategy in community settings, it requires an approach involving a greater program offers. Given the limited resources in Portugal, it is likely that potential users will become unmotivated after realising that the resources are scarce and scattered.

A theme articulated amongst participants was the lack of personalised interventions. The identification of this barrier may reflect the value attributed by participants in maintaining their personhood and usual routines. Further, previous studies have shown that older adults may value the affective characteristics of care as much as achieving better health outcomes [23]. It has been known for a long time that intervention strategies should be tailored to the cultural and socioeconomic context. There are no strategies that have universal applicability [24]. There is a growing body of evidence demonstrating that personalised interventions should be applied to each person to achieve positive clinical outcomes and increase their satisfaction [25]. This type of care can be the path to include the person at the centre of care and improve older adults' adherence to falls prevention strategies. Despite this acknowledgment, reports from participants revealed that in the programs they engaged in, this did not happen.

Another barrier highlighted in this study is the social context, namely the stigma associated with falls and social awkwardness. According to participants, older adults perceived falling as a stigma as they related falls with declining capabilities and loss of independence and consequently with the need to be admitted in a residential or nursing home. Many older adults feel embarrassed and stigmatised about their falls, and consequently choose not to show their weakness [26].

Similar findings have been identified among older adults in Eastern Culture. In older Chinese people, there was a refusal to use walking aids as they perceived them as a bad omen and carried stigma [27].

It is necessary to remove the stigma associated with falling so that older adults can get the help they need to promote healthy and active aging. Therefore, fall prevention strategies should convey the message of positive health and social benefits, such as improving muscle strength and body balance rather than focusing on reducing falls [28].

Participation in group programs can lead to social benefits and often act as an enabler for continued participation, although the transition to new groups could be challenging [29]. In this study, the participants considered the group environment as socially awkward because they felt out of place in that environment. This barrier can be linked closely to an individual's preference as in other researches the group environment was appointed either as an enabler or a barrier to continuing with a fall prevention program [29].

Another identified barrier is the economic context. This barrier has a crucial preponderance for older adults' participation in falls prevention strategies, because if they do not have the financial capacity to support their daily expenses, they will not consider undertaking any other activities. Other studies also identified the financial situation as a barrier to participate in a fall prevention strategy [30,31]. However, there seems to be a consensus in the literature that the cost associated with intervention may not be perceived as a barrier, as long as the cost is fair and reasonable enough [26].

Regarding the health status, participants reported their experience of facing physical challenges. Other researchers also identified the lack of physical fitness and impaired mobility as major barriers to undertake a falls prevention strategy [32,33]. In addition, they identified that previous habits and perceived value of physical activity can be an important factor to older adults' participation in exercise programs [32].

To undertake a falls prevention strategy participants must change their behaviour in the same manner as a sedentary person needs to be supported and encouraged to take an exercise program [34]. Physical training must be a progressive and adaptive process to allow the body to adapt to the stress of exercise with greater fitness [33]. Apparently, in the programs attended by participants, the exercise routines were not tailored to their needs and health status, and, therefore, they were not able to perform well. As mentioned previously, fall prevention strategies must be tailored to the context and the participants in order to increase their adherence. Furthermore, fall prevention programs must be multidimensional, combining a wide range of specific interventions that go beyond physical exercise [18,33].

The fear of falling was perceived as a barrier that leads older adults to feel physically limited and consequently have to protect themselves against dangers, by delegating their care to others, and ultimately denying their own autonomy and physical independence. In other researches, older adults with previous falls were more prone to undertake a falls prevention strategy, and those who were afraid of falling were four times more likely to enrol in these types of strategies [18].

The underestimation of risk and falls being perceived as inevitable and not preventable are lined up with the conviction that falls are part of ageing. These findings may suggest that falls prevention strategy are not effective and emphasise the vital need that older adults have to acquire more knowledge to demystify myths and misconceptions about falls. Educational or awareness strategies must be part of a multidimensional falls preventions strategy to counteract the common misconception that falls are simply an issue for older and frail adults as a result of accidents and, therefore, not preventable [18,33].

Limitations and Trustworthiness

Researchers carried out 18 interviews, which is considered sufficient for data saturation to occur. Data were collected by semi-structured interview during which participants described their experiences. The overall results illuminate variations in older adults' perspectives on barriers to undertake a falls prevention strategy.

In this study, participants' mental and physical status were not assessed. This is a limitation as active depression and sever physical illness could potentially influence the participants' answers. Additionally, similar to previous studies that depend on data collected from interviews, actual reports may diverge from what participants revealed due to biases such as lack of confidence in guaranteeing anonymity or protection of identity, values, or beliefs. We collected data from the reports of various participants to reduce this bias.

The study's trustworthiness was confirmed through credibility, transferability, dependability, and confirmability as described by Nowell, Norris, White, and Moules [35]. To increase credibility researchers debated each phase of analysis. Disagreements were solved by discussion until achieving consensus. To ensure its transferability, the researchers provide descriptions with appropriate quotations so that those who seek to transfer the findings to different sittings can judge transferability. To achieve dependability, researchers detailed every phase of the decision-making process so that others can follow the research. To ensure confirmability, external observers search for inconsistencies by comparing the similarity of their perceptions with the ones from the researchers.

5. Conclusions

In conclusion, this research has shown that older adults identify different key barriers to engage in a fall prevention strategy. According to participants' narratives, we identified six categories of barriers, namely healthcare system gaps, social context, economic context, health status, psychological capability, and lack of knowledge.

From our point of view, some barriers need urgently to be addressed for older adults to participate in a falls prevention strategy. The healthcare system gaps and social context are major barriers that highlight the critical need to develop and disseminate fall prevention strategies through public and private partnerships and social marketing.

These programs should be structured based on personalised interventions for each person, as scientific evidence shows that tailored interventions can lead to positive clinical outcomes and increase personal satisfaction.

Another barrier and perhaps the most important is the economic context because if the person does not have the financial capacity to support the fees to carry out the program, they will certainly not engage in these activities. Falls prevention strategies must be low cost because falls are a public health problem, with impact on economic costs for healthcare systems worldwide, so prevention must be a priority. Thus, fall prevention strategies should have a minimal cost for users and ultimately be supported by the healthcare systems.

Further research is needed to better understand the relationships and impact of these barriers, also it would be valuable to study which barriers are the drives of success to participation in a falls prevention strategy.

Author Contributions: J.B.F.: Conceptualization; Data curation; Formal analysis; Investigation; Methodology; Project administration; Writing Reviewing and Editing. S.B.F.: Conceptualization; Formal analysis; Investigation; Methodology; Writing and Reviewing. A.S.A.: Conceptualization; Formal analysis; Investigation; Writing and Reviewing. D.A.V.: Formal analysis; Investigation; Methodology; Writing and Reviewing. C.A.M.: Conceptualization; Methodology; Writing and Reviewing. All authors have read and agreed to the published version of the manuscript.

Funding: This research did not receive any specific grant from funding agencies in the public, commercial, or not-for-profit sectors.

Institutional Review Board Statement: The study was conducted according to the guidelines of the Declaration of Helsinki, and approved by the Institutional Review Board of CAS (ID/02-06.19, approved on 10 June 2019).

Informed Consent Statement: Informed consent was obtained from all subjects involved in the study.

Data Availability Statement: The data presented in this study are available on request from the corresponding author. The data are not publicly available due to participants´privacy.

Acknowledgments: This work is financed by national funds through the FCT—Foundation for Science and Technology, I.P., under the project UIDB/04585/2020. The researchers would like to thank the Centro de Investigação Interdisciplinar Egas Moniz (CiiEM) for the support provided for the publication of this article.

Conflicts of Interest: The authors declare that they have no conflict of interests.

Ethical Approval: Before conducting the study, a research protocol was analysed and approved by the CAS Institutional Review Board (Date: 10 June 2019; ID/02-06.19).

References

1. World Health Organization. Falls—Key Facts. 2018. Available online: https://www.who.int/news-room/fact-sheets/detail/falls (accessed on 22 January 2021).
2. Bergen, G.; Stevens, M.R.; Burns, E.R. Falls and fall injuries among adults aged ≥65 Years—United States, 2014. *Morb. Mortal. Wkly. Rep.* **2016**, *65*, 993–998. [CrossRef]
3. Haagsma, J.A.; Olij, B.F.; Majdan, M.; van Beeck, E.F.; Vos, T.; Castle, C.D.; Dingels, Z.V.; Fox, J.T.; Hamilton, E.B.; Liu, Z.; et al. Falls in older aged adults in 22 European countries: Incidence, mortality and burden of disease from 1990 to 2017. *Inj. Prev.* **2020**, *26*, 67–74. [CrossRef]
4. Heron, M. Deaths: Leading causes for 2016. national vital statistics reports: From the Centers for Disease Control and Prevention. National Center for Health Statistics. *Natl. Vital Stat. Syst.* **2018**, *67*, 1–77.
5. Hoffman, G.J.; Liu, H.; Alexander, N.B.; Tinetti, M.; Braun, T.M.; Min, L.C. Posthospital fall injuries and 30-day readmissions in adults 65 years and older. *J. Am. Med. Assoc. Netw. Open* **2019**, *2*, e194276. [CrossRef] [PubMed]
6. Burns, E.; Kakara, R. Deaths from falls among persons aged ≥65 years—United States, 2007–2016. *Morb. Mortal. Wkly. Rep.* **2018**, *67*, 509–514. [CrossRef]
7. Hefny, A.F.; Abbas, A.K.; Abu-Zidan, F.M. Geriatric fall-related injuries. *Afr. Health Sci.* **2016**, *16*, 554–559. [CrossRef] [PubMed]
8. Pi, H.; Hu, M.; Zhang, J.; Peng, P.; Nie, D. Circumstances of falls and fall-related injuries among frail elderly under home care in China. *Int. J. Nurs. Sci.* **2015**, *2*, 237–242. [CrossRef]
9. Loganathan, A.; Ng, C.J.; Tan, M.P.; Low, W.Y. Barriers faced by healthcare professionals when managing falls in older people in Kuala Lumpur, Malaysia: A qualitative study. *BMJ Open* **2015**, *5*, e008460. [CrossRef]
10. National Institute for Health and Care Excellence. Falls in Older People. 2015. Available online: www.nice.org.uk/guidance/qs86 (accessed on 20 January 2021).
11. Cameron, I.D.; Gillespie, L.D.; Robertson, M.C.; Murray, G.R.; Hill, K.D.; Cumming, R.G.; Kerse, N. Interventions for preventing falls in older people in care facilities and hospitals. *Cochrane Database Syst. Rev.* **2012**, *12*, CD005465. [CrossRef] [PubMed]
12. Miake-Lye, I.M.; Hempel, S.; Ganz, D.A.; Shekelle, P.G. Inpatient fall prevention programs as a patient safety strategy: A systematic review. *Ann. Intern. Med.* **2013**, *158*, 390–396. [CrossRef]
13. Thomas, E.; Battaglia, G.; Patti, A.; Brusa, J.; Leonardi, V.; Palma, A.; Bellafiore, M. Physical activity programs for balance and fall prevention in elderly: A systematic review. *Medicine* **2019**, *98*, e16218. [CrossRef] [PubMed]
14. Kim, K.I.; Jung, H.K.; Kim, C.O.; Kim, S.K.; Cho, H.H.; Kim, D.Y.; Ha, Y.C.; Hwang, S.H.; Won, C.W.; Lim, J.Y.; et al. Korean Association of Internal Medicine, The Korean Geriatrics Society evidence-based guidelines for fall prevention in Korea. *Korean J. Intern. Med.* **2017**, *32*, 199–210. [CrossRef]
15. Panel on prevention of falls in older persons, American Geriatrics Society and British Geriatrics Society summary of the updated American Geriatrics Society/British Geriatrics Society clinical practice guideline for prevention of falls in older persons. *J. Am. Geriatr. Soc.* **2011**, *59*, 148–157. [CrossRef] [PubMed]
16. Sazlina, S.; Krishnan, R.; Shamsul, A.; Zaiton, A.; Visvanathan, R. Prevalence of falls among older people attending a primary care clinic in Kuala Lumpur, Malaysia. *J. Community Health* **2008**, *14*, 11–16.
17. Coe, L.J.; St John, J.A.; Hariprasad, S.; Shankar, K.N.; MacCulloch, P.A.; Bettano, A.L.; Zotter, J. An integrated approach to falls prevention: A model for linking clinical and community interventions through the Massachusetts Prevention and Wellness Trust Fund. *Front. Public Health* **2017**, *5*, 38. [CrossRef] [PubMed]
18. Kiami, S.R.; Sky, R.; Goodgold, S. Facilitators and barriers to enrolling in falls prevention programming among community dwelling older adults. *Arch. Gerontol. Geriatr.* **2019**, *82*, 106–113. [CrossRef]
19. Tong, A.; Sainsbury, P.; Craig, J. Consolidated criteria for reporting qualitative research (COREQ): A 32-item checklist for interviews and focus groups. *Int. J. Qual. Health Care* **2007**, *19*, 349–357. [CrossRef]
20. Veiligheid, N.L. Valanalyse screeningstool valrisico voor de eerstelijnszorg fall analysis. Fall risk screening tool for primary care. 2017. Available online: https://intranet.onzehuisartsen.nl/file/download/default/A0990575496919D58AF03796C9263DFC/VNL-valanalyse-2017-ONLINE.pdf (accessed on 15 July 2019). (In Dutch).
21. Braun, V.; Clarke, V.; Hayfield, N.; Terry, G. Thematic analysis. In *Handbook of Research Methods in Health Social Sciences*; Liamputtong, P., Ed.; Springer: Singapore, 2019; pp. 843–860.
22. Naseri, C.; McPhail, S.M.; Haines, T.P.; Morris, M.E.; Shorr, R.; Etherton-Beer, C.; Netto, J.; Flicker, L.; Bulsara, M.; Lee, D.A.; et al. Perspectives of older adults regarding barriers and enablers to engaging in fall prevention activities after hospital discharge. *Health Soc. Care Community* **2020**, *28*, 1710–1722. [CrossRef]
23. Byrne, K.; Frazee, K.; Sims-Gould, J.; Martin-Matthews, A. Valuing the older person in the context of delivery and receipt of home support: Client perspectives. *J. Appl. Gerontol.* **2012**, *31*, 377–401. [CrossRef]
24. Siddiqi, K.; Newell, J.; Robinson, M. Getting evidence into practice: What works in developing countries? *Int. J. Qual. Health* **2005**, *17*, 447–454. [CrossRef]

25. Kuipers, S.J.; Cramm, J.M.; Nieboer, A.P. The importance of patient-centered care and co-creation of care for satisfaction with care and physical and social well-being of patients with multi-morbidity in the primary care setting. *BMC Health Serv. Res.* **2019**, *19*, 13. [CrossRef]
26. Horton, K.; Dickinson, A. The role of culture and diversity in the prevention of falls among older Chinese people. *Can. J. Aging* **2011**, *30*, 57–66. [CrossRef] [PubMed]
27. Kong, K.S.; Lee, F.K.; Mackenzie, A.E.; Lee, D.T. Psychosocial consequences of falling: The perspective of older Hong Kong Chinese who had experienced recent falls. *J. Adv. Nurs.* **2002**, *37*, 234–242. [CrossRef] [PubMed]
28. Stevens, J.A.; Noonan, R.K.; Rubenstein, L.Z. Older adult fall prevention: Perceptions, beliefs, and behaviors. *Am. J. Lifestyle Med.* **2010**, *4*, 16–20. [CrossRef]
29. Finnegan, S.; Bruce, J.; Seers, K. What enables older people to continue with their falls prevention exercises? A qualitative systematic review. *BMJ Open* **2019**, *9*, e026074. [CrossRef] [PubMed]
30. Barmentloo, L.M.; Dontje, M.L.; Koopman, M.Y.; Olij, B.F.; Oudshoorn, C.; Mackenbach, J.P.; Polinder, S.; Erasmus, V. Barriers and facilitators for screening older adults on fall risk in a hospital setting: Perspectives from patients and healthcare professionals. *Int. J. Environ. Res. Public Health* **2020**, *17*, 1461. [CrossRef]
31. Child, S.; Goodwin, V.; Garside, R.; Jones-Hughes, T.; Boddy, K.; Stein, K. Factors influencing the implementation of fall-prevention programmes: A systematic review and synthesis of qualitative studies. *Implement. Sci.* **2012**, *7*, 2–14. [CrossRef]
32. Olanrewaju, O.; Kelly, S.; Cowan, A.; Brayne, C.; Lafortune, L. Physical activity in community dwelling older people: A systematic review of reviews of interventions and context. *PLoS ONE* **2016**, *11*, e0168614. [CrossRef]
33. Sherrington, C.; Tiedemann, A. Physiotherapy in the prevention of falls in older people. *J. Physiother.* **2015**, *61*, 54–60. [CrossRef]
34. Whitehead, C.H.; Wundke, R.; Crotty, M. Attitudes to falls and injury prevention: What are the barriers to implementing falls prevention strategies? *Clin. Rehabil.* **2006**, *20*, 536–542. [CrossRef]
35. Nowell, L.S.; Norris, J.M.; White, D.E.; Moules, N.J. Thematic analysis: Striving to meet the trustworthiness criteria. *Int. J. Qual. Methods* **2017**, *16*, 1–13. [CrossRef]

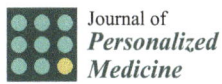

Article

Effect of a Music Therapy Intervention Using Gerdner and Colleagues' Protocol for Caregivers and Elderly Patients with Dementia: A Single-Blind Randomized Controlled Study

Guido Edoardo D'Aniello [1,*], Davide Maria Cammisuli [2], Alice Cattaneo [1], Gian Mauro Manzoni [1,3], Enrico Molinari [1,2] and Gianluca Castelnuovo [1,2]

[1] Istituto Auxologico Italiano IRCCS, Psychology Research Laboratory, 20122 Milan, Italy; al.cattaneo@auxologico.it (A.C.); gianmauro.manzoni@uniecampus.it (G.M.M.); molinari@auxologico.it (E.M.); gianluca.castelnuovo@unicatt.it (G.C.)
[2] Department of Psychology, Catholic University of the Sacred Heart, 20123 Milan, Italy; dm.cammisuli@gmail.com
[3] Faculty of Psychology, eCampus University, 20060 Novedrate, Italy
* Correspondence: g.daniello@auxologico.it; Tel.: +39-328-0326424

Abstract: Music therapy (MT) is considered one of the complementary strategies to pharmacological treatment for behavioral and psychological symptoms (BPSD) of dementia. However, studies adopting MT protocols tailored for institutionalized people with dementia are limited and their usefulness for supporting caregivers is under investigated to date. Our study aimed at evaluating the effects of an MT intervention according to Gerdner and colleagues' protocol in a sample of 60 elderly people with moderate-to-severe dementia of the Auxologico Institute (Milan, Italy) and associated caregivers, randomly assigned to an Experimental Group (EG) (n = 30) undergoing 30 min of MT two times a week for 8 weeks and to a Control Group (n = 30) (CG) receiving standard care. Before and after the intervention, residents-associated caregivers were administered the Caregiver Burden Inventory (CBI) and the Neuropsychiatric Inventory (NPI). Depression and worry were also assessed in caregivers prior to the intervention, by the Beck Depression Inventory-II and the Penn State Worry Questionnaire, respectively. A mixed model ANCOVA revealed a Time*Group effect (p = 0.006) with regard to CBI decreasing after the intervention for the EG and Time*Group effects (p = 0.001) with regard to NPI_frequencyXseverity and NPI_distress, with a greater effect for the EG than the CG. Implications for MT protocols implementations are discussed.

Keywords: music therapy; dementia; caregiver; RCT

1. Introduction

Behavioral and psychological symptoms of dementia (BPSD) refer to the spectrum of non-cognitive and non-neurological features significantly impacting on prognosis and patient management and constitute a major component of the disease, irrespective of its subtypes [1]. As dementia is a progressive disease, BPSD worsen over time, requiring higher support and increased sanitary and care costs [2]. The BPSD improve caregivers' burden and distress [3] and are related to an increased level of dependence according to the progression of the disease [4]. Indeed, many studies have focused on the stressors associated with caregivers' support. Remarkably, caregivers' coping strategies and personality factors seem to play a critical role towards controlling BPSD [5]. Further, BPSD increasing causes higher caregiver distress [3].

It has been estimated that the prevalence of BPSD in people with dementia living in institutional settings is approximately 91–96% [1] and the majority of patients mainly present with an outcome of neuropsychiatric symptoms such as depression, apathy, irritability, anxiety, euphoria, hallucination and disinhibition [6]. One of the most extensively used instruments to assess BPSD is the Neuropsychiatric Inventory (NPI) [7]. Validity

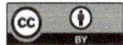

and reliability of the NPI have been established in different languages; it can evaluate 12 symptoms based on a caregiver's interview about patient (i.e., delusions, hallucinations, agitation, depression, anxiety, apathy, irritability, euphoria, disinhibition, aberrant motor behavior, night-time behavior disturbances, and eating behavior abnormalities) covering a wide range of symptoms associated with progressive dementia states. Treatment of BPSD currently represents a relevant therapeutic challenge for patients with moderate-to-severe dementia because of their difficulty in explaining feeling and emotions and agitation reported in the course of the disease [8]. Particularly, people with moderate-to-severe dementia are at higher risk of developing aggression [9], in terms of violent behavior and physically/verbally inappropriate responses to environmental stimuli [10].

Pharmacological treatment usually constitutes the primary approach to excessive behaviors but adverse effects of medication (e.g., speech inhibition, diminished language skills, altered gait and falls, and even a more severe cognitive deterioration) may occur in the treatment course [11], with negative consequences on patients' global status. Non-specific experiences such as music listening, touch therapy, and hand massage may be beneficial for calming neuropsychiatric symptoms presented by patients with moderate-to-severe dementia [12]. Specifically, Music Therapy (MT) represents a non-pharmacological complementary strategy to pharmacological treatment for dealing with neuropsychiatric symptoms of people with dementia [13]. Recent advancements improving personalized medicine in research, diagnosis and treatment of dementia have sustained a more comprehensive approach for patients, with the aim of better finalizing scientific knowledge to tailored interventions starting from data integration about an individual's specific pattern of genetic variability, environment and lifestyle factors [14].

Through non-verbal behavior and sound-music performances, MT allows participants to convey their emotions and feelings, establish a contact with significant others and modify their affective status and interpersonal communication, with a positive adaptation to their social environment. In particular, Gerdner and colleagues' protocol [15,16] supports the fact that archaic expressive and relational non-verbal abilities persist across a person's life span and may be reactivated by MT as interpersonal modalities of relationship. More specifically, Gerdner outlined a specific theoretical framework in order to formalize and refine an individualized music listening for patients with dementia through the "*Mid-range theory of individualized music intervention for agitation*" (IMIA) [17]. The first factor on which IMIA is based concerns the perception of music by the person with dementia. Although the pathology may drastically reduce the ability to understand and produce language, the receptive and expressive skills concerning music are generally preserved much longer and beyond the severity of cognitive decline. For this reason, although the literature has not yet come to a univocal and solid explanation, we tend to consider music processing as partially independent from cognitive efficiency [18]. The second factor concerns the ability of music to elicit memories. As a powerful means of reminiscence, music can produce both pleasant and unpleasant memories, depending on the type of evoked stimuli, images and sensations linked to the person's private experience [19]. In order to avoid the possibility that music may elicit negative memories, it must be selected (i.e., an "*individualized approach*"). It has to be part of the patient's positive experience and should be based on his/her personal preferences (for example, popular music at the time of patient's adulthood, or songs offered during religious or other services followed, etc.). As specified by Gerdner [16], the assessment must cover individual songs as well as preferred instruments and genres; if cognitive impairment affects the ability of the person to select music, it is possible to interview the caregiver to find this information.

Given these characteristics, such a kind of protocol seems to be promising as a complementary strategy to pharmacological treatment for people with dementia living in institutional settings. Starting from this assumption, the aim of our study was to evaluate the effect of an MT intervention adopting Gerdner and colleagues' protocol in reducing neuropsychiatric symptoms reported by dementia patients and in ameliorating the caregiver's burden.

2. Materials and Methods

2.1. Participants

A randomized controlled trial (RCT) was conducted at the RSA *Monsignor Bicchierai* in the Istituto Auxologico (Milan, Italy). A total of 60 residents and associated caregivers were randomly assigned to the Experimental Group (EG) (n = 30) and to the Control Group (CG) (n = 30). The residents underwent a complete psychogeriatric and neurological examination at the Institute, including the administration of the Mini Mental State Examination (MMSE). Inclusion criteria to the study for residents encompassed: (i) a diagnosis of dementia, according to the Diagnostic and Statistical Manual of Mental Disorders, Fourth Edition; (ii) age over 80 years; (iii) an MMSE score < 20, ranging from moderate to severe dementia [20]. The residents were excluded if they report: (i) a severe psychiatric condition; (ii) a hearing impairment; (iii) any other inability that may interfere in attending a 20-minute MT intervention; (iv) absence of a reliable informant caregiver. No restriction was applied for residents-associated caregivers. Eligible participants and their caregivers were provided with a detailed explanation of the study. All the patients signed an informed consent and for those with a severe cognitive deterioration, the consent was provided by the caregivers who were reassured of confidentiality and anonymity of the data collected during the study. Participants could withdraw from the study at any time without any effect on their usual care at the Facility.

2.2. Clinical Measures and Outcomes

Caregivers were administered the Caregiver Burden Inventory (CBI) [21] by a trained clinical psychologist dedicated to elderly care in the Facility. In addition, the Beck Depression Inventory-II [22] and the Penn State Worry Questionnaire [23] were used prior to the intervention. The caregivers were also interviewed about associated residents' neuropsychiatric symptoms by the Neuropsychiatric Inventory (NPI) (Cummings et al., 1994) [7] reporting two main scores (NPI_aXb = frequency for severity; NPI_distress = caregiver's distress). The effectiveness of the MT was expected as an improvement in the following outcome measures after the intervention: CBI total score, NPI_aXb and NPI_distress scores.

2.3. MT Intervention

The residents and associated caregivers were allocated to the EG and the CG using a predetermined list of randomization, with 1:1 allocation ratio and they were blinded towards the intervention (Figure 1). All the participants completed the study protocol. In both cases, caregivers were considered part of the Facility staff signing the *Individualized Care Plan* designed by the multidisciplinary group (i.e., geriatrician, nursing coordinator, educator, social assistant, and clinical psychologist) for each resident and agreed to attend the Facility activities program during the intervention. While residents and associated caregivers of the CG followed the usual care provided by the Assisted Healthcare Residence staff (i.e., educational support and entertainment activities), residents and associated caregivers of the EG underwent an intervention of music listening strictly respecting Gerdner and colleagues' protocol [24], as follows: (1) music selection according to patient's preference by caregivers [25]; (2) music material file (i.e., Mp3) preparation for each resident, as a result of the collaboration between caregiver and psychologist; (3) MT intervention on residents' room at the Facility as a quiet and comfortable environment (i.e., 30 min 2 times a week for 8 weeks, for a total of 16 sessions); (4) information provided to caregivers by the psychologist on patient's monitoring during sessions (in case of agitation, music listening was interrupted).

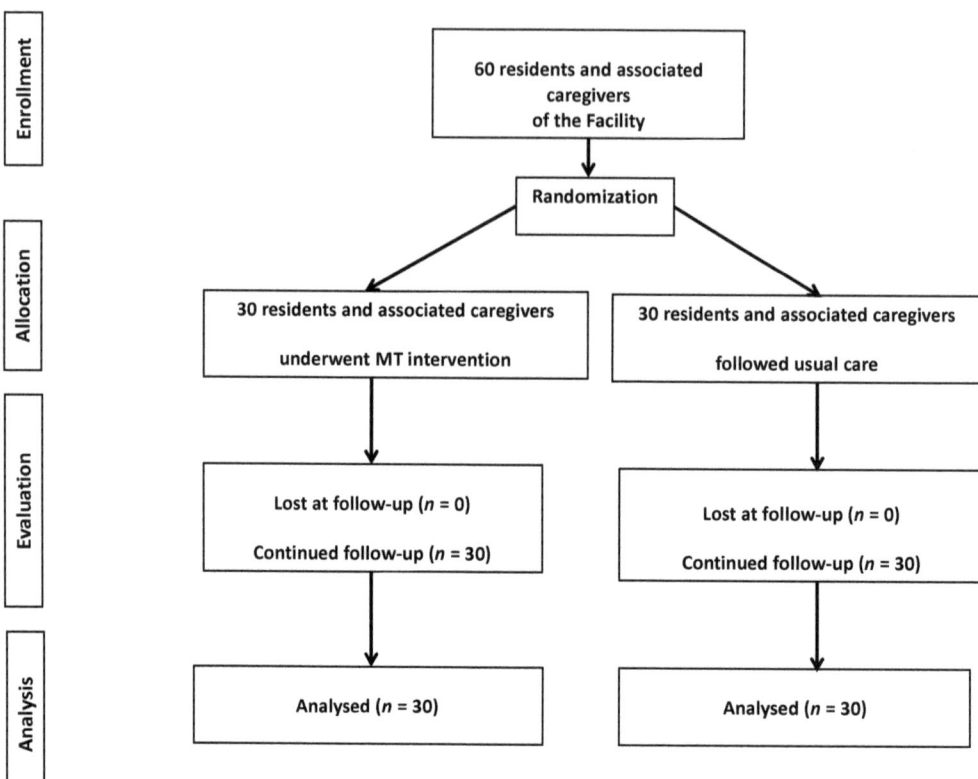

Figure 1. The study flow chart.

2.4. Statistical Analysis

The collected data passed the Shapiro–Wilk test for normality distribution and Levene test for variances homogeneity. The comparability of the two study groups was first determined using T-tests for independent samples for continuous variables. Then, changes between groups after the intervention were compared by a mixed model ANCOVA by controlling for significant differences that resulted after the T-tests at baseline (Dependent variables: CBI; NPI_aXb; NPI distress; Factors: Time and Groups, EG vs. CG; Covariates: BDI; PSWQ). The effect size was calculated by the eta squared.

3. Results

3.1. Descriptive Analysis of the Whole Sample

Age and education of the residents were 89.50($\pm$6.96) and 9.68($\pm$5.20) years, respectively, 41.7% male and 58.3% female, with an MMSE of 9.45 $\pm$ 6.66. Age and education of the caregivers were of 61.7($\pm$7.67) and of 11.5($\pm$7.66) years, respectively. Descriptive statistics of clinical measures are shown in Table 1.

Table 1. Clinical measures of the EG and the CG prior and after the intervention.

	EG (n = 30)	CG (n = 30)
BDI-II	9.23 ± 1.68	6.15 ± 1.12
PSWQ	49.80 ± 12.44	40.10 ± 15.39
CBI (baseline)	27.26 ± 13.37	24.06 ± 10.51
CBI (follow-up)	19.53 ± 10.40	30.53 ± 11.69
NPI_aXb (baseline)	20.46 ± 9.00	22.46 ± 12.96
NPI_aXb (follow-up)	6.70 ± 5.17	18.70 ± 8.65
NPI_distress (baseline)	10.66 ± 6.07	12.96 ± 6.21
NPI_distress (follow-up)	2.46 ± 2.06	10.66 ± 5.31

Data are expressed as mean ± standard deviation; EG: Experimental Groups; CG: Control Group; BDI-II: Beck Depression Inventory-II; PSWQ: Penn State Worry Questionnaire; CBI: Caregiver Burden Inventory; NPI_aXb: Neuropsychiatric Inventory_frequency for serverity; NPI_distress: Neuropsychiatric Inventory_distress.

3.2. Comparison of the EG and the CG

The T-tests for independent samples revealed that groups did not differ in terms of CBI (t(58) = 1.019, p = 0.313), NPI_aXb (t(58) = 1.715, p = 0.490) and NPI_distress (t(58) = 0.025, p = 0.156) dimensions at baseline. Conversely, significant differences were found in terms of depression severity (BDI-II) (t(58) = 3.768, p = 0.044), and worry (PSWQ) (t(58) = 0.678, p = 0.009).

3.3. CBI Results

As shown in Figure 2, a Time*Group effect (λ = 0.872; $F(1,56)$ = 8.038; p = 0.006; η^2 = 0.128) was found with regard to CBI that decreases after the intervention in the EG while this trend was not shown for the CG.

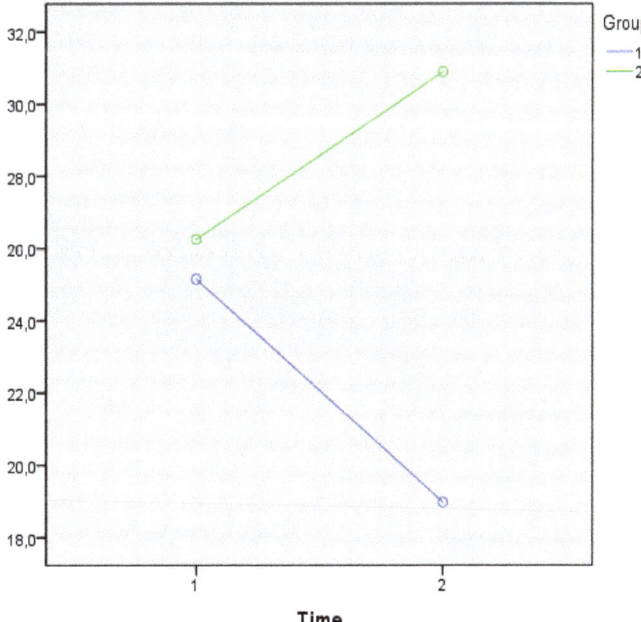

Figure 2. Comparison of the average CBI global scores in the EG (purple line) and in the CG over time (green line).

3.4. NPI Results

As shown in Figure 3, a Time*Group effect ($\lambda = 0.740$; $F(1,56) = 20.343$, $p = 0.001$; $\eta^2 = 0.260$) was also found with regard to NPI_aXb, with a greater effect for the EG. Likewise, as shown in Figure 4, a Time*Group effect ($\lambda = 0.779$; $F(1,56) = 16,165$, $p = 0.001$; $\eta^2 = 0.221$) was found with regard to NPI_distress, with a greater effect for the EG.

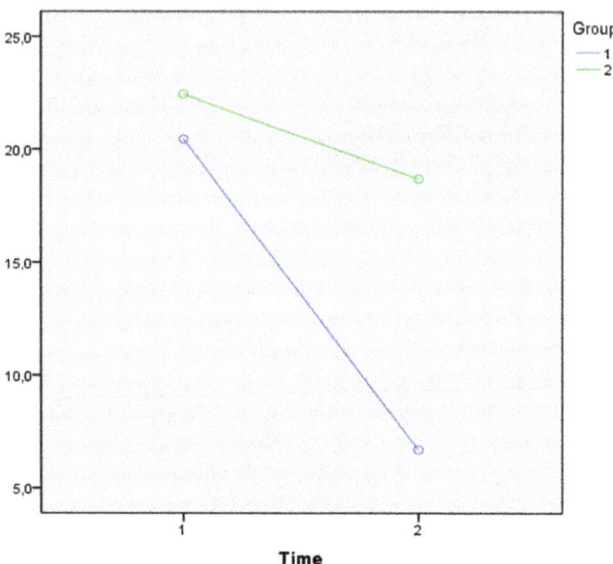

Figure 3. Comparison of the average NPI_aXb in the EG (purple line) and in the CG (green line) over time.

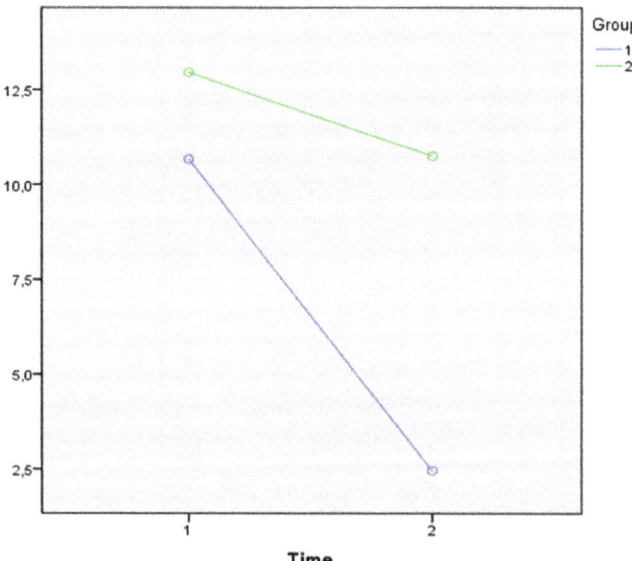

Figure 4. Comparison of the average NPI_distress in the EG (purple line) and in the CG over time (green line).

4. Discussion

We demonstrated that a structured MT intervention (i.e., 30 min two times a week for 8 weeks) based on Gerdner and colleagues' protocol [24] ameliorates caregivers' burden and reduces neuropsychiatric symptoms reported in assisted elderly residents with dementia better than usual care, both for their frequency/severity and perceived distress by caregivers. According to a recent 12-year longitudinal cohort study [26], understanding the natural course of neuropsychiatric symptoms in dementia is important for patient care planning and trial design. Remarkably, starting from a previous systematic literature review [27] highlighting how depression, agitation/aggression and apathy are the most distressing symptoms for caregivers assisting people with dementia, the MT intervention adopted reported an effect on neuropsychiatric symptoms as a whole, suggesting how it may be beneficial for a large spectrum of dimensions potentially impacting on patients' behavior and caregivers' health.

Other investigations have already shown a reduction in some neuropsychiatric symptoms associated with dementia after MT interventions. In detail, Garland et al. [28] showed that both listening to audiotapes with a conversation about positive experiences from the past and the exposure to a selection of songs that the individual used to enjoy in their youth are effective in reducing agitation. Holmes et al. [29] revealed that live interactive music is more effective than pre-recorded music in reducing apathy in moderate and severe dementia. Moreover, a case–control study [30] concluded that MT sessions consisting of singing songs chosen by the group accompanied by instruments significantly reduce agitation and anxiety in a sample of people suffering from moderate-to-severe Alzheimer's dementia. More recently, Raglio and colleagues [31] completed a Randomized Controlled Trial (RCT) reporting that consecutive cycles of 12 active MT sessions three times a week is sufficient for observing a significant reduction in behavioral disorders in severely impaired patients with dementia. Finally, Sung et al. [32] investigated the effects of group music sessions of 30 min, twice a week for 6 weeks in institutionalized elders with dementia (i.e., five-minute warm-up session with movements and breathing; 20-minute session of active participation using percussion instruments; five minutes of soft music listening) founding that such a type of intervention is effective for anxiety reduction. Our study added a few thoughts on MT protocols highlighting the potential role of music in evoking emotional response associated with personal memories (i.e., autobiographical events) thanks to an individualized approach able to bypass cognitive impairment severity.

Further, our findings are in line with the latest published Cochrane review [33] reporting that providing people with dementia with at least five sessions of a music-based therapeutic intervention improves overall behavioral and psychological problems at the end of treatment. According to the guidelines of the *Italian Psychogeriatric Association* [34] highlighting the necessity to produce RCTs based on structured evidence-based music protocols for people with dementia, we would stress that Gerdner and colleagues' schema represents an effective way to improve wellbeing both for people with dementia living in institutional settings and for their caregivers. Gerdner and colleagues' protocol for the usage of personal music materials to evoke past memories of the patients may represent an original application of personalized medicine in dementia, even if more efforts are necessary to meet the clinical complexity of the disease and to build stronger evidence able to address rehabilitation practice.

However, our study had some limitations. In order to reach a better generalizability of results, larger randomized *double-blind* controlled trials with follow-up measuring maintenance effects are encouraged in the future. Indeed, interventions based on listening to the music usually present the greatest effect at the end of the intervention, without maintenance effect [35]. It is also necessary to develop clinical trials aiming to design standardized protocols depending on etiology and stage of dementia so they can be applied alongside psychological intervention (e.g., cognitive-behavioral therapy) or pharmacological treatment. In addition, the CBI includes items referred to daily living and it does not fulfil criteria to specifically evaluate residents at institutional settings. In order to implement future RCTs, researchers should also assume measures such as the Revised Scale for Caregiving Self Efficacy [36] with the scope of facilitating the development of improved caregiver strategies for dealing with stressors form care. Potential effects of medication received by patients with dementia that may influence results were also not taken into account.

5. Conclusions

We documented that a structured MT intervention administered for 8 weeks (20 min a day) in a relaxing way for patients with moderate-to-severe dementia living in institutional settings is able to reduce BPSD and ameliorate caregivers' burden. Such an intervention was brief, safe, low-cost and can be replicated in similar contexts, without spending in excessive sanitary and human resources. A caregiver's efficacy for managing BPSD is an important determinant of familiar stress and plays a pivotal role with regard to patients' management. Implementing MT interventions with a more comprehensive assessment of caregivers' profile may be advantageous in supporting institutionalized elderly people with dementia.

Author Contributions: Conceptualization, G.E.D. and G.C.; methodology, G.E.D. and G.M.M.; formal analysis, D.M.C.; investigation, G.E.D.; resources, G.E.D.; data curation, A.C.; writing—original draft preparation, D.M.C.; writing—review and editing, E.M. and G.C.; visualization, A.C.; supervision, E.M. and G.C.; project administration, G.C. All authors have read and agreed to the published version of the manuscript.

Funding: This research received no external funding.

Institutional Review Board Statement: The study was conducted according to the guidelines of the Declaration of Helsinki and approved by the Ethics Committee of the Istituto Auxologico Italiano, (Milan, Italy) (Protocol number: "Interventions for Dementia 04/2018").

Informed Consent Statement: Informed consent was obtained from all subjects involved in the study.

Data Availability Statement: Details regarding data supporting results can be found at: http://tesionline.unicatt.it/handle/10280/59475, Accessed date: 11 April 2021.

Conflicts of Interest: The authors declare no conflict of interest.

References

1. Bessey, L.J.; Walaszek, A. Management of behavioral and psychological symptoms of dementia. *Curr. Psychiatry Rep.* **2019**, *21*, 1–11. [CrossRef] [PubMed]
2. Oliveira, A.M.D.; Radanovic, M.; Mello, P.C.H.D.; Buchain, P.C.; Vizzotto, A.D.B.; Celestino, D.L.; Celestino, D.L.; Florindo, S.; Piersol, C.V.; Forlenza, O.V. Nonpharmacological interventions to reduce behavioral and psychological symptoms of dementia: A systematic review. *BioMed Res. Int.* **2015**, *2015*, 218980. [CrossRef] [PubMed]
3. Mukherjee, A.; Biswas, A.; Roy, A.; Biswas, S.; Gangopadhyay, G.; Das, S.K. Behavioural and psychological symptoms of dementia: Correlates and impact on caregiver distress. *Dement. Geriatr. Cogn. Dis.* **2017**, *7*, 354–365. [CrossRef]
4. Moyle, W.; Murfield, J.E.; Griffiths, S.G.; Venturato, L. Assessing quality of life of older people with dementia: A comparison of quantitative self-report and proxy accounts. *J. Adv. Nurs.* **2012**, *68*, 2237–2246. [CrossRef] [PubMed]
5. Baharudin, A.D.; Din, N.C.; Subramaniam, P.; Razali, R. The associations between behavioral-psychological symptoms of dementia (BPSD) and coping strategy, burden of care and personality style among low-income caregivers of patients with dementia. *BMC Public Health* **2019**, *19*, 447. [CrossRef]
6. Lanctôt, K.L.; Amatniek, J.; Ancoli-Israel, S.; Arnold, S.E.; Ballard, C.; Cohen-Mansfield, J.; Ismail, Z.; Lyketsos, C.; Miller, D.S.; Musiek, E.; et al. Neuropsychiatric signs and symptoms of Alzheimer's disease: New treatment paradigms. *Alzheimers Dement.* **2017**, *3*, 440–449. [CrossRef]
7. Cummings, J.L. The Neuropsychiatric Inventory: Assessing psychopathology in dementia patients. *Neurology* **1997**, *48* (Suppl. 6), 10S–16S. [CrossRef]
8. Alsawy, S.; Mansell, W.; McEvoy, P.; Tai, S. What is good communication for people living with dementia? A mixed-methods systematic review. *Int. Psychogeriatr.* **2017**, *29*, 1785–1800. [CrossRef]
9. Gerdner, L.A. Effects of individualized versus classical "relaxation" music on the frequency of agitation in elderly persons with Alzheimer's disease and related disorders. *Int. Psychogeriatr.* **2000**, *12*, 49–65. [CrossRef] [PubMed]
10. Cipriani, G.; Danti, S.; Carlesi, C.; Di Fiorino, M. Old and dangerous: Prison and dementia. *J. Forensic Leg. Med.* **2017**, *51*, 40–44. [CrossRef]

11. Barry, H.E.; Bedford, L.E.; McGrattan, M.; Ryan, C.; Passmore, A.P.; Robinson, A.L.; Molloy, G.J.; Darcy, C.M.; Buchanan, H.; Hughes, C.M. Improving medicines management for people with dementia in primary care: A qualitative study of healthcare professionals to develop a theory-informed intervention. *BMC Health Serv. Res.* **2020**, *20*, 120. [CrossRef]
12. Viggo Hansen, N.; Jørgensen, T.; Ørtenblad, L. Massage and touch for dementia. *Cochrane Database Syst. Rev.* **2006**, *2006*, CD004989.
13. Cammisuli, D.M.; Danti, S.; Bosinelli, F.; Cipriani, G. Non-pharmacological interventions for people with Alzheimer's disease: A critical review of the scientific literature from the last ten years. *Eur. Geriatr. Med.* **2016**, *7*, 57–64. [CrossRef]
14. Reitz, C. Toward precision medicine in Alzheimer's disease. *Ann. Transl. Med.* **2016**, *4*, 107. [CrossRef]
15. Gerdner, L.A. Use of individualized music by trained staff and family: Translating research into practice. *J. Gerontol. Nurs.* **2005**, *31*, 22–30. [CrossRef]
16. Gerdner, L.A.; Buckwalter, K.C. Clarification: Research and Associated Evidence-Based Protocol for Individualized Music in Persons with Dementia. *Am. J. Geriatr. Psychiatry* **2017**, *25*, 1289–1291. [CrossRef]
17. Gerdner, L.A. Individualized music intervention protocol. *J. Gerontol. Nurs.* **1999**, *25*, 10–16. [CrossRef] [PubMed]
18. Schellenberg, E.G.; Weiss, M.W. Music and cognitive abilities. In *The Psychology of Music*; Deutsch, D., Ed.; Elsevier Academic Press Cambridge: Cambridge, UK, 2013; Volume 1, pp. 499–550.
19. Ratovohery, S.; Baudouin, A.; Palisson, J.; Maillet, D.; Bailon, O.; Belin, C.; Narme, P. Music as a mnemonic strategy to mitigate verbal episodic memory in Alzheimer's disease: Does musical valence matter? *J. Clin. Exp. Neuropsychol.* **2019**, *41*, 1060–1073. [CrossRef] [PubMed]
20. Perneczky, R.; Wagenpfeil, S.; Komossa, K.; Grimmer, T.; Diehl, J.; Kurz, A. Mapping scores onto stages: Mini-mental state examination and clinical dementia rating. *Am. J. Geriatr. Psychiatry* **2006**, *14*, 139–144. [CrossRef] [PubMed]
21. Novak, M.; Guest, C. Application of a multidimensional caregiver burden inventory. *Gerontologist* **1989**, *29*, 798–803. [CrossRef]
22. Beck, A.T.; Steer, R.A.; Brown, G.K. *Manual of the Beck Depression Inventory-II*; Psychological Corporation: San Antonio, TX, USA, 1996.
23. Meyer, T.J.; Miller, M.L.; Metzger, R.L.; Borkovec, T.D. Development and validation of the Penn State Worry Questionnaire. *Behav. Res. Ther.* **1990**, *28*, 487–495. [CrossRef]
24. Gerdner, L.A. Individualized music for dementia: Evolution and application of evidence-based protocol. *World J. Psychiatry* **2012**, *2*, 26–32. [CrossRef] [PubMed]
25. Gerdner, L.A.; Hartsock, J.; Buckwalter, K.C. *Assessment of Personal Music Preference (Family Version)*; The University of Iowa College of Nursing Gerontological Nursing Interventions Research Center, Research Dissemination Core: Iowa City, IA, USA, 2000.
26. Vik-Mo, A.O.; Giil, L.M.; Borda, M.G.; Ballard, C.; Aarsland, D. The individual course of neuropsychiatric symptoms in people with Alzheimer's and Lewy body dementia: 12-year longitudinal cohort study. *Br. J. Psychiatry* **2020**, *216*, 43–48. [CrossRef]
27. Feast, A.; Moniz-Cook, E.; Stoner, C.; Charlesworth, G.; Orrell, M. A systematic review of the relationship between behavioral and psychological symptoms (BPSD) and caregiver well-being. *Int. Psychogeriatr.* **2016**, *28*, 1761–1774. [CrossRef] [PubMed]
28. Garland, K.; Beer, E.; Eppingstall, B.; O'Connor, D.W. A comparison of two treatments of agitated behavior in nursing home residents with dementia: Simulated family presence and preferred music. *Am. J. Geriatr. Psychiatry* **2007**, *15*, 514–521. [CrossRef]
29. Holmes, C.; Knights, A.; Dean, C.; Hodkinson, S.; Hopkins, V. Keep music live: Music and the alleviation of apathy in dementia subjects. *Int. Psychogeriatr.* **2006**, *18*, 623–630. [CrossRef]
30. Svansdottir, H.B.; Snaedal, J. Music therapy in moderate and severe dementia of Alzheimer's type: A case–control study. *Int. Psychogeriatr.* **2006**, *18*, 613–621. [CrossRef]
31. Raglio, A.; Bellandi, D.; Baiardi, P.; Gianotti, M.; Ubezio, M.C.; Zanacchi, E.; Granieri, E.; Imbriani, M.; Stramba-Badiale, M. Effect of Active Music Therapy and Individualized Listening to Music on Dementia: A Multicenter Randomized Controlled Trial. *JAGS* **2015**, *63*, 1534–1539. [CrossRef] [PubMed]
32. Sung, H.C.; Lee, W.L.; Li, T.L.; Watson, R. A group music intervention using percussion instruments with familiar music to reduce anxiety and agitation of institutionalized older adults with dementia. *Int. J. Geriatr. Psychiatry* **2012**, *27*, 621–627. [CrossRef]
33. Van der Steen, J.T.; Smaling, H.J.A.; van der Wouden, J.C.; Bruinsma, M.S.; Scholten, R.; Vink, A.C. Music-based therapeutic interventions for people with dementia. *Cochrane Database Syst. Rev.* **2017**, *2*, CD003477. [CrossRef] [PubMed]
34. Raglio, A.; Bellelli, G.; Mazzola, P.; Bellandi, D.; Giovagnoli, A.R.; Farina, E.; Stramba-Badiale, M.; Gentile, S.; Gianelli, M.V.; Ubezio, M.C.; et al. Music, music therapy and dementia: A review of literature and the recommendations of the Italian Psychogeriatric Association. *Maturitas* **2012**, *72*, 305–310. [CrossRef] [PubMed]
35. Moreno-Morales, C.; Calero, R.; Moreno-Morales, P.; Pintado, C. Music Therapy in the Treatment of Dementia: A Systematic Review and Meta-Analysis. *Front. Med.* **2020**, *7*, 160. [CrossRef] [PubMed]
36. Steffen, A.M.; McKibbin, C.; Zeiss, A.M.; Gallagher-Thompson, D.; Bandura, A. The revised scale for caregiving self-efficacy: Reliability and validity studies. *J. Gerontol. B Psychol. Sci. Soc. Sci.* **2002**, *57*, 74–86. [CrossRef] [PubMed]

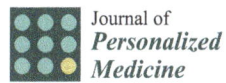

Article

Complexity of Nurse Practitioners' Role in Facilitating a Dignified Death for Long-Term Care Home Residents during the COVID-19 Pandemic

Shirin Vellani [1,2], Veronique Boscart [1,3], Astrid Escrig-Pinol [1,4], Alexia Cumal [1,2], Alexandra Krassikova [1,5], Souraya Sidani [6], Nancy Zheng [1], Lydia Yeung [1] and Katherine S. McGilton [1,2,*]

[1] KITE, Toronto Rehabilitation Institute–University Health Network, Toronto, ON M5G 2A2, Canada; shirin.vellani@mail.utoronto.ca (S.V.); vboscart@conestogac.on.ca (V.B.); aescrig@esimar.edu.es (A.E.-P.); alexia.cumal@mail.utoronto.ca (A.C.); alexandra.krassikova@mail.utoronto.ca (A.K.); nancy.zheng@mail.utoronto.ca (N.Z.); Lydia.yeung@uhn.ca (L.Y.)
[2] Lawrence S. Bloomberg, Faculty of Nursing, University of Toronto, Toronto, ON M5T 1P8, Canada
[3] Canadian Institute for Seniors Care, Conestoga College, Kitchener, ON N2G 4M4, Canada
[4] Mar Nursing School, Universitat Pompeu Fabra, 08002 Barcelona, Spain
[5] Rehabilitation Sciences Institute, Faculty of Medicine, University of Toronto, Toronto, ON M5G 1V7, Canada
[6] Daphne Cockwell School of Nursing, Ryerson University, Toronto, ON M5B 1Z5, Canada; ssidani@ryerson.ca
* Correspondence: Kathy.mcgilton@uhn.ca

Abstract: Due to the interplay of multiple complex and interrelated factors, long-term care (LTC) home residents are increasingly vulnerable to sustaining poor outcomes in crisis situations such as the COVID-19 pandemic. While death is considered an unavoidable end for LTC home residents, the importance of facilitating a good death is one of the primary goals of palliative and end-of-life care. Nurse practitioners (NPs) are well-situated to optimize the palliative and end-of-life care needs of LTC home residents. This study explores the role of NPs in facilitating a dignified death for LTC home residents while also facing increased pressures related to the COVID-19 pandemic. The current exploratory qualitative study employed a phenomenological approach. A purposive sample of 14 NPs working in LTC homes was recruited. Data were generated using semi-structured interviews and examined using thematic analysis. Three categories were derived: (a) advance care planning and goals of care discussions; (b) pain and symptom management at the end-of-life; and (c) care after death. The findings suggest that further implementation of the NP role in LTC homes in collaboration with LTC home team and external partners will promote a good death and optimize the experiences of residents and their care partners during the end-of-life journey.

Keywords: nurse practitioners; nursing home; COVID-19; palliative care; end-of-life; dignified death; older adults

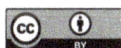

1. Introduction

Individuals transition into long-term care (LTC) homes closer to the end of their life, often with multiple comorbid conditions, higher levels of frailty and complex care needs [1,2]. Within two years of admittance to LTC homes, most residents die [3,4]. As such, integrating a palliative approach to care would be the best practice, yet this approach is not implemented in the majority of LTC homes [5]. A palliative approach consists of four central components: advance care planning (ACP); optimization of pain and symptom management; psychosocial and spiritual support for patients and their care partners such as friends and relatives; as well as shared decision-making [6]. While death is an unavoidable ending for LTC residents, promoting a good death is an important goal of palliative and end-of-life (EOL) care [7,8]. This has become even more pressing during the SARS Coronavirus Disease-2019 (COVID-19) pandemic, where a large percentage of deaths were among LTC home residents, ranging from 8% in South Korea, 39% in the

United States [9] to 69% in Canada [10]. A good death is characterized by freedom from preventable distress in a dying person, their care partners, and healthcare providers; being in harmony with the wishes of the dying person and their family; and following clinical, cultural, and ethical principles [8].

Sufficient staffing is critical for integrating a palliative approach to care and to achieve a good death in LTC settings [11]. However, the LTC sector continues to suffer from chronic staff shortages. Furthermore, to optimize the infection prevention and control measures, LTC home residents have been forced to isolate in their own spaces with visitation restrictions from informal care partners [12]. Traditionally, care partners served as a means for socialization and comfort for residents and also assisted them with activities of daily living [13] and EOL care. During the pandemic, there was also a shift in physicians' presence in LTC homes, where many only worked virtually because of their multiple responsibilities across different sites [14], limiting the planning and implementation of palliative care. In contrast, nurse practitioners (NPs) in Ontario were able to work on-site [15] and provide palliative and EOL care by functioning closely with the registered nurses, registered practical nurses, and personal support workers in LTC homes [16]. In Ontario, Canada, NPs are advanced practice registered nurses, who can autonomously assess, diagnose, and treat patients [17,18] and are well situated to optimize the palliative and EOL care needs of LTC home residents. Empirical evidence demonstrates that palliative care provided by NPs in various settings was effective in improving persons' emotional and mental wellbeing as well as their quality of life [19]. NPs also increase ACP [20–22] and provide effective management of EOL symptoms [23,24].

There is limited knowledge of the role of NPs in delivering and coordinating EOL care and facilitating a "dignified death" for LTC home residents during the COVID-19 pandemic. The term "dignified death" is used in this study as the pandemic has hampered the staff's ability to ensure a good death by exposing the entire LTC sector to a myriad of challenges such as understaffing, limited family contacts and a lack of palliative care supplies in some LTC homes [25,26]. In this study, we focused on NPs' perspectives and aimed to explore their role and experiences in facilitating a dignified death for LTC home residents, while also facing the increased pressures related to the COVID-19 pandemic. The findings will provide more insight and understanding into the roles NPs can play in integrating a palliative approach to care in LTC settings. Additionally, they will highlight knowledge gaps in optimizing resident-centered palliative care in LTC homes and yield implications for policy makers, researchers and clinicians.

2. Methods

2.1. Study Design and Participants

We designed an exploratory qualitative study to examine the role and experiences of NPs in supporting a dignified death during the COVID-19 pandemic, as the phenomenon is not yet well-observed or understood [27]. The study used a phenomenological approach, which is valuable in revealing shared and divergent experiences among participants [28]. We conducted telephone-based semi-structured interviews with NPs providing care to LTC home residents during the pandemic. Recruitment of NPs was assisted by the Nurse Practitioners Association of Ontario (npao.org). An email with information about the project, inclusion criteria, and an invitation to connect with the Research Coordinator (RC) was sent out to all NPAO members by their Practice and Policy Manager. The inclusion criteria were NPs who worked at least three days a week in an LTC home that had experienced positive cases of COVID-19.

The final sample included 14 NPs from 14 separate LTC homes, representing approximately 13% of all NPs working in the province of Ontario LTC home sector. The recruited NPs worked in both rural and urban settings, as well as in an even mix of profit and not-for-profit homes. This sample size was determined by reaching data saturation, i.e., information became repetitious from one interview to the next [29]. The characteristics of the participating NPs and their respective LTC homes are summarized in Table 1.

Table 1. Characteristics of study participants and their workplace.

Participant Characteristics	
Average Age (range)	45 (28–66)
Gender (%)	
Men	3 (21%)
Women	11 (79%)
Years of work experience (range)	9.3 (2–21)
Group (%)	
Attending NP	8 (57%)
NP outreach team	6 (43%)
LTC home Ownership (%)	
For-profit	6 (43%)
Not-for-profit	8 (57%)
Beds in LTC homes where participants work	182 (62–302)

Most participants were employed full-time and experienced an increase in work hours during the pandemic. Most NPs were females, with an average of nine years of experience in the NP role. Eight were attending NPs and six were outreach NPs. Attending NPs provide direct primary health care to residents, work to increase the knowledge and skills of LTC staff and participate in administrative and leadership activities to improve resident outcomes and reduce pressures on acute care services [30]. The outreach NP role was created to provide comprehensive acute and episodic care to LTC home residents in order to avoid transfers to the emergency department, facilitate hospital transfers where necessary and reduce hospital stays through early repatriation back to LTC homes [31].

2.2. Procedures

After receiving approval from the Research Ethics Board at the participating institution, we obtained informed written consent from participants. In order to maintain their privacy, each participant was assigned a unique identification number and all their identifying information (e.g., name of the LTC home) was anonymized in the interview transcripts. Furthermore, the research team had considered potential emotional distress for the participants with sharing their experiences during the pandemic. Therefore, participants were offered breaks, opportunity to reschedule or drop out and resources for emotional support during the interview, when appropriate. Telephone interviews were conducted by the RC (AK), while a note-taker (LY or AC) recorded the topics conversed and other relevant information. We audio-recorded the interviews, which, on average, lasted 50 min and took place between August and October 2020. Participants were provided a CAD 50 gift card as an honorarium serving as a token of appreciation for their time and effort to participate during these extremely busy and challenging times imposed by the pandemic. Most NPs participated in the study after their regular work hours to prevent any work-time lost deserving recognition from the research team and the honorarium may have served as an incentive to participate. However, gift card was only introduced after NPs had expressed desire to participate to prevent the risk of undue inducement as suggested by other authors [32]. Additionally, participants had the option of leaving the study at any time.

Semi-structured interviews were designed to prompt NPs to elaborate and reflect on their experiences [33] related to EOL care before and during the pandemic, their thoughts on their roles and responsibilities, and how they adapted in the context of the crisis. The interview guide was piloted for clarity and relevance with an NP experienced in LTC homes, but this was not included as a part of the study. The interview guide is in Supplementary Material Table S1.

2.3. Data Analysis

The RC reviewed and anonymized the professionally transcribed interviews by using participant ID numbers, guaranteeing confidentiality. Data were exported into NVIVO12 to be managed, organized, and coded. This provided the research team a greater degree of transparency and integrity as members were able to create notes on their thoughts alongside the participant data. It also allowed for tracking the analysis process efficiently and mapping the relationship between data. However, some team members had no prior experience of using the NVIVO software, which required more time to train members on its features before starting the analysis process. There were also issues with software compatibility with different operating systems.

We employed an inductive thematic analysis strategy adapted from Braun and Clark [34]. The analysis was conducted in five steps. The first step involved familiarization with the data, which involved the research team reading the interview transcripts multiple times and writing down ideas as they arose in the due process. Debrief sessions were held after each interview to discuss and record emerging topics. In the second step, the initial themes were generated in a systematic manner across all the interviews. Two analysts (a primary analyst (AK) and a secondary analyst (either SV/AC/LY/NZ)) independently coded each transcript into initial themes and met regularly to compare and reconcile coding divergences. The third step involved the identification of broader categories by collating the codes and gathering data appropriate to each category. Preliminary themes were used as a point of departure and evolved as analysts generated additional themes during the coding stage. We organized these topics into 10 preliminary themes. Initial themes were grouped into three broad categories. In the fourth stage, broader categories were reviewed by the full research team to reach a consensus on these categories. Once the consensus was reached, the analysis team verified the coherence of categories and themes by reading all collated extracts for each theme, while also confirming that they were sufficiently and meaningfully different from each other [34]. This strategy allowed for refinement of the themes and categories. In the final step, the research team generated clear definitions and names of the categories and themes [34,35], as presented in Table 2 below.

Table 2. Categories and themes related to the Nurse Practitioners' role in facilitating a dignified death in long-term care homes during the COVID-19 pandemic using Thematic Analysis [34].

Thematic Analysis Steps	Codes, Categories and Themes
1. Familiarization with data	1.1. The full corpus of interviews was transcribed by a professional transcription service and reviewed for accuracy against the recordings by the RC. 1.2. The primary (AK) and secondary analysts (SV, AC, LY, NZ) created a list of 10 initial themes: NP Clinical Responsibilities, NP Leadership Responsibilities, NP Educational Responsibilities, NP Administrative Responsibilities, Staffing, Infection Control and Prevention, Resident Care, Assuming Multiple Roles, Pandemic Preparedness, Interprofessional Collaboration.
2. Generation of initial themes	2.1. Additional themes generated included: ACP; palliative and EOL care; virtual care; resident outcomes; death and dying; confinement and isolation. 2.2. If an analyst identified a new topic in a transcript, they would engage in discussion with other analysts to see if the topic fit into one of the previously identified themes or a new theme was required to be generated.

Table 2. Cont.

Thematic Analysis Steps	Codes, Categories and Themes
3. Identification of broader categories	3.1. The research team reviewed the full list of themes to identify sub-categories. For example, when participants talked about palliative care, an initial theme, they did so in the context of how they carried out ACP and goals of care conversations, so we included this theme in the sub-category, "Taking a proactive approach to facilitate mass ACP conversations". 3.2. Upon review of sub-categories, the research team then aggregated them into three broader categories. For example, sub-categories "Taking a proactive approach to facilitate mass ACP conversations" and "Connecting with care partners for difficult yet critical discussions (goals of care)" were grouped into one category, "ACP and goals of care discussion". 3.3. The initial themes were collated into the agreed upon categories and sub-categories by the analysis team.
4. Review of categories and consensus	4.1. The team checked each sub-category against the organized, coded data to ensure internal consistency and polished them as needed. For example, two sub-categories were merged, i.e., "Keeping a vigil at the time death" and "psychosocial needs of residents", into a single sub-category, "Addressing psychosocial needs of residents and care partners". 4.2. The analysis team reviewed all identified categories against the developing topics to make sure that they correctly represented the meanings manifest in the dataset as a whole. 4.3. All identified categories and sub-categories were discussed by the research team to draw mutual links between them and devise an outline that tells the story of the data.
5. Defining and naming final categories	5.1. Using a consensus approach, the research team generated names and definitions for the final categories and sub-categories listed below: A. ACP and goals of care discussion A.1. Taking a proactive approach to facilitate mass ACP conversations A.2. Connecting with care partners for difficult yet critical discussions (goals of care) B. Pain and symptom management at the EOL B1. Optimizing emergency supplies B2. Prescribing anticipatory medications to aid symptom management B3. Consulting with experts where needed B4. Addressing psychosocial needs of residents and care partners C. Care after death C1. Being present with staff for the dignified performance of last offices C2. Providing emotional support to staff and family upon death

Credibility was ensured by conducting systematic peer debriefing sessions, incorporating researcher reflexivity and triangulation, keeping an exhaustive record of the process and decisions made, managing data systematically, and analyzing opposing accounts [33,36]. Discussions during these peer debriefing sessions resulted in adjustments in the order and phrasing of questions to improve the flow and clarity during subsequent interviews, and in a list of preliminary themes appearing on each interview. For example, while we initially thought there was a sub-category related to how NPs partnered with families to ensure a dignified death, with more debriefing sessions and subsequent interviews, we realized that NPs reached out to family members for different purposes along the journey. Thus, the specific reasons for reaching out to families were included as themes within each category to better represent the important role NPs had related to connecting with families in all aspects of EOL care. The Standards for Reporting Qualitative Research guidelines were followed [37].

3. Results

Three categories were derived in relation to the NPs' roles and responsibilities in facilitating a dignified death for LTC home residents under their care: (a) ACP and goals of care discussions; (b) pain and symptom management at the EOL; and (c) care after death. The categories are presented in Table 2 and detailed below.

3.1. ACP and Goals of Care Discussions

NPs described this responsibility as engaging with residents and more frequently with their health care proxies, who were often care partners, by taking a proactive approach to facilitate ACP and goals of care conversations. They connected with care partners for difficult, yet critical, discussions when the residents appeared to be nearing the EOL. During the pandemic, these conversations with care partners usually happened virtually over the telephone or through video calls. NPs attested to the importance of implementing a palliative approach to care where the focus is on the residents' quality of life, while also adhering to the safety requirements necessitated by the COVID-19 pandemic. Many highlighted the complexity of these discussions in light of care partners' inability to see firsthand the residents' decline due to the physical distancing restrictions. One NP explained:

> *This was time-consuming, but we were very successful in bringing families into sort of an understanding of reality and acceptance of end-of-life issues ... advance-care planning was a huge, huge part of my time–helping families to move along that continuum.* (NP 13)

NPs explained that, generally, ACP and goals of care conversations are carried out with care partners and residents at the time of admission to the LTC home, and regularly thereafter, particularly when any acute changes in condition arise. However, during the pandemic, the need and frequency of these conversations increased markedly, as explained by this NP:

> *If there's a change in the resident's condition, I would be the one in touch with the families. It was a bit more fast-forwarded (during the pandemic). I just had so many of them. So, I would have daily conversations with probably five to 10 families about goals of care.* (NP 3)

Some LTC homes did not have the resources to tackle these discussions in a timely way. Therefore, several NP participants were specifically assigned by their LTC home management to support LTC staff in holding ACP and goals of care discussions with families, given the constant risk of a sudden decline in residents' condition. In addition, several NPs organized and chaired virtual care conferences linking families with the care team and physicians, involving residents whenever possible. One NP (*NP 8*) noted that their team was called "palliative rescue", alluding to the fact that when there was a COVID-19 outbreak, several residents became sick very fast, potentially needing life-sustaining treatments and goals of care discussions. This NP explained:

> *One of my homes I was supporting virtually and via telephone had a COVID outbreak. They started with 10 cases, and then within three days, they had 30, and then it was escalating, and then by the end of the week, they had over 77 cases. So, at that point, we spoke with the DOC [director of care] and were asked to support goals of care discussions with the families because the home had not done them and so the entire outreach team started calling families to discuss goals of care.* (NP 8)

Many NPs noted that communication with families was a responsibility that frequently fell upon them during the pandemic. Several NPs indicated that although these conversations were lengthy, they were gratifying. NPs engaged in difficult conversations with care partners regarding prior requests for life-sustaining treatments, such as resuscitation, in light of the inherent risk of aerosolizing COVID-19 viral particles during such interventions, and the impact of these treatments on residents' quality of life and wellbeing. These interactions provided care partners the opportunity for shared decision-making to devise a plan of care, whether that involved comfort care in the LTC home or transfer to a hospital, which was not always possible due to the pandemic and restrictions imposed by the acute care hospitals, making these conversations even more difficult. In terms of restrictions, some NPs indicated that in order to prepare for the surge of patients with COVID-19 in acute care, some administrators within LTC homes were informed to avoid hospital transfers by managing their residents' acute changes in condition within their homes. As such, NPs needed to make decisions on how to balance the needs of the residents and potential outcomes of life-sustaining treatments. Some NPs made these difficult decisions in consultation with emergency department physicians, which was often made possible based on a history of working together.

NPs were sensitive to the fact that care partners could not be present physically due to the social distancing measures when the residents were dying. As such, in many cases, NPs helped family members appreciate the inevitable nearing of the EOL and also provided much needed emotional support. One participant explained:

Yes, communicating with families was my big responsibility really. It sort of just fell upon me, explaining to the families what was happening and if it looked like the person was at the end-of-life, then I would be talking to them about palliative care and what things we could do for the person in the home in order for them to have a dignified death in the home. (NP 12)

Overall, NPs made it their duty to keep the families abreast of the residents' condition, such as how COVID-19 was affecting them and what the care options were for the day, which served as a lifeline for the families given their inability to be physically present with the resident. They served as a link between the family and the residents, listened to the families' fears and concerns, and answered their questions.

3.2. Pain and Symptom Management at the EOL

The NPs' second responsibility consisted of optimizing comfort for residents who were at the EOL and where death was imminent, through pain and symptom management. This involved working closely with LTC home staff and management teams in optimizing emergency supplies and planning ahead for emergencies; prescribing anticipatory medications to aid EOL symptom management; consulting with expert clinicians where needed; and addressing the psychosocial needs of residents and families. Some NPs played an instrumental role in creating the EOL order sets with input from palliative care physicians in their local hospital. They also updated these order sets regularly to include relevant symptom management for residents dying of COVID-19 infection due to its unique symptom profile because the appearance and progression of symptoms such as respiratory distress can be rapid and fulminant, intensifying over a short period of time; and shared them with clinicians at other LTC homes. Additionally, NPs led educational initiatives to prepare and guide staff on interventions pertaining to intravenous therapy and hypodermoclysis. Moreover, NPs became involved in sourcing an optimal stock of emergency supplies such as oxygen, parenteral antibiotics and analgesics in the event that they were needed after hours. One NP explained:

We had a lot more End-of-Life meds in the building. We had more oxygen concentrators. We had more IM antibiotics, more Hydromorphone ... we did increase our emergency stock med, so that we could ... like at 2:00 a.m. if we needed to. So, I guess that's the other thing we did plan. (NP 6)

In general, NPs were instrumental in ensuring that analgesics and other medications were available when needed for palliative and EOL care needs. Many NPs stressed the importance of collaborative teamwork involving LTC home nurses and other staff to optimize residents' care given the scarcity of resources and shortage of staff.

NPs expressed that it was difficult to complete timely in-person assessments given the challenges associated with insufficient staffing and the time required to don and doff the personal protective equipment (PPE) with each resident interaction. Despite this, they tried their best and worked with other staff for ongoing identification of distressing symptoms, prescribing anticipatory and emergent treatments to address them, specifically in cases where EOL order sets had not been implemented. Many referred to the fact that LTC home physicians were generally not present in person during the pandemic, requiring NPs to manage this limitation in medical management. Therefore, NPs also assisted staff in the safe and timely delivery and assessment of prescribed therapies, including opioids. Ultimately, together, the teams ensured that residents died peacefully. Several NPs expressed that EOL care was most challenging because of the physical/social isolation, whereby direct contact with residents was more limited, in addition to family and friends not being able to visit. Many NPs found that working closely with the LTC staff and connecting with other NPs working in the LTC sector served as sources of strength to deal with challenges they experienced during these times. NPs ensured that staff and residents' care partners had their direct numbers to reach out any time of the day. Moreover, they worked hard to identify residents close to the EOL and ensured that symptom management was provided, as this quote exemplifies:

> We just really wanted to identify the residents who were unfortunately really sick or passing away from COVID. Because we didn't want them to die uncomfortably and alone and without any support and care. And that was probably the most emotional because you find residents with a respiratory rate of 50 and they're diaphoretic and they're struggling to breathe and they're alone. And so, we did provide our assessments and we tried to give the residents the treatment that they needed to die comfortably. (NP 10)

NPs talked about the complexity of LTC home resident care associated with their advanced age and multimorbidities, sometimes requiring consultation with expert clinicians and services to optimize pain and symptom management at the EOL. NPs consulted physicians with expertise in nephrology, palliative care, and geriatrics mostly virtually when they were unable to visit in-person. Furthermore, to address situations when they were not available, NPs developed algorithms for LTC home staff on how to consult with specialists. In some LTC homes, palliative care physicians provided expert consultations to NPs in order to facilitate a dignified death for residents with more complex needs, as is highlighted in this quote:

> So, the ten residents that died, I provided their palliative care, their end-of-life symptom management. And if there was a resident that I was having difficulty managing their symptoms, I would call and consult with a palliative care physician to get those symptoms under control. (NP 1)

Therefore, NPs' resourcefulness in consulting with clinical experts helped to ensure the better control of symptoms for residents who were nearing death.

Many NPs also addressed the psychosocial needs of residents and their families, particularly when the residents were nearing the EOL. They expressed that sitting vigil at the time of death is considered a norm in LTC homes; however, this was challenging during the pandemic. They felt a sense of responsibility to promote human connection in these difficult circumstances as best as possible, through creative means, with support from LTC home staff. Several NPs pointed out that compassionate visits were offered to care partners when their residents were imminently dying, allowing them to stay as long as possible while making sure that their PPE remained safely usable. This was illustrated by NPs in the following quotes:

> When we were talking about comfort or end-of-life, then we were offering compassionate visits. So essentially once I was in contact with the families, then I would put them on the list of allowed visitors. (NP 3)

> As soon as we possibly could, if people were dying, knowing they were clearly at the end-of-life, then families could come in–one person at a time with full PPE. (NP 13)

In cases where families could come but were unable to be at the bedside due to the active risk of exposure to the aerosolized virus, NPs and LTC home staff tried unprecedented and creative ways to allow families and residents to see and hear each other through a window or virtual means. One NP shared her experience with a resident that involved juggling with safety procedures while also enabling family connection in the last moments of life:

> I feel at peace at least with what we were able to do for her ... her oxygen requirements were going up fast ... potentially aerosolizing the COVID virus. ... we knew she was

> *going to pass away from COVID ... and she was on the main floor so the family was able to come to her window. We were able to sort of set up the phone on our end and then call their cell phone on the other side, so it kind of looked like you were talking to each other ... it was very sad but it was also, you know, the quote "good death" if you will.* (NP 5)

Finding creative ways to promote connection and support the psychological needs of the resident and care partners at the last moments of life highlights the critical role the NPs played.

Moreover, in many cases, NPs collaborated with LTC home staff such as personal support workers to keep vigil at the time of residents' death so that they would not die alone. They held residents' hands or played a musical instrument when the care partner could not be at their bedside. This was believed to be a source of comfort for residents as well as staff, and in line with enabling a dignified death given the restrictions imposed by the COVID-19 pandemic.

3.3. Care after Death

The third NP role responsibility involved being present with the staff for the dignified performance of last offices and providing emotional support to staff and care partners upon residents' death. Care after death also included informing the care partners of the death, upholding the pandemic-related policy of allowing only one grieving care partner at a time, and completing death certificates, sometimes after hours. Several NPs expressed feeling significant moral distress as the pandemic led to losing several residents under their care in a short period of time, in addition to seeing care partners lose time for genuine human connections that will not be replaced. One NP explained:

> *It was very difficult to watch families come in one at a time and try to manage their grieving by themselves, with their other family in the parking lot. That's what's changed at end-of-life; that's what made it so difficult. Calling a resident's family to say that they passed away, and they weren't there.* (NP 1)

Despite their own high emotional burden, NPs worked hard to provide emotional support to grieving care partners.

NPs also worked closely with LTC home nurses and the administrators in devising and implementing new policies related to the care after death. To contain the potential spread of the COVID-19 virus, they had a very restricted amount of time to pronounce death, inform the family, perform the last offices (previously performed by the funeral homes), and hand over the body to the funeral home staff, who were not allowed to come into the building; all of this while avoiding the omnipresent media. NPs identified that they were under a great deal of pressure to prevent the accumulation of bodies in LTC homes. NPs took on the leadership role in identifying the best practices in performing the last offices with dignity and care as well as instituting specific considerations for those who died with COVID-19 infection. They educated staff on COVID-19-focused care after death through demonstrations and hands-on help. As, many unregistered staff had no previous experience of performing last offices. One NP describes their post-death experience as follows:

> *The other thing that we had a lot of policy around, this sounds horrible, but on pronouncing death and removing bodies from the home. This was a nightmare. We got this thing that said nobody could come in the home to take them out—I'm going to cry ... but we had to do all of the post-mortem care and the nurses found that so hard. So again, we needed to look at how it was done, how do you transport people out. How do we keep the media from photographing people that died as they're being taken out of the home? It was brutal.* (NP 13)

Given that NPs in the province of Ontario have the ability to complete the death certificates if they had the primary responsibility of the patient, they were responsible for completing them as soon as the residents passed. This NP describes her experience below:

> *All the death certificates were completed online. I would often get a phone call in the middle of the night to do a death certificate, like at 2:00 a.m. to complete one, where those could have waited 'till the next morning, previously.* (NP 6)

As such, NPs worked beyond normal hours to fulfill their duties that also involved administrative tasks post residents' death, highlighting the significance of their role and the added stress.

NPs described challenges encountered by the LTC home staff after any resident's death due to experiencing pandemic-based disenfranchised grief. For example, novel and continuously changing COVID-19 policies affected how LTC home staff would traditionally perform care after death. As a result, NPs had to meet the pandemic-imposed demands while also mindfully allocating large amounts of time and effort in working closely with nurses and other staff to adapt new policies and providing them emotional support to recognize and process the losses. One participant stated:

> *Because normally the way nursing homes deal with resident death is the funeral home would come and prepare the body and whatnot. And there's actually a ceremony, not a real ceremony, but all the staff lines up at the front entrance and it's more of a respectful send-off to the resident, whereas this is kind of like "OK, let's just get the body ready and take them outside." And no one was allowed to be there to witness all of this stuff. So, it just doesn't feel as humanistic as how it was done pre-COVID.* (NP 2)

NPs provided emotional support to staff, especially after the changes to the processes after death were made, which often left little room for staff's own grieving. As one NP noted:

> *What I learned very quickly is she [staff] just needed to be listened to, and just needed to have someone who could validate her fears and say yeah, we don't know all the answers but we're going to get through this, and we're going to do it together ... mostly it was listening, listening, listening, and modeling. And trying–and not appearing fearful yourself.* (NP 13)

Many NPs expressed that given the challenges associated with working during the pandemic, they had minimal time to focus on in their own self-care; however, they found communication exchanges with other staff helpful. NPs relayed a sense of accomplishment and gratitude to be a part of the healthcare workforce during this pandemic. They highlighted that their work was complemented by the LTC home staff and administrators, all of whom were devoted to doing their best to provide person-centered care during this time of crisis when much was unknown. It appears that NPs served as a binding force that played a crucial role in holding together the staff and residents in facilitating a dignified death for the residents.

4. Discussion

SARS COVID-19-related adverse events and mortality have been the highest in the LTC sector globally [38,39]. This is because of a complex interplay of multiple intricate and inextricably connected factors that increase the vulnerability of LTC home residents to not only contract COVID-19 infection but also to sustain poor outcomes, including death [40,41]. Amidst this unprecedented crisis, there has been a further decline in already limited human and material resources in LTC homes to optimally provide for the needs of the residents and the workforce, who continued to care for their residents with threadbare resources [42].

Residents admitted to LTC homes are increasingly complex, with high care needs [1,2]. Death is a critical juncture for not only the residents but also their care partners and LTC home staff [3,4]. However, the COVID-19 pandemic brought a variety of challenges in the achievement of a good death. This study demonstrated that NPs, along with staff within LTC home teams, collaborated and worked tirelessly to support a dignified death experience for residents. NPs and staff assisted in ACP and goals of care discussions with residents and care partners, both proactively and when residents showed signs of acute changes in condition. This, in turn, helped care partners move forward in accepting the impending EOL. Findings from our study correlate with other studies that demonstrated an increase in ACP discussion where NPs were involved in the residents' care team [20–22], with one study showing a 300% increase in the number of residents with ACP discussions [20]. Similar to the findings in our study, Campbell and colleagues also found that NPs were part of the collective approach in ensuring residents were frequently assessed, especially those in the last stage of their life [43]. NPs worked hard so that residents' distressing symptoms were addressed, that they were comfortable, and died in their familiar surroundings rather than a hospital, when appropriate. NPs helped LTC home staff and administrators implement new policies and procedures related to post-death care, such as dignified care of the deceased, while maintaining the infection prevention and control measures, in addition to catering to the emotional needs of the staff and grieving care partners.

Our study demonstrated that NPs played a vital role in promoting a dignified death for LTC home residents while navigating the challenges of the COVID-19 pandemic. Based on previous studies, a good death is a broad construct where multiple factors can play a role to achieve it [44]. These factors can be related to the individual experiencing the death, their care partners as well as healthcare providers. Allison and O'Connor describe a 6-step framework used by clinical nurse specialists to facilitate a good death in residential aged care facilities [45]. The framework involved (1) responding within 24–48 h of a referral; (2) visiting the residential aged care setting to assess the resident and train the staff; (3) developing a care plan; (4) encouraging staff to proactively request medications for pain, respiratory secretion, and nausea from the general practitioner; (5) liaising with management and ensuring support for staff; and (6) involving the family in care planning and preparing them for death. The findings from our study suggest that NPs were able to faciliate a dignified death which appeared to be aligned with the 6-step framework provided by Allison and O'Connor, but also did more due to their expanded scope of practice. For example, some NPs were available 24 h a day either in person or over the phone, not only to staff but also to residents' care partners. Additionally, they were able to prescribe medications including opioids in order to maximize comfort in the last moments of life.

In addition to pain control, peace, and dignity, the presence of care partners, and being surrounded by familiar people and things have also been identified as sources promoting a good death in those dying with dementia [46]. Though people's preferences for the presence of others may vary, having someone present at the time of death can serve to address the primal need for companionship and is seen as a closing chance to display comfort and affection to the resident [47]. Whereas COVID-19 stripped the care partners of these opportunities, NPs collaborated with LTC home staff in identifying ways to connect them through virtual and other creative means. NPs or the staff also sat vigil by the residents' bedside of those who were in the last moments of their life. However, there remains a need for further initiatives and research on how to best care for residents' spiritual and cultural needs as well as the needs of the bereaved in light of the strange circumstances imposed by the COVID-19 pandemic [48].

This study highlights several research, policy, and clinical implications. NPs fostered interdisciplinary collaboration for in-house care that embraced an integrated palliative approach with chronic disease management. However, a palliative approach to care is not a norm in the LTC sector and regular ACP discussions are not a standard of practice [49]. ACP discussions are generally held in the form of level of care documentation to identify residents' and their proxy's wishes related to hospital admission and resuscitation at the time of admission to the LTC home and do not necessarily identify their values and wishes such as for their EOL care. Furthermore, previous research has identified that non-palliative specialist NPs who have provided palliative care to people under their care have also expressed the need for education in palliative care [50], highlighting a gap in relevant training and education. A recent work commissioned by the Alzheimer

Society of Canada on Improving End-of-Life Care for People with Dementia in LTC homes during the COVID-19 pandemic and beyond proposes three strategies to implement a palliative approach [49]. These include (a) adopting it in the whole home; (b) education and training of all staff on a palliative approach to care; and (c) implementing policies and tools that assist staff to use their knowledge about a palliative approach to enhance resident care [49]. Some LTC homes have successfully implemented a palliative approach through initiatives such as the Strengthening a Palliative Approach in Long Term Care Model (SPA-LTC) [51,52]. Hence, there is much to learn from their experiences in order to successfully implement this approach in other homes and to increase the capacity of LTC home staff, including the NPs as well as external consultants. Additionally, there is a need to implement the same palliative care standards of practice across all practice settings, appreciating the highly complex resident population served by LTC homes.

NPs working collaboratively with their team members have demonstrated the ability to provide high quality palliative and EOL care [19,23,53]. Countries and regions where the role of NPs is either non-existent or in infancy can learn from the experiences of various regions in Canada, the USA and the UK, where the role of the NP has been successfully implemented [18] to be able to autonomously assess, diagnose, order, and interpret diagnostic tests and treat their patients with full prescriptive authority. In addition, they are able to collaborate with other healthcare practitioners including primary care physicians and palliative care specialists and seek further advice when required. Furthermore, they embrace shared decision-making and serve as a link bringing the healthcare team, residents and their care partners together for coordinated care planning [43,54]. As a result, NPs globally can be in a better position to deliver timely and person-centered care to LTC home residents, which includes the provision of a dignified death.

Although this study provides new insights into the evidence involving the role of NPs in the integration of a palliative approach, it has limitations. It is an exploratory study involving a small sample of NPs; hence, the findings may not be transferable to other regions. However, the NPs included in our study worked in geographically diverse regions of Ontario, including both private and not-for-profit homes serving a wide range in the number of residents. In addition, we did not compare the experiences of NPs working in different models, i.e., attending or outreach and in different types of LTC homes. This was due to them all having performed similar functions and conveying the same sense of duty in caring for their residents who are experiencing the EOL. However, future research should explore the differences between the roles, responsibilities, and outcomes associated with the two groups of NPs working in LTC settings. Finally, the study did not include other LTC home staff such as nurses and administrators. This results in missing insights into their role in implementing an integrated palliative approach and supporting a dignified death to their residents during the pandemic.

5. Conclusions

Despite numerous challenges, the NPs played a critical role in facilitating a dignified death for LTC residents through ACP and goals of care discussions, EOL pain and symptom management and care measures after the death of residents. A dignified death for residents was accomplished in close collaboration with LTC home staff. The COVID-19 pandemic has emphasized the need to take an upstream approach in implementing an integrated palliative approach to care for residents and their care partners that focuses on the needs of the whole person while acknowledging their mortality. While LTC homes need to implement this approach, in light of the exceptional circumstances imposed by the pandemic, it is critical that interventions are in place to address complicated bereavement in care partners and moral distress in LTC home staff.

Supplementary Materials: The following are available online at https://www.mdpi.com/article/10.3390/jpm11050433/s1, Table S1: Semi-Structured Interview Guide with Nurse Practitioners.

Author Contributions: All authors have contributed substantially to the work reported. Conceptualization, K.S.M. and S.V.; methodology, A.E.-P., and K.S.M.; validation, K.S.M., A.E.-P., S.V. and A.K.; formal analysis, S.V., A.K., A.C., N.Z., L.Y., A.E.-P. and K.S.M.; investigation, A.K., A.C. and L.Y.; resources, K.S.M.; data curation, A.K., K.S.M. and S.V.; writing—original draft preparation, S.V.; writing—review and editing, S.V., K.S.M., V.B., A.E.-P., A.C., S.S., A.K., L.Y., N.Z.; visualization, A.K.; supervision, K.S.M.; project administration, L.Y. and A.K.; funding acquisition, K.S.M. All authors have read and agreed to the published version of the manuscript.

Funding: This research was funded by Maria and Walter Schroeder Institute for Brain Innovation and Recovery.

Institutional Review Board Statement: The study was conducted according to the guidelines of the Declaration of Helsinki and approved by the Research Ethics Board of the Toronto Rehabilitation Institute-University Health Network (protocol code: 20-5652; date of approval: 20 July 2020).

Informed Consent Statement: Informed consent was obtained from all participants involved in the study.

Data Availability Statement: Not applicable.

Acknowledgments: We would like to acknowledge the NPs who took time to participate in the study.

Conflicts of Interest: The authors declare no conflict of interest. The funders had no role in the design of the study; in the collection, analyses, or interpretation of data; in the writing of the manuscript, or in the decision to publish the results.

References

1. Kelly, A.; Conell-Price, J.; Covinsky, K.; Cenzer, I.S.; Chang, A.; Boscardin, W.J.; Smith, A.K. Length of Stay for Older Adults Residing in Nursing Homes at the End of Life. *J. Am. Geriatr. Soc.* **2010**, *58*, 1701–1706. [CrossRef]
2. Hirdes, J.P.; Mitchell, L.; Maxwell, C.J.; White, N. Beyond the 'Iron Lungs of Gerontology': Using Evidence to Shape the Future of Nursing Homes in Canada. *Can. J. Aging/La Rev. Can. du Vieil.* **2011**, *30*, 371–390. [CrossRef]
3. Hoben, M.; Chamberlain, S.A.; Gruneir, A.; Knopp-Sihota, J.A.; Sutherland, J.M.; Poss, J.W.; Doupe, M.B.; Bergstrom, V.; Norton, P.G.; Schalm, C.; et al. Nursing Home Length of Stay in 3 Canadian Health Regions: Temporal Trends, Jurisdictional Differences, and Associated Factors. *J. Am. Med. Dir. Assoc.* **2019**, *20*, 1121–1128. [CrossRef]
4. Boyle, T. Death rates higher in for-profit nursing homes, report says. In *Toronto Star*; Jordan Bitove: Toronto, ON, Canada, 2015.
5. Touzel, M.; Shadd, J. Content Validity of a Conceptual Model of a Palliative Approach. *J. Palliat. Med.* **2018**, *21*, 1627–1635. [CrossRef]
6. Vellani, S.; Puts, M.; Iaboni, A.; McGilton, K. Integration of a palliative approach in the care of older adults with dementia in primary care settings: A scoping review. *Can. J. Aging* **2021**, in press.
7. Smith, A.K.; Periyakoil, V.S. Should We Bury "The Good Death"? *J. Am. Geriatr. Soc.* **2018**, *66*, 856–858. [CrossRef] [PubMed]
8. Vanderveken, L.; Schoenmakers, B.; De Lepeleire, J. A Better Understanding of the Concept "A Good Death": How Do Healthcare Providers Define a Good Death? *Am. J. Geriatr. Psychiatry* **2019**, *27*, 463–471. [CrossRef] [PubMed]
9. Comas-Herrera, A.; Zalakaín, J.; Lemmon, E.; Henderson, D.; Litwin, C.; Hsu, A.T.; Schmidt, A.E.; Arling, G.; Kruse, F.; Fernández, J.-L. *Mortality Associated with COVID-19 in Care Homes: International Evidence*; International Long-Term Care Policy Network: London, UK, 2020.
10. Canadian Institute for Health Information. *The Impact of COVID-19 on Long-Term Care in Canada: Focus on the First 6 Months*; CIHI: Ottawa, ON, Canada, 2021.
11. Froggatt, K.A.; Moore, D.C.; Block, L.V.D.; Ling, J.; Payne, S.A.; Arrue, B.; Baranska, I.; Deliens, L.; Engels, Y.; Finne-Soveri, H.; et al. Palliative Care Implementation in Long-Term Care Facilities: European Association for Palliative Care White Paper. *J. Am. Med. Dir. Assoc.* **2020**, *21*, 1051–1057. [CrossRef] [PubMed]
12. Armitage, R.; Nellums, L.B. COVID-19 and the consequences of isolating the elderly. *Lancet Public Health* **2020**, *5*, e256. [CrossRef]
13. Williams, S.W.; Zimmerman, S.; Williams, C.S. Family Caregiver Involvement for Long-Term Care Residents at the End of Life. *J. Gerontol. Ser. B* **2012**, *67*, 595–604. [CrossRef]
14. Ministry of Health. *COVID-19 Guidance: Primary Care Providers in a Community Setting*; Ministry of Health: Toronto, ON, Canada, 2020.
15. Government of Ontario. *Emergency Management and Civil Protection Act*; Government of Ontario: Toronto, ON, Canada, 2020.
16. McGilton, K.S.; Krassikova, A.; Boscart, V.; Sidani, S.; Iaboni, A.; Vellani, S.; Escrig-Pinol, A. Nurse Practitioners Rising to the Challenge during the Coronavirus Disease 2019 Pandemic in Long-Term Care Homes. *Gerontologist* **2021**, gnab030. [CrossRef] [PubMed]
17. Maier, C.B.; Batenburg, R.; Birch, S.; Zander, B.; Elliott, R.; Busse, R. Health workforce planning: Which countries include nurse practitioners and physician assistants and to what effect? *Health Policy* **2018**, *122*, 1085–1092. [CrossRef] [PubMed]

18. International Council of Nurses [ICN]. *Nurse Practitioner/Advance Practice Nurse Network: Country Specific Practice Profiles*; International Council of Nurses: Geneva, Switzerland, 2020.
19. Dyar, S.; Lesperance, M.; Shannon, R.; Sloan, J.; Colon-Otero, G. A nurse practitioner directed intervention improves the quality of life of patients with metastatic cancer: Results of a randomized pilot study. *J. Palliat. Med.* **2012**, *15*, 890–895. [CrossRef] [PubMed]
20. Craswell, A.; Wallis, M.; Coates, K.; Marsden, E.; Taylor, A.; Broadbent, M.; Nguyen, K.-H.; Johnston-Devin, C.; Glenwright, A.; Crilly, J. Enhanced primary care provided by a nurse practitioner candidate to aged care facility residents: A mixed methods study. *Collegian* **2020**, *27*, 281–287. [CrossRef]
21. Acorn, M. Nurse Practitioners as Most Responsible Provider: Impact on Care for Seniors Admitted to an Ontario Hospital. *Int. J. Nurs. Clin. Pract.* **2015**, *2*, 1–11. [CrossRef]
22. Mullaney, S.E.; Melillo, K.D.; Lee, A.J.; MacArthur, R. The association of nurse practitioners' mortality risk assessments and advance care planning discussions on nursing home patients' clinical outcomes. *J. Am. Assoc. Nurse Pract.* **2016**, *28*, 304–310. [CrossRef]
23. Kaasalainen, S.; Ploeg, J.; McAiney, C.; Martin, L.S.; Donald, F.; Martin-Misener, R.; Brazil, K.; Taniguchi, A.; Wickson-Griffiths, A.; Carter, N.; et al. Role of the nurse practitioner in providing palliative care in long-term care homes. *Int. J. Palliat. Nurs.* **2013**, *19*, 477–485. [CrossRef] [PubMed]
24. Miller, S.C.; Lima, J.C.; Intrator, O.; Martin, E.; Bull, J.; Hanson, L.C. Palliative Care Consultations in Nursing Homes and Reductions in Acute Care Use and Potentially Burdensome End-of-Life Transitions. *J. Am. Geriatr. Soc.* **2016**, *64*, 2280–2287. [CrossRef]
25. Arya, A. *Palliative Care has been Lacking for Decades in Long-Term Care*; Institute for Research on Public Policy: Montreal, QC, Canada, 2021.
26. Ontario Health Coalition. *Situation Critical, Planning, Access, Levels of Care and Violence in Ontario's Long-Term Care*; Ontario Health Coalition: Toronto, ON, Canada, 2019.
27. Creswell, J.W. *Qualitative Inquiry & Research Design*; Sage Publications: Thousand Oaks, CA, USA, 2007.
28. Brink, H.; Van Der Walt, C.; Van Rensburg, G. *Fundamentals of Research Methodology for Health Care Professionals*, 2nd ed.; Juta Academic: Cape Town, South Africa, 2006.
29. Strauss, A.; Corbin, J. *Basics of Qualitative Research: Techniques and Procedures for Developing Grounded Theory*, 2nd ed.; Sage: London, UK, 1998.
30. Willging, P.R. Better geriatric care isn't an 'impossible dream'. *Nurs. Homes* **2004**, *53*, 16.
31. El-Masri, M.M.; Omar, A.; Groh, E.M. Evaluating the Effectiveness of a Nurse Practitioner-Led Outreach Program for Long-Term-Care Homes. *Can. J. Nurs. Res.* **2015**, *47*, 39–55. [CrossRef]
32. Grady, C. Payment of clinical research subjects. *J. Clin. Investig.* **2005**, *115*, 1681–1687. [CrossRef] [PubMed]
33. Patton, M.Q. *Qualitative Research & Evaluation Methods*; Sage Publications: Thousand Oaks, CA, USA, 2001.
34. Braun, V.; Clarke, V. Using thematic analysis in psychology. *Qual. Res. Psychol.* **2006**, *3*, 77–101. [CrossRef]
35. Höbler, F.; Argueta-Warden, X.; Rodríguez-Monforte, M.; Escrig-Pinol, A.; Wittich, W.; McGilton, K.S. Exploring the sensory screening experiences of nurses working in long-term care homes with residents who have dementia: A qualitative study. *BMC Geriatr.* **2018**, *18*, 235. [CrossRef]
36. Lincoln, Y.S.; Guba, E.G. *Naturalistic Injury*; Sage Publications: Newbury Park, CA, USA, 1985.
37. O'Brien, B.C.; Harris, I.B.; Beckman, T.J.; Reed, D.A.; Cook, D.A. Standards for reporting qualitative research: A synthesis of recommendations. *Acad. Med.* **2014**, *89*, 1245–1251. [CrossRef]
38. Hirdes, J.P.; Declercq, A.D.; Finne-Soveri, H.; Fries, B.E.; Geffen, L.; Heckman, G.; Lum, T.; Meehan, B.; Millar, N.; Morris, J.N. *The Long-Term Care Pandemic: International Perspectives on COVID-19 and the Future of Nursing Homes*; Balsillie School of International Affairs: Waterloo, ON, Canada, 2020.
39. Canadian Institute for Health Information. *Pandemic Experience in the Long-Term Care Sector: How Does Canada Compare with Other Countries?* CIHI: Ottawa, ON, Canada, 2020.
40. Andrew, M.; Searle, S.D.; E McElhaney, J.; A McNeil, S.; Clarke, B.; Rockwood, K.; Kelvin, D.J. COVID-19, frailty and long-term care: Implications for policy and practice. *J. Infect. Dev. Ctries.* **2020**, *14*, 428–432. [CrossRef]
41. Ritchie, H.; Ortiz-Ospina, E.; Beltekian, D.; Mathieu, J.; Hasell, J.; Macdonald, B.; Giattino, C.; Appel, C.; Roser, M. *Coronavirus Pandemic (COVID-19)*; OurWorldInData.org: Oxford, UK, 2020.
42. Casey, L. Staffing shortages, absentee leaders linked to high mortality in Ontario long-term care homes. In *The Globe and Mail*; The Canadian Press: Toronto, ON, Canada, 2021.
43. Campbell, T.D.; Bayly, M.; Peacock, S. Provision of Resident-Centered Care by Nurse Practitioners in Saskatchewan Long-Term Care Facilities: Qualitative Findings from a Mixed Methods Study. *Res. Gerontol. Nurs.* **2020**, *13*, 73–81. [CrossRef] [PubMed]
44. Munday, D.; Petrova, M.; Dale, J. Exploring preferences for place of death with terminally ill patients: Qualitative study of experiences of general practitioners and community nurses in England. *BMJ* **2009**, *339*, b2391. [CrossRef] [PubMed]
45. Allison, M.; O'Connor, M. Facilitating a good death in residential aged care settings, with support from community palliative care (FOCUS: PRIMARY HEALTHCARE). *Aust. Nurs. Midwifery J.* **2020**, *26*, 41.
46. Takahashi, Z.; Yamakawa, M.; Nakanishi, M.; Fukahori, H.; Igarashi, N.; Aoyama, M.; Sato, K.; Sakai, S.; Nagae, H.; Miyashita, M. Defining a good death for people with dementia: A scoping review. *Jpn. J. Nurs. Sci.* **2021**, *18*, e12402. [CrossRef]

47. Thompson, G.; Shindruk, C.; Wickson-Griffiths, A.; Sussman, T.; Hunter, P.; McClement, S.; Chochinov, H.; McCleary, L.; Kaasalainen, S.; Venturato, L. "Who would want to die like that?" Perspectives on dying alone in a long-term care setting. *Death Stud.* **2019**, *43*, 509–520. [CrossRef]
48. Bolt, S.R.; van der Steen, J.T.; Mujezinović, I.; Janssen, D.J.; Schols, J.M.; Zwakhalen, S.M.; Khemai, C.; Knapen, P.A.G.M.; Dijkstra, L.; Meijers, J.M. Practical nursing recommendations for palliative care for people with dementia living in long-term care facilities during the COVID-19 pandemic: A rapid scoping review. *Int. J. Nurs. Stud.* **2021**, *113*, 103781. [CrossRef]
49. Kaasalainen, S.; Mccleary, L.; Vellani, S.; Pereira, J. Improving End-of-Life Care for People with Dementia in LTC Homes during the COVID-19 Pandemic and Beyond. *Can. Geriatr. J.* **2021**, in press.
50. Collins, C.M.; Small, S.P. The nurse practitioner role is ideally suited for palliative care practice: A qualitative descriptive study. *Can. Oncol. Nurs. J.* **2019**, *29*, 4–9. [CrossRef]
51. Kaasalainen, S. Current issues with implementing a palliative approach in long-term care: Where do we go from here? *Palliat. Med.* **2020**, *34*, 555–557. [CrossRef]
52. Kaasalainen, S.; Sussman, T.; McCleary, L.; Thompson, G.; Hunter, P.V.; Wickson-Griffiths, A.; Cook, R.; Bello-Haas, V.D.; Venturato, L.; Papaioannou, A.; et al. Palliative Care Models in Long-Term Care: A Scoping Review. *Can. J. Nurs. Leadersh.* **2019**, *32*, 8–26. [CrossRef]
53. Mileski, M.; Pannu, U.; Payne, B.; Sterling, E.; McClay, R. The Impact of Nurse Practitioners on Hospitalizations and Discharges from Long-term Nursing Facilities: A Systematic Review. *Healthcare* **2020**, *8*, 114. [CrossRef]
54. Donald, F.; Martin-Misener, R.; Carter, N.; Donald, E.E.; Kaasalainen, S.; Wickson-Griffiths, A.; Lloyd, M.; Akhtar-Danesh, N.; DiCenso, A. A systematic review of the effectiveness of advanced practice nurses in long-term care. *J. Adv. Nurs.* **2013**, *69*, 2148–2161. [CrossRef]

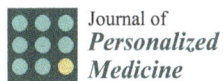

Article

The Development of a Personalized Symptom Management Mobile Health Application for Persons Living with HIV in China

Shuyu Han [1], Yaolin Pei [2], Lina Wang [3], Yan Hu [1,4,*], Xiang Qi [2], Rui Zhao [1,5], Lin Zhang [6], Wenxiu Sun [6], Zheng Zhu [1,4] and Bei Wu [2,*]

1. School of Nursing, Fudan University, Shanghai 200032, China; 18111170001@fudan.edu.cn (S.H.); zhruicc@foxmail.com (R.Z.); zhengzhu@fudan.edu.cn (Z.Z.)
2. Rory Meyers College of Nursing, New York University, New York, NY 10010, USA; yp22@nyu.edu (Y.P.); xq450@nyu.edu (X.Q.)
3. School of Medicine, Huzhou University, Huzhou Central Hospital, Huzhou 313000, China; 13587278357@163.com
4. Fudan University Centre for Evidence-Based Nursing: A Joanna Briggs Institute Centre of Excellence, Shanghai 200032, China
5. Children's Hospital of Fudan University, Shanghai 201102, China
6. Shanghai Public Health Clinical Center Affiliated with Fudan University, Shanghai 201508, China; zhanglin@shphc.org.cn (L.Z.); sunwenxiu@shphc.org.cn (W.S.)
* Correspondence: huyan@fudan.edu.cn (Y.H.); bei.wu@nyu.edu (B.W.); Tel.: +86-13651860058 (Y.H.); +86-2129925951 (B.W.)

Citation: Han, S.; Pei, Y.; Wang, L.; Hu, Y.; Qi, X.; Zhao, R.; Zhang, L.; Sun, W.; Zhu, Z.; Wu, B. The Development of a Personalized Symptom Management Mobile Health Application for Persons Living with HIV in China. *J. Pers. Med.* **2021**, *11*, 346. https://doi.org/10.3390/jpm11050346

Academic Editor: Riitta Suhonen

Received: 28 March 2021
Accepted: 23 April 2021
Published: 25 April 2021

Publisher's Note: MDPI stays neutral with regard to jurisdictional claims in published maps and institutional affiliations.

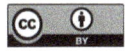

Copyright: © 2021 by the authors. Licensee MDPI, Basel, Switzerland. This article is an open access article distributed under the terms and conditions of the Creative Commons Attribution (CC BY) license (https://creativecommons.org/licenses/by/4.0/).

Abstract: Persons living with HIV (PLWH) continuously experience symptom burdens. Their symptom prevalence and severity are also quite different. Mobile health (mHealth) applications (apps) offer exceptional opportunities for using personalized interventions when and where PLWH are needed. This study aimed to demonstrate the development process of the symptom management (SM) app and the structure and content of it. Our research team systematically searched for evidence-based resources and summarized up-to-date evidence for symptom management and health education. Our multidisciplinary research team that included physicians, nurses, software engineers, and nursing professors, evaluated the structure and content of the drafted app. Both quantitative data and qualitative results were collected at a group discussion meeting. Quantitative data were scores of sufficient evidence, situational suitability, practicability, cost-effectiveness, and understandability (ranged from one to four) for 119 items of the app contents, including the health tracking module, the self-assessment module, coping strategies for 18 symptoms (80 items), medication management, complementary therapy, diet management, exercise, relaxation techniques, and the obtaining support module. The SM app was comprised of eight modules and provided several personalized symptom management functions, including assessing symptoms and receiving different symptom management strategies, tracking health indicators, and communicating with medical staff. The SM app was a promising and flexible tool for HIV symptom management. It provided PLWH with personalized symptom management strategies and facilitated the case management for medical staff. Future studies are needed to further test the app's usability among PLWH users and its effects on symptom management.

Keywords: HIV; mobile health; smartphone application; symptom management

1. Introduction

Since the development of antiretroviral therapy (ART), persons living with HIV (PLWH) can achieve a relatively satisfying life expectancy [1]. However, symptoms and related health outcomes have brought significant challenges and distress to the quality of life for PLWH. Many factors such as HIV infection, opportunistic infections and comorbidities,

ART toxicity, and social discrimination contribute to the onset and progression of symptoms among PLWH [2,3]. Although ART helps to decrease symptom intensity [4], it also brings on additional symptoms such as lipodystrophy, insomnia, and rash [3]. Evidence showed that both the number and frequency of symptoms were not associated with CD4 count levels, which indicated that those symptoms persisted throughout the HIV infection trajectory in PLWH [4]. PLWH usually suffer from physical and psychological symptoms simultaneously [5]. Common symptoms of PLWH include fatigue, depression, pain, rash, and insomnia. The average symptom counts can be as high as 8–17 [6–8]. Previous studies reported a different but high prevalence of these common symptoms, with a range of 43–78% [6–8]. PLWH are burdened with multiple symptoms. They also have different symptoms of distress and unmet needs further exacerbate their situations. Therefore, the long-term and complexity of HIV symptoms call for more personalized and sustainable symptoms management strategies.

Chinese PLWH receive free ART based on the National Strategies of Four Frees and One Care for HIV/AIDS [9]. However, only publicly-funded domestic antiretroviral medications are free of charge. The integrase strand transfer inhibitors (INSTIs), which are the internationally recommended first-line treatment medication for PLWH [10], by contrast, are imported and needed to be paid out-of-pocket. Therefore, due to the issue of affordability, instead of taking these imported INSTIs, most Chinese PLWH choose to take free ART medications, e.g., efavirenz (EFV) or lopinavir/ritonavir (LPV/r). These medications may increase their risks for medication toxicity and symptoms of distress (EFV may lead to rash and sleep disorders, LPV/r may lead to diarrhea [11]). Evidence also showed that PLWH in developing countries were disproportionally affected by mental symptoms compared to their counterparts in developed countries [12]. The prevalence of depression and anxiety symptoms among Chinese PLWH is 61% and 43%, respectively [13]. The symptom burden may seriously affect PLWH's ART medication adherence, clinical prognosis, and quality of life [3,8,14]. Furthermore, Chinese PLWH's needs for symptom management are unmet due to their severe symptom burden, fear of asking for help because of HIV-related stigma, and difficulties in getting timely assistance for symptom management from medical staff [15,16]. Therefore, the development of symptom management for Chinese PLWH is urgently needed.

Smartphone use has been increasing and popularizing rapidly in the last two decades [17]. The health education and self-management strategies provided by the mobile health (mHealth) applications (apps) benefit both PLWH and medical professionals [18]. Several mHealth apps designed for PLWH provide functionalities, including medication reminders, communication to peers or providers, medical information searching engine and resources, and laboratory reports [19]. Although one app was previously developed to facilitate symptom management among PLWH [20], culturally tailored symptom management tools and suitable strategies for Chinese PLWH are still limited. Our research team developed a mHealth app to provide PLWH with a more convenient tool for personalized symptom management. This study aimed to demonstrate the development process of the symptom management (SM) app and its structure and content.

2. Framework

Our study was guided by a framework (Figure 1) informed by the University of California, San Francisco (UCSF) Symptom Management Model [21] and the Self-regulatory HIV/AIDS Symptom Management Model (SSMM-HIV) [14]. Three key components of symptom management are symptom experience, management strategies, and outcomes. Symptom experience focuses on symptom occurrence (the cognitive pathway) and symptom distress (the emotional pathway). Symptom management strategies consider who, what (the nature of the strategy), when, where, how (delivered), to whom (the recipient of intervention), how much (the intervention dose) and why. Outcomes involve symptom outcomes and clinical outcomes. Social support, ART medication adherence, and quality of life are equally essential components of HIV/AIDS symptom management. Guided by this framework, we designed the main functions and content of the SM app.

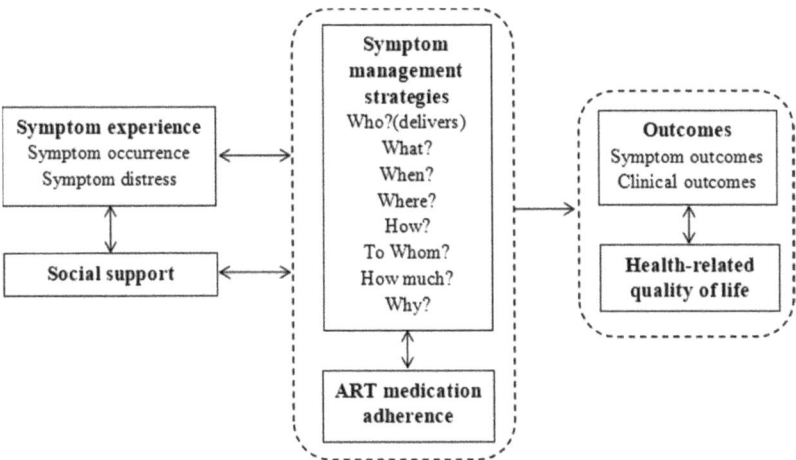

Figure 1. Symptom Management Framework.

3. Materials and Methods

According to the Good Practice Guidelines on Health Apps and Smart Devices [22], it was important to collect health content information from evidence-based resources and the opinions from multidisciplinary experts (healthcare professionals, engineers, professional bodies, patient or consumer associations, etc.). Therefore, the development of the SM app included two phrases. Nursing researchers first systematically searched for evidence-based resources to summarize up-to-date evidence for symptom management and health education and then completed the app's first draft. At the next step, the multidisciplinary research team including physicians, nurses, software engineers, and nursing researchers, evaluated the quality of the app through a group meeting.

3.1. Drafting the Structure and Content of the App

Our research team designed the overall structure of the SM app according to the symptom management framework and determined the symptoms based on the modified sign and symptom checklist for HIV (SSC-HIV rev) [23] and self-completed HIV symptom index [24]. These two tools reflected common symptoms of PLWH and had been applied among Chinese PLWH in previous studies [16,25]. Then nursing researchers searched health education and coping strategies for each symptom.

Our research team developed the Chinese culturally adapted AIDS Clinical Nursing Practice Guidelines in 2014, which contained comprehensive evidence for common symptoms [26]. Given this important previous work, we only searched for literature that stood in the high hierarchy of the evidence pyramid, i.e., guidelines rather than original studies and systematic reviews. We also included clinical manuals and books in both English and Chinese concerning PLWH treatment and care that focused on symptom evaluation, symptom treatment, and symptom management strategies. We thoroughly searched evidence-based resources at various websites, including the World Health Organization, UNAIDS, the Centers for Disease Control and Prevention, Association of Nurses in AIDS Care, European AIDS Clinical Society Department of Health and Human Services, U.S. Department of Health and Human Services, International Association of Providers of AIDS Care, British HIV Association, New York State Department of Health AIDS Institute,

Office of the AIDS Research Advisory Council (OARAC), and Canadian AIDS Treatment Information Exchange (CATIE).

3.2. Group Discussion and Written Feedback from the Multidisciplinary Research Team

We drafted the structure and content of the app from the review of the evidence-based resource. A group discussion meeting with the multidisciplinary research team was conducted in November 2017 in a conference room at the Shanghai Public Health Center (SPHC) affiliated with Fudan University. The handbook and checklist that quantitatively evaluated the quality of the app were sent to each expert by email in advance. During this 150 min group discussion meeting, a researcher (the sixth author) introduced the framework and contents of the app, and experts individually gave their suggestions and feedback. A total of 119 items, including the health tracking module, the self-assessment module, coping strategies for 18 symptoms (80 items), medication management, complementary therapy, diet management, exercise, relaxation techniques, and the obtaining support module were evaluated in terms of sufficient evidence, situational suitability, practicability, cost-effectiveness, and understandability (scores from 1 to 4). The group discussion was recorded and analyzed within 24 h. Members could also communicate with the researcher staff for additional suggestions after the meeting. Informed consent was obtained from all group members.

4. Results

4.1. Suggestions and Feedback from the Group Discussion

After systematically searching and summarizing evidence-based resources for symptom management (Supplementary Material Table S1 presents the detailed sources), we drafted the structure and content of the app and then conducted the multidisciplinary group meeting. Ten experts, including hospital managers, nursing professors, physicians, nurses, and software engineers, gave their suggestions and feedback. Among them, three had Ph.D. degrees, three had master's degrees, and six had bachelor's degrees. All experts completed the evaluation checklist. They generally agreed with the framework and content of the app and gave high scores on the questionnaire. Supplementary Material Table S2 presents the detailed scores for each item. The qualitative suggestions were as follows:

The health tracking module operated convenient and attractive functions of checking laboratory tests. However, this model needed to be enhanced with data visualization. Tables or trend charts were recommended to help users track their health indicators. According to this suggestion, the revised app added the indicator trend submodule in the health tracking module. When an indicator had more than two times of data, this submodule could generate a trend chart.

Experts strongly recommended simplifying the assessment tools in the self-assessment module. For instance, we could apply the two-item Patient Health Questionnaire (PHQ-2) instead of the nine-item Patient Health Questionnaire (PHQ-9) to assess depression. According to this suggestion, all symptom assessment tools were simplified to less than four items (Supplementary Material Table S3).

We revised or deleted some details of the symptom management coping strategies according to the experts' suggestions to make the strategies applicable in the local context. For example, (a) the experts thought that some complementary therapies for fatigue and diet therapies for depression were not suitable for the recommendation. Therefore, we deleted the following: "Taking vitamin or mineral supplements, such as vitamin B12, can help relieve fatigue. Some traditional Chinese medicines, such as rhodiola, ginseng, and licorice, may also help relieve fatigue." and "We suggest consuming more vitamin-D-rich foods, such as eggs, and vitamin B, such as blueberries and bamboo shoots to ameliorate depressive symptoms. Additionally, food rich in Omega-3 and tryptophan may help improve moods." (b) Symptom diaries (sleep diary and emotion diary) were recommended for deletion. One expert (E8) thought they were complicated and increased the amount of reading for users. (c) The deletion of some medication advice for symptom management was suggested. For example, some listed medicines for diarrhea were not available in China and should be deleted (E1 and E3). Medication for perianal neoplasms should be used under particular conditions. The listing of these medications in the app, which might be misleading and cause clinical risks, was suggested to be deleted (E10). One of the headache management strategies was as follows: "Herbal short-toned chrysanthemum may be effective in relieving headache. It is recommended to take it more than two hours apart from the ART medication and under the guidance of medical staff." Short-toned chrysanthemum was not commonly prescribed clinically and ought to be deleted (E2). (d) One item for fever management was as follows: "Fever may occur at any stage of the disease. It is an indicator of the disease and a process by which the immune system reacts to outside pathogens. When experiencing a fever, you should focus on cooling down, identifying the cause of your fever, preventing chills, and consuming enough water." The experts suggested revising and adding the following expression: "When experiencing a fever, you should visit a doctor as soon as possible." (E3)

In order to provide more comprehensive medication guidance, experts recommended adding a table of ART medication interactions with other medications in the app. We accepted this suggestion and added the table in the medication management submodule in the coping strategies module.

Stigma might discourage PLWH from downloading and using this app. Logo and homepage should not show HIV. In addition, data security and confidentiality should be strengthened to reduce patients' concerns. The following measures were conducted to address these issues: (a) We removed all HIV-related information in the app logo and homepage. (b) To ensure internal network security, we could use virtual local area network (VLAN) technology and logical isolation strategies. Using the latest firewall technology and packet filtering or proxy technologies could allow data to pass through selectively, making it possible to effectively monitor any activity between the internal network and the external network and prevent malicious and illegal access. (c) All data were recommended to be transmitted on the Web API (application programming interface) to ensure data transmission security. Encrypting sensitive data during the transmission process was recommended. An application authentication and authorization mechanism were also established. (d) Users could set a login password and/or gesture password. The screen would be locked if no operations were performed in the last 5 min. (e) To prevent data leakage, we transmitted the patient's laboratory test data directly from the hospital's health information system (HIS) to the mobile terminal of the app. The web-based administration portal could not acquire any user's medical or identity information.

It would be user-friendly to provide a communication platform between medical staff and PLWH. Thus, medical staff could give personalized information support according to the patients' questions. We accepted this suggestion and designed a question and answers (Q&As) submodule in the obtaining support module (the staff answered questions from users on the web-based administration portal). Medical staff should answer users' questions on the web-based administration portal within 48 h.

In order to strengthen the sustainability of the SM app, experts recommended designing neat and aesthetically pleasing app interfaces and providing various forms of information, including text, pictures, audio, and videos, to attract more users. They also recommended embedding the app into the routine process of clinical follow-ups, such as case management in SPHC.

4.2. Structure and Key Functions of the App

Based on all our previous work, the final app structure and functions in the mobile terminal include eight modules. Users see the home page as Figure 3a after opening the SM app (Figure 2). Four major modules are shown on the home page, including health tracking, self-assessment, coping strategies, and obtaining support. Other modules with smaller logos are newly registered user, regular user, symptom history, and reminders and settings. By clicking the round blue button at the top left of the home page, users can connect their personal information with the HIS of SPHC through the Certification Information button (Figure 3c). Technicians check users' ID numbers and names within 48 h and give user's permission to browse their medical reports in the web-based administration portal. If users have had visits in SPHC, they can see all the information, including their prescriptions and laboratory reports, in the SM app.

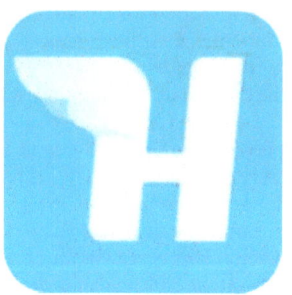

Figure 2. Logo of the SM app.

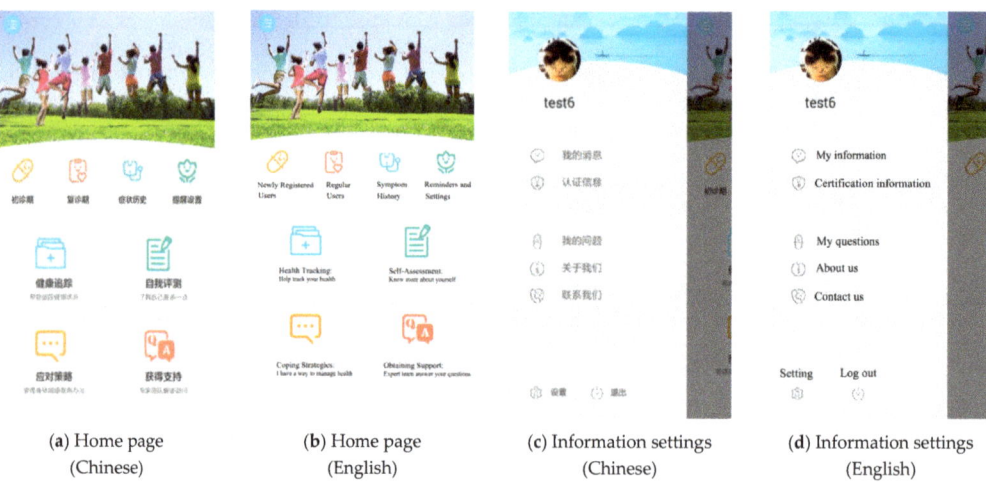

(**a**) Home page (Chinese)   (**b**) Home page (English)   (**c**) Information settings (Chinese)   (**d**) Information settings (English)

Figure 3. Screenshot of the home page and information settings.

4.2.1. Self-Assessment Module

By clicking the self-assessment module on the home page, users can see symptom assessment options as in Figure 4a. Symptom assessment includes two mental symptoms (depression and anxiety) and 16 physical symptoms (fatigue, headache, muscle and joint pain, fever, sleep disorder, diarrhea, nausea or vomiting, shortness of breath or cough, numbness/tingling of hands or feet, perianal neoplasms, fat redistribution, weight loss, rash, oral leukoplakia or ulcers, memory loss, and blurred vision). By clicking on one of the symptom buttons (such as depression), users can see the assessment tools as in Figure 4c. We applied PHQ-2 to screen depression [27] and the Generalized Anxiety Disorder scale (GAD-2) to screen anxiety [28]. Both PHQ-2 and GAD-2 are widely used valid screening tools. There were no available validated and widely-used screening tools for each physical symptom. Therefore, we designed screening tools for 16 physical symptoms. According to the symptom management framework, symptom experience focuses on symptom occurrence (the cognitive pathway) and symptom distress (the emotional pathway), i.e., symptom severity and symptom distress. Therefore, all the physical symptoms were assessed from these two aspects. For example, the two items for fatigue: (1) If a score of 0 means no fatigue at all, and a score of 10 means the worst fatigue you can imagine, how much do you rate your fatigue over the past 2 weeks? (2) How much does fatigue affect your daily life (0 = not at all, 1 = a little, 2 = a moderate amount, 3 = very much, 4 = extremely)? All the brief self-reported tools that assess each symptom are available in Supplementary Material Table S3.

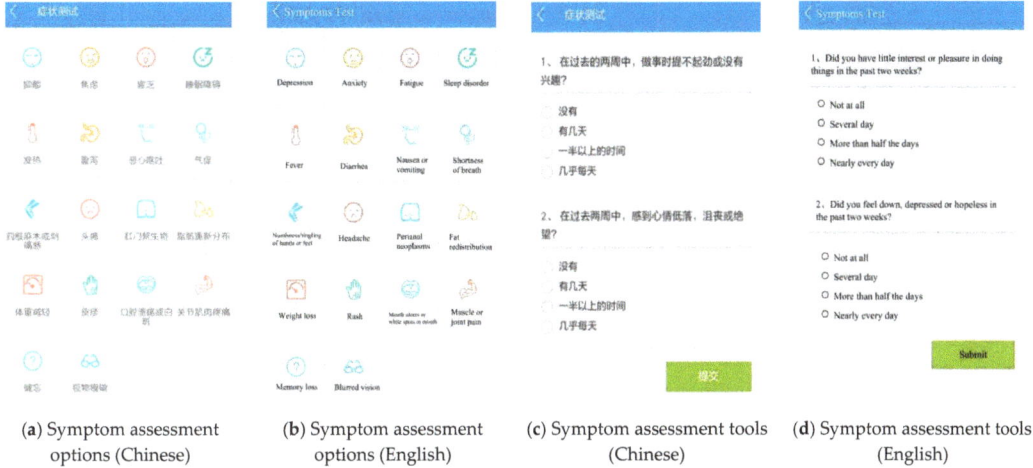

(**a**) Symptom assessment options (Chinese) (**b**) Symptom assessment options (English) (**c**) Symptom assessment tools (Chinese) (**d**) Symptom assessment tools (English)

Figure 4. Screenshot of symptom assessment options and symptom assessment tools.

A total of 80 symptom management strategies are available in the SM app. Users receive personalized result interpretations and strategies (Figure 5a) according to their assessment submission and cutoffs. Appendix 3 also presents all the cutoffs for each assessment tool.

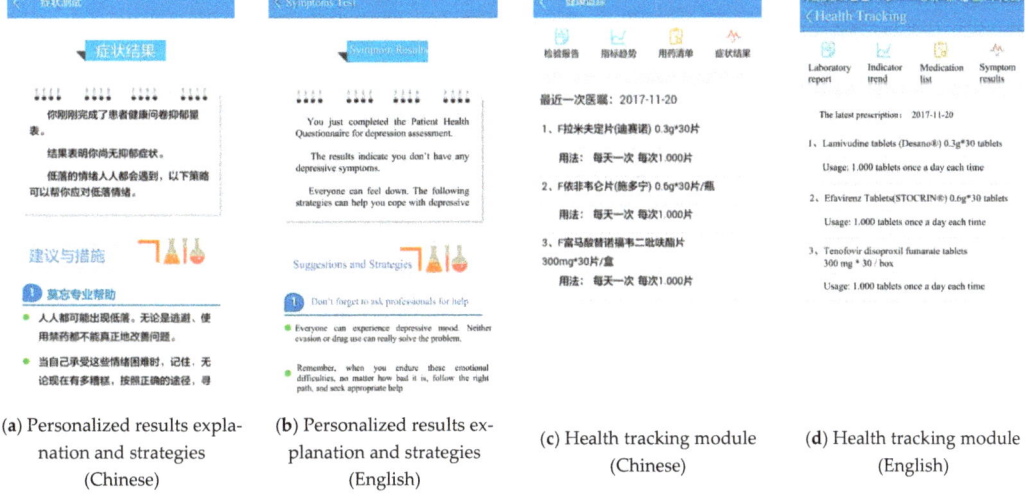

(**a**) Personalized results explanation and strategies (Chinese) (**b**) Personalized results explanation and strategies (English) (**c**) Health tracking module (Chinese) (**d**) Health tracking module (English)

Figure 5. Personalized results explanation and strategies, and the health tracking module.

4.2.2. Health Tracking Module

By clicking the health tracking module on the home page, users can see their latest prescription and four submodules on the screen, i.e., laboratory report, indicator trend, medication list, and symptoms results (Figure 5c). By clicking the laboratory report button, users can see their lab report results transferred from the HIS system (Figure 6a). If they have not visited SHPC before, they can input blood test results themselves. The indicator trend button in the health tracking module can generate tables and trend charts to help users track their health indicators, including their viral load, CD4+ T cell count, body temperature, body weight, pain, fatigue, and ART medication adherence (Figure 6c).

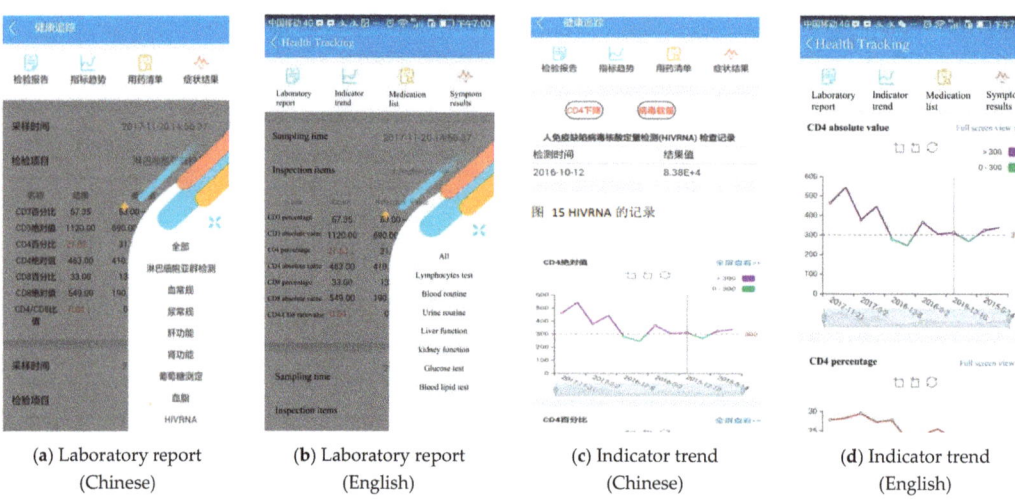

(**a**) Laboratory report (Chinese) (**b**) Laboratory report (English) (**c**) Indicator trend (Chinese) (**d**) Indicator trend (English)

Figure 6. Screenshot of laboratory report and indicator trend.

4.2.3. Coping Strategy Module

The coping strategy module on the home page provides basic knowledge and coping strategies, including medication management (ART medication introduction, the principles of taking ART medication, taking medicine under particular circumstances, the interaction of ART medication with other medication, and coping strategies for the side effects of ART medication), the principles of using a complementary therapy, diet adjustment (balanced diet, safe diet, and diet under special circumstances), exercise (exercise principles, exercise choice, exercise plan, and precautions), and relaxation training (mindfulness, deep breathing, image guidance, body scan, and activating events–beliefs–consequences (ABC) rational-emotive behavior therapy).

4.2.4. Obtaining Support Module

The obtaining support module on the home page has four submodules including, health care support, peer support, information support, and Q&As. Any questions left on the Q&As submodule are answered by medical staff within 48 h.

4.2.5. Other Modules

The newly registered user module on the home page provides knowledge patients who took ART medication for less than six months needed to know, including an introduction to HIV, an introduction to ART, ART medication adherence, timely follow-up, safety measures, and a healthy lifestyle. The regular user module on the home page provides knowledge and topics designed for patients who have taken ART medication for more than six months, including treatment goals, treatment progress, medication resistance, medication side effects, healthy lifestyle, and fertility options.

4.2.6. Web-Based Administration Portal Functions

The web-based administration portal for medical staff and technical staff includes five functions:

1. The user management function manages all registered account information.
2. The information publishing function can push or edit health education content.
3. The content management function can summarize user assessment data and provide reminders for outliers. Case managers contact and provide personalized interventions based on their lab tests.
4. The Q&A function can answer user questions.
5. Other functions include basic statistical functions such as analyzing users' login numbers and viewing each module's number.

4.3. Privacy and Confidentiality

The following design helps users understand that the SM app protects users' privacy and confidentiality. Firstly, people cannot distinguish from the logo (Figure 2) and homepage (Figure 3a) that the SM app was designed for PLWH. Secondly, it is not mandatory for users to provide their personal information. If they do not provide their ID number, they can still use all the functions of the app. The only advantage for connecting their ID number with our hospital is that they can check and look up all the medical prescriptions, laboratory tests through the app as Figures 5c and 6a. If users do not provide personal information but still want to see the generated trend of their health status based on the health indicators, such as CD4 + T cell count (Figure 6c), they can input data by themselves. Thirdly, users can set a login password and/or guest password. The screen is locked if no operations are performed in the last 5 min.

5. Discussion

To our knowledge, the SM app was the first attempt to develop a mHealth app for personalized symptom management for PLWH in China. It was developed based on evidence-based resource reviews and input from our multidisciplinary research team. The SM app can be operated on both Android and iOS systems. It also has a web-based administration portal managed by medical staff and technicians.

mHealth technology has been developing rapidly in recent years. Given the potential to improve access to care by reducing geographical and financial barriers, mHealth apps provide feasible, accessible, and effective platforms for self-management of many chronic diseases, including hypertension [29], diabetes [30], and cancer [31]. They are also increasingly being used for the care of PLWH [19]. HIV infection is a lifelong chronic disease. After HIV infection, symptom management is a long-term task for PLWH. PLWH also have different symptom prevalence and severity. Therefore, mHealth apps are promising choices for expanding the HIV personalized symptom management interventions.

The SM app provides reliable symptom management knowledge from evidence-based resources that are recommended by researchers. The multidisciplinary group discussion was an efficient way to collect opinions from different areas and perspectives and played an important role in ensuring the accuracy and cultural adaptability of the app's content and promoting the app's acceptability. After the input from the multidisciplinary research group, the app could meet PLWH's personalized needs for symptom management and became a promising tool to promote case management for medical professionals.

One symptom management app for PLWH in the United States of America (mVIP) provides symptom management strategies for 13 symptoms [20]. Our app has a bigger symptom pool (18 symptoms), which may cover more PLWH's symptom issues. Guided by a symptom management framework, the SM app also includes health contents and functions about improving medication adherence and social support. General health contents are provided for newly registered users and regular users and may improve the quality of life outcome. Particularly, the SM app has several personalized symptom management functions. Firstly, PLWH can assess their symptoms and receive different symptom management strategies according to their assessment results. Secondly, the health tracking module provides PLWH with a convenient tool to track their health indicators. Thirdly, PLWH can communicate with medical staff to gain support through the SM app. These personalized functions can meet personalized needs and may encourage more usage.

Several limitations of this study should be noted. Firstly, the SM app currently only connects with the HIS of the SPHC, and users can only check prescriptions and laboratory tests from SPHC. Secondly, PLWH did not participate in the development process of the app. Future research is needed to examine whether the SM app meets the expectations of PLWH and medical staff and evaluate the app's usability. The app will be revised and updated according to the user feedback. When the SM app is determined to be user-friendly and suitable to be promoted to a larger group of PLWH, its effects on symptom management for PLWH will be tested and open access to HIS in other hospitals.

6. Conclusions

The SM app was developed based on evidence-based resource reviews and the input from our multidisciplinary research team. It provided PLWH with reliable symptom management knowledge and personalized symptom management functions. The web-based administration portal also provided the medical staff with convenient functions for case management. Future studies are needed to further test the app's usability and effectiveness on symptom management. We will refine the SM app based on users' experience and the collected data.

7. Patents

The SM app, which was developed for both iOS and Android, applied for a patent (National Copyright Administration of the People's Republic of China: No.02700189).

Supplementary Materials: The following are available online at https://www.mdpi.com/article/10.3390/jpm11050346/s1, Table S1: Symptom management app content source; Table S2: Scores in terms of evidence-based, situational suitability, practicability, cost-effectiveness, and understandability in the group discussion; Table S3: Assessment tool and cutoff in the symptom management app.

Author Contributions: Conceptualization, Y.H.; methodology, Y.H.; software, S.H.; validation, S.H.; formal analysis, R.Z.; investigation, R.Z.; resources, L.Z. and W.S.; data curation, R.Z.; writing—original draft preparation, S.H.; writing–review & editing, Y.P., L.W., X.Q., and B.W.; visualization, S.H.; supervision, Z.Z.; project administration, R.Z. and W.S.; funding acquisition, Y.H. and Z.Z. All authors have read and agreed to the published version of the manuscript.

Funding: This research was funded by the National Natural Science Foundation of China (Grant Number 71673057) and the China Scholarship Council (No. 201906100135).

Institutional Review Board Statement: The study was conducted according to the guidelines of the Declaration of Helsinki and approved by the Research Ethical Committee of the School of Nursing, Fudan University (IRB#TYSA2016-3-1) and the Shanghai Public Health Center (SPHC) affiliated with Fudan University (2019-S036-02).

Informed Consent Statement: Informed consent was obtained from all subjects involved in the study.

Data Availability Statement: All the raw data are available in the Supplementary Materials.

Acknowledgments: The authors would like to appreciate all the staff who helped us complete this project. They are: Hongzhou Lu, Yinzhong Shen, Renfang Zhang, Jiangrong Wang, the physicians at the Shanghai Public Health Center Affiliated with Fudan University; Meijuan Bao, Lijun Zha, Yanjuan Gan, the nurses at the Shanghai Public Health Center Affiliated with Fudan University; Mingcheng Zhu, software engineer at the Shanghai Public Health Center affiliated with Fudan University.

Conflicts of Interest: The authors declare no conflict of interest.

References

1. Yoshimura, K. Current status of HIV/AIDS in the ART era. *J. Infect. Chemother.* **2017**, *23*, 12–16. [CrossRef]
2. Román, E.; Chou, F.-Y. Development of a Spanish HIV/AIDS symptom management guidebook. *J. Transcult. Nurs.* **2011**, *22*, 235–239. [CrossRef] [PubMed]
3. Zhu, Z.; Hu, Y.; Li, H.-W.; Bao, M.-J.; Zhang, L.; Zha, L.-J.; Hou, X.-H.; Lu, H.-Z. The implementation and evaluation of HIV symptom management guidelines: A preliminary study in China. *Int. J. Nurs. Sci.* **2018**, *5*, 315–321. [CrossRef] [PubMed]
4. Willard, S.; Holzemer, W.L.; Wantland, D.J.; Cuca, Y.P.; Kirksey, K.M.; Portillo, C.J.; Corless, I.B.; Rivero-Méndez, M.; Rosa, M.E.; Nicholas, P.K.; et al. Does "asymptomatic" mean without symptoms for those living with HIV infection? *AIDS Care.* **2009**, *21*, 322–328. [CrossRef]
5. Namisango, E.; Harding, R.; Katabira, E.T.; Siegert, R.J.; Powell, R.A.; Atuhaire, L.; Moens, K.; Taylor, S. A novel symptom cluster analysis among ambulatory HIV/AIDS patients in Uganda. *AIDS Care.* **2015**, *27*, 954–963. [CrossRef] [PubMed]
6. Chen, W.-T.; Shiu, C.; Yang, J.P.; Tun, M.M.M.; Zhang, L.; Wang, K.; Chen, L.-C.; Aung, M.N.; Lu, H.; Zhao, H. Tobacco use and HIV symptom severity in Chinese people living with HIV. *AIDS Care.* **2020**, *32*, 217–222. [CrossRef]
7. Lee, K.A.; Gay, C.; Portillo, C.J.; Coggins, T.; Davis, H.; Pullinger, C.R.; Aouizerat, B.E. Symptom experience in HIV-infected adults: A function of demographic and clinical characteristics. *J. Pain Symptom Manag.* **2009**, *38*, 882–893. [CrossRef] [PubMed]
8. Olson, B.; Vincent, W.; Meyer, J.P.; Kershaw, T.; Sikkema, K.J.; Heckman, T.G.; Hansen, N.B. Depressive symptoms, physical symptoms, and health-related quality of life among older adults with HIV. *Qual. Life Res.* **2019**, *28*, 3313–3322. [CrossRef]
9. Li, L.; Ji, G.; Lin, C.; Liang, L.J.; Lan, C.W. Antiretroviral therapy initiation following policy changes: Observations from China. *Asia-Pac. J. Public Health.* **2016**, *28*, 416–422. [CrossRef]
10. Saag, M.S.; Gandhi, R.T.; Hoy, J.F.; Landovitz, R.J.; Thompson, M.A.; Sax, P.E.; Smith, D.M.; Benson, C.A.; Buchbinder, S.P.; del Rio, C.; et al. Antiretroviral drugs for treatment and prevention of HIV infection in adults: 2020 recommendations of the International Antiviral Society-USA Panel. *JAMA.* **2020**, *324*, 1651–1669. [CrossRef] [PubMed]
11. AIDS and Hepatitis C Professional Group, Society of Infectious Disease, Chinese Medical Association; Chinese Center for Disease Control and Prevention. Chinese guidelines for diagnosis and treatment of HIV/AIDS (2018). *Chin. J. Intern. Med.* **2018**, *57*, 1–18. [CrossRef]
12. Rezaei, S.; Ahmadi, S.; Rahmati, J.; Hosseinifard, H.; Dehnad, A.; Aryankhesal, A.; Shabaninejad, H.; Ghasemyani, S.; Alihosseini, S.; Bragazzi, N.L.; et al. Global prevalence of depression in HIV/AIDS: A systematic review and meta-analysis. *BMJ Support. Palliat. Care.* **2019**, *9*, 404–412. [CrossRef]
13. Niu, L.; Luo, D.; Liu, Y.; Silenzio, V.M.; Xiao, S. The mental health of people living with HIV in China, 1998–2014: A systematic review. *PLoS ONE* **2016**, *11*, e0153489. [CrossRef]
14. Spirig, R.; Moody, K.; Battegay, M.; De Geest, S. Symptom management in HIV/AIDS: Advancing the conceptualization. *ANS Adv. Nurs. Sci.* **2005**, *28*, 333–344. [CrossRef]
15. Dong, N.; Chen, W.-T.; Lu, H.; Zhu, Z.; Hu, Y.; Bao, M. Unmet needs of symptom management and associated factors among the HIV-positive population in Shanghai, China: A cross-sectional study. *Appl. Nurs. Res.* **2020**, *54*, 151283. [CrossRef] [PubMed]
16. Zhu, Z.; Hu, Y.; Guo, M.; Williams, A.B. Urban and rural differences: Unmet needs for symptom management in people living with HIV in China. *J. Assoc. Nurses AIDS Care.* **2019**, *30*, 206–217. [CrossRef] [PubMed]
17. ITU. Statistics. Available online: https://www.itu.int/en/ITU-D/Statistics/Pages/stat/default.aspx (accessed on 18 July 2020).
18. Baig, M.M.; GholamHosseini, H.; Connolly, M.J. Mobile healthcare applications: System design review, critical issues and challenges. *Australas. Phys. Eng. Sci. Med.* **2015**, *38*, 23–38. [CrossRef] [PubMed]
19. Schnall, R.; Mosley, J.P.; Iribarren, S.J.; Bakken, S.; Carballo-Diéguez, A.; Brown, W., III. Comparison of a user centered design, self-management app to existing mHealth apps for persons living with HIV. *JMIR mHealth uHealth.* **2015**, *3*, e91. [CrossRef] [PubMed]
20. Schnall, R.; Cho, H.; Mangone, A.; Pichon, A.; Jia, H. Mobile health technology for improving symptom management in low income persons living with HIV. *AIDS Behav.* **2018**, *22*, 3373–3383. [CrossRef] [PubMed]
21. Dodd, M.; Janson, S.; Facione, N.; Faucett, J.; Froelicher, E.S.; Humphreys, J.; Lee, K.; Miaskowski, C.; Puntillo, K.; Rankin, S.; et al. Advancing the science of symptom management. *J. Adv. Nurs.* **2001**, *33*, 668–676. [CrossRef]
22. Haute Autorité de Santé. Good Practice Guidelines on Health Apps and Smart Devices (Mobile Health or mHealth). 2016. Available online: https://www.has-sante.fr/upload/docs/application/pdf/2017-03/dir1/good_practice_guidelines_on_health_apps_and_smart_devices_mobile_health_or_mhealth.pdf (accessed on 26 October 2016).
23. Holzemer, W.L.; Hudson, A.; Kirksey, K.M.; Hamilton, M.J.; Bakken, S. The revised sign and symptom check-list for HIV (SSC-HIVrev). *J. Assoc. Nurses AIDS Care.* **2001**, *12*, 60–70. [CrossRef]
24. Justice, A.C.; Holmes, W.; Gifford, A.L.; Rabeneck, L.; Zackin, R.; Sinclair, G.; Weissman, S.; Neidig, J.; Marcus, C.; Chesney, M.; et al. Development and validation of a self-completed HIV symptom index. *J. Clin. Epidemiol.* **2001**, *54* (Suppl. 1), S77–S90. [CrossRef]
25. Zhu, Z.; Hu, Y.; Xing, W.; Guo, M.; Zhao, R.; Han, S.; Wu, B. Identifying symptom clusters among people living with HIV on antiretroviral therapy in China: A network analysis. *J. Pain Symptom Manag.* **2019**, *57*, 617–626. [CrossRef] [PubMed]
26. Fu, L. *Development of the HIV/AIDS Clinical Nursing Practice Guidelines*; Fudan University: Shanghai, China, 2014.
27. Kroenke, K.; Spitzer, R.L.; Williams, J.B.W. The patient health questionnaire-2: Validity of a two-item depression screener. *Med. Care.* **2003**, *41*, 1284–1292. [CrossRef] [PubMed]

28. Kroenke, K.; Spitzer, R.L.; Williams, J.B.W.; Monahan, P.O.; Löwe, B. Anxiety disorders in primary care: Prevalence, impairment, comorbidity, and detection. *Ann. Intern. Med.* **2007**, *146*, 317–325. [CrossRef] [PubMed]
29. Mohammadi, R.; Ayatolahi Tafti, M.; Hoveidamanesh, S.; Ghanavati, R.; Pournik, O. Reflection on mobile applications for blood pressure management: A systematic review on potential effects and initiatives. *Stud. Health Technol. Inform.* **2018**, *247*, 306–310.
30. Brzan, P.P.; Rotman, E.; Pajnkihar, M.; Klanjsek, P. Mobile applications for control and self management of diabetes: A systematic review. *J. Med. Syst.* **2016**, *40*, 210. [CrossRef]
31. Cannon, C. Telehealth, mobile applications, and wearable devices are expanding cancer care beyond walls. *Semin. Oncol. Nurs.* **2018**, *34*, 118–125. [CrossRef]

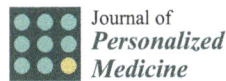

Article

Personalized Healthcare: The Importance of Patients' Rights in Clinical Practice from the Perspective of Nursing Students in Poland, Spain and Slovakia—A Cross-Sectional Study

Ewa Kupcewicz [1,*], Elżbieta Grochans [2], Helena Kadučáková [3], Marzena Mikla [4,5], Aleksandra Bentkowska [6], Adam Kupcewicz [7], Anna Andruszkiewicz [8] and Marcin Jóźwik [9]

1. Department of Nursing, Collegium Medicum, University of Warmia and Mazury in Olsztyn, 14 C Zolnierska Street, 10-719 Olsztyn, Poland
2. Department of Nursing, Pomeranian Medical University in Szczecin, 48 Zolnierska Street, 71-210 Szczecin, Poland; grochans@pum.edu.pl
3. Department of Nursing, Faculty of Health, Catholic University in Ruzomberok, 48 A. Hlinku Street, 034-01 Ruzomberok, Slovakia; helena.kaducakova@ku.sk
4. Department of Nursing, Campus de Espinardo, University of Murcia, Edificio 23, 30100 Murcia, Spain; marmikla@yahoo.com
5. Murcian Institute of Biosanitary Research (IMIB), 30120 Murcia, Spain
6. Oncological and General Surgery Clinic, University Clinical Hospital in Olsztyn, 30 Warszawska Street, 10-900 Olsztyn, Poland; a.bentkowska.kruszwicka@gmail.com
7. Faculty of Law and Administration, University of Warmia and Mazury in Olsztyn, 2 Oczapowskiego Street, 10-719 Olsztyn, Poland; adam.kupcewicz@gmail.com.pl
8. Department of Basic Clinical Skills and Postgraduate Education for Nurses and Midwifes, Nicolaus Copernicus University in Toruń, Łukasiewicza 1 Street, 85-821 Bydgoszcz, Poland; anna.andruszkiewicz@cm.umk.pl
9. Department of Gynecology and Obstetrics, Faculty of Medicine, Collegium Medicum, University of Warmia and Mazury in Olsztyn, 44 Niepodleglosci Street, 10-045 Olsztyn, Poland; marcin.jozwik@uwm.edu.pl
* Correspondence: ekupcewicz@wp.pl; Tel.: +48-696-076-764

Abstract: Background: This study aimed to define the role and importance of patients' rights in personalized healthcare from the perspective of nursing students in Poland, Spain and Slovakia. Methods: The research was carried out by means of a diagnostic survey, using the survey technique, with the participation of 1002 nursing students attending a full-time undergraduate study program at three European countries. The "Patients' rights" questionnaire was used as a research tool. The average age of students was 21.6 years (±3.4). The empirical material collected was subjected to a statistical analysis. Results: The study demonstrated that 72.1% of nursing students from Spain, 51.2% from Poland and 38.5% from Slovakia believe that patients' rights are respected at a good level in their country. Significant intergroup differences (F = 67.43; $p < 0.0001$) were observed in the self-assessment of students' knowledge of patients' rights. The highest average values were obtained by students from Spain (3.54 ± 0.92), while 35.9% of students from Slovakia and 25.5% from Poland were quite critical and pointed to their low level of knowledge of patients' rights in their self-assessment. When ranking patients' rights related to respecting dignity, students from Spain obtained much higher average values (4.37 ± 0.92) than students from the other two countries. Conclusions: The level of students' knowledge of patients' rights and the respect for patients' rights by medical personnel is, in the opinion of the respondents, quite diverse and requires in-depth educational activities among nursing students at the university level in respective countries.

Keywords: patients' rights; student; nursing; personalized medicine

1. Introduction

Personalized medicine is a model in which disease prevention and treatment is based on the patient's unique clinical, genetic and environmental characteristics [1–3]. Personalized healthcare, providing opportunities for a more precise approach to individual medical

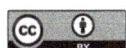

care, is of particular benefit to the patients. It also poses a unique challenge in terms of its holistic approach to health and sickness. This approach assumes that it is a person who should be treated, not just an illness, since a strong link exists among body, soul and mind; they form one entity and only a balance among them can ensure the state of health [4].

Personalized healthcare involves the important issue of patients' rights, which determine the status of the patient during the provision of health services and the obligations of the medical personnel towards the patients as well as towards their relatives [5]. Consequently, the observance of patients' rights by medical personnel in clinical practice is regarded as an ethical obligation and a legal obligation [6]. The concept of patients' rights was developed on the basis of the Universal Declaration of Human Rights adopted in 1948 by the United Nations (UN) General Assembly, which explicitly states that every human being has an inherent right to life, freedom, privacy, free development in society and respect for their dignity [6–8]. The aim of the concept of patients' rights is to protect the autonomy of the patient from interference by others, as well as the right to demand the rightful conditions for the exercise of those rights [6].

According to the World Health Organization (WHO), patients' rights vary from country to country, and it is often the prevailing cultural and social norms that determine the catalogue of patients' rights applicable in a given country [7]. However, there is international consensus that all patients have a fundamental right to privacy, to the confidentiality of their medical data, to consent or refuse treatment and to information about the risks associated with medical procedures [7].

In Europe, the observance of patients' rights is guaranteed, among others, by the Convention on Human Rights and Biomedicine of 1997 (also referred to as the European Bioethics Convention or the Oviedo Convention) [9]. Another document is the European Charter of Patients' Rights, issued in 2002 by the Active Citizenship Network, which governs basic issues concerning patients' rights [10]. The charter mentions, among others, the right of access to health services and the right to respect of patients' time, regardless of the phase or place of treatment, which states that every person has the right to receive the necessary treatment within a swift, predetermined period [10]. Such a guarantee has been introduced in selected European countries, e.g., Sweden, Denmark, Finland, Norway, England, Scotland, Wales, Ireland, Portugal, Spain and the Netherlands [11]. The European Parliament and the Council of the European Union have played a significant role in protecting patients' rights, recognizing that the Member States of the European Union have a responsibility to provide citizens in their territory with safe, efficient, high-quality and quantitatively adequate medical care. The undertaken actions resulted in the introduction of Directive 2011/24/EU of the European Parliament and of the Council of 9 March 2011 on the application of patients' rights in cross-border healthcare [12–16]. As numerous studies have shown, the management of patient care with regard to personal needs, rights and duties requires a certain degree of personalization [17,18]. It is connected with the theoretical and clinical preparation of students of nursing studies for future work related to patient care [19]. Nursing program curricula provide students with the opportunity to achieve learning outcomes in terms of knowledge of human rights, children's rights and patients' rights [19,20]. In the process of socialization under the guidance of academic teachers, nursing students, as future nurses, acquire social competences to be guided in their future work by professional values when making decisions in the face of emerging, healthcare-related ethical challenges [21]. In terms of social competence, a graduate of nursing studies is ready to respect the rights of the patient, to respect the dignity and autonomy of the persons under their care, to be guided by the welfare of the patient and to show understanding for differences in worldview and culture and empathy in relation to the patient and their family [19,20].

The aim of this study was to define the role and importance of patients' rights in personalized healthcare from the perspective of nursing students in Poland, Spain and Slovakia.

The following research problems were formulated:
- Are there differences in the observance of patients' rights in healthcare-providing institutions in the opinion of nursing students in Poland, Spain and Slovakia and to what extent?
- To what extent does knowledge of selected patients' rights in clinical practice regarding an ill or healthy person differ among nursing students in Poland, Spain and Slovakia?

2. Materials and Methods

2.1. Settings and Design

The study was carried out between May 2018 and April 2019 by means of a diagnostic survey, using the survey technique, with the participation of 1002 nursing students, studying in first degree (bachelor's degree) programs in a full-time system at the University of Warmia and Mazury in Olsztyn and the Pomeranian Medical University in Szczecin (Poland), the University of Murcia in Murcia (Spain) and the Catholic University in Ružomberok (Slovakia). The surveys were carried out at the place where the didactic classes for students were conducted, and the distribution of the prepared sets of paper questionnaires to a given university was handled by one of the researchers. Upon obtaining permission from the academic teacher to conduct the survey, students were informed of the purpose and the scope of the study and provided with instructions on how to complete the questionnaire. Students had the opportunity to ask questions and receive comprehensive explanations. The survey was anonymous and voluntary; the time taken to complete the questionnaires in person was approximately 20 min. The inclusion criterion for the students in the study was the age of the subjects up to 30 years, while the exclusion criterion was the absence of informed consent to participate in the study. Students could also opt-out of the study at any time without providing a reason. In total, 1017 survey forms were distributed among students. After collecting data and eliminating defective questionnaires, 1002 (i.e., 98.5%) correctly completed paper version questionnaires were accepted for the final statistical analysis. The collected data were entered into a spreadsheet in Excel software and the results were analyzed collectively.

2.2. Participants

The investigated group included 404 (40.3%) students from Poland, 208 students (20.8%) from Spain and 390 students (38.9%) from Slovakia. The mean age for all subjects was 21.6 years (± 3.4). Among the students, women accounted for 91.3% ($n = 915$), men for 8.7% ($n = 87$). The distribution of first-, second- and third-year students across the universities was similar. The most numerous group were second-year students ($n = 458$; 45.71%), while 329 (32.83%) studied in the first year and 215 (21.46%) in the third year. The age of the students was analyzed in three age groups, assuming the following ranges: ≤ 20 years ($n = 401$; 40.02%), 21–22 years ($n = 410$; 40.92%) and ≥ 23 years ($n = 191$; 19.06%). The presented data are part of a larger international project and detailed sociodemographic characteristics are also included in other publications [22,23].

2.3. Research Instruments

A structured survey questionnaire created by the authors, entitled "Patients' Rights", was used to measure the variables of the study. The questionnaire consisted of two parts. The first part contained subjective questions to determine the structure of the surveyed group of students in terms of sociodemographic variables such as place of residence (country), gender, age, level of education and mode and year of studies. These questions included five closed questions, including all possible answer options, and one open question to determine the age of the respondents. The second part of the questionnaire contained 14 questions of an objective or subjective nature, which made it possible to determine the level of students' knowledge of patients' rights and selected aspects related to their observance in personalized healthcare addressed to sick and healthy people. The questions included two so-called "ranking" questions, to self-assess students' level of knowledge of patients' rights and to prioritize the patient's right to dignity. In the first ranked question, the respondent could choose from a rating scale from 2 to 5, reflecting the level of their current knowledge of patients' rights, where "2" and "3" indicated a low level of knowledge, "4" an average level and "5" a high level. Similarly, in the second question concerning the ranking of the importance of the patient's right to respect for dignity, the respondent indicated on a rating scale from 2 to 5, the rank given to the patients' right, where "2" and "3" indicated a low rank, "4" an average rank and "5" a high rank. In the remaining questions, the respondent was asked to mark one of four or five possible answers for each question.

The process of constructing the applied tool involved the development of a set of statements concerning the studied variables using information retrieved from the literature on the subject. Once the final set of questions in the Polish language was established, it was translated into the Spanish and Slovak languages. The research tool in equivalent language versions was subjected to a psychometric assessment. The reliability of the questionnaire was assessed through the internal consistency estimation, which was established based on Cronbach's alpha coefficients. When estimating the internal consistency degree, two of the questions from the second part of the questionnaire were rejected due to only slight thematic coherence. The reliability of all the other questions, measured by the value of the Cronbach's alpha coefficient, ranged from 0.60 to 0.71 [24].

2.4. Statistical Analysis

Statistical analyses were performed using the Polish version of STATISTICA 13 (TIBCO, Palo Alto, CA, USA). The mean, standard deviation and confidence interval for the mean ±95%, median, minimum and maximum were used to describe some of the analyzed variables. The ANOVA analysis of variance (F-test) comparing multiple samples of independent groups was used to investigate the significance of differences in the ranking of the subjective assessment of students' level of knowledge and in the ranking of the patients' right to respect for dignity. The significance of variation in the knowledge of patients' rights was assessed with the chi-square test (χ^2). For all tests, a significance level of $p < 0.05$ was assumed. The analyses of the results are presented in descriptive, tabular and graphical forms [24]. The research meets the criteria for a cross-sectional study [25].

3. Results

Students participating in the survey were given the opportunity to express their opinion on selected patients' rights in personalized healthcare based on their own experience of staying in a healthcare facility as a patient and as a nursing student, deepening their knowledge during clinical activities. The majority of nursing students (79.8%; $n = 800$) had used medical services as a patient in a hospital or clinic/outpatient clinic in the last three years preceding the survey. Their level of satisfaction with the quality of the medical services provided at that time significantly varied ($\chi^2 = 45.53$; $p < 0.0001$). The majority of students expressed a positive opinion on the overall quality of the medical services provided. However, only 33.9% of respondents reported that they had been informed about their rights and that information about patients' rights and the Patient Ombudsman was posted in a publicly accessible place. Taking into account the cultural background and the organization of the healthcare system in the different countries, a significant variation in results was observed ($\chi^2 = 124.26$; $p < 0.0001$) as regards the provision of information to patients concerning their rights. As analyses show, significantly more respondents in Poland (62.4%) than in Slovakia (37.7%) and Spain (16.5%) were informed about their rights when using medical services. When assessing the observance of patients' rights in personalized medical care, the results of the answers to the question concerning the provision of a sufficient level of intimacy to the patient during the provision of medical services were also sought. As indicated by the data, 60.5% of respondents confirmed that they were ensured good conditions when receiving medical services that minimized the feeling of embarrassment and reduced privacy.

3.1. Observance of Patients' Rights in Personalized Healthcare as Perceived by Nursing Students

In the opinion of nursing students, respect for the patients' right to receive comprehensive information about their own health condition and planned medical treatment in personalized healthcare significantly varied ($\chi^2 = 315.61$; $p < 0.0001$) in the analyzed subgroups. A high percentage (92.8%) of nursing students from Spain indicated that the right in question is respected in their country. However, around half of the respondents (51%) in the Slovak group and only 28.5% in the Polish group were of the same opinion. Further analysis involving the issue of compliance with the patients' right to receive pastoral care during the hospital stay showed statistically significant differences ($\chi^2 = 122.24$; $p < 0.0001$). More than half of the respondents confirmed this possibility and one in three Spanish students had no opinion about it, while in the Polish group 16.6% ($n = 67$) and in the Slovak group 13.6% ($n = 68$) of nursing students declared that they had no knowledge about it (Table 1).

Table 1. Distribution of answers to questions on patients' rights-a comparative analysis.

No.	Patients' Rights	Answer Scale	Responses-Number (%)			Chi-Squared Test (χ^2)	p
			Poland $n = 404$	Spain $n = 208$	Slovakia $n = 390$		
1	The right to obtain comprehensive and understandable information on their health condition	Yes	115 (28.5)	193 (92.8)	199 (51.0)	315.61	0.0001 ***
		No	92 (22.8)	9 (4.3)	109 (28.0)		
		I have no opinion	133 (32.9)	6 (2.9)	32 (8.2)		
		I don't know	64 (15.8)	0 (0.0)	50 (12.8)		
2	The patient's right to pastoral care while staying in hospital	Yes	262 (64.9)	118 (56.7)	210 (58.9)	122.24	0.0001 ***
		No	13 (3.2)	22 (10.6)	62 (9.7)		
		I have no opinion	62 (15.4)	67 (32.2)	50 (17.9)		
		I don't know	67 (16.6)	1 (0.5)	68 (13.6)		
3	The right to deposit valuables in a hospital depository during on-site (stationary) treatment	Yes	310 (76.7)	130 (62.5)	356 (91.3)	121.64	0.0001 ***
		No	26 (6.4)	19 (9.1)	13 (3.3)		
		I have no opinion	43 (10.6)	59 (28.4)	10 (2.6)		
		I don't know	25 (6.2)	0 (0.0)	11 (2.8)		
4	Data protection and confidentiality of patient information by healthcare professionals	Yes	346 (85.6)	165 (79.3)	356 (91.3)	66.13	0.0001 ***
		No	14 (3.5)	37 (17.8)	11 (2.8)		
		I have no opinion	29 (7.2)	4 (1.9)	9 (2.3)		
		I don't know	15 (3.7)	2 (1.0)	14 (3.6)		
5	Disclosure of information subject to professional secrecy by healthcare professionals	I don't know	59 (14,6)	20 (9.6)	89 (22.8)	36.78	0.0001 ***
		Yes, if the information covered could contribute to a risk to the health and life of others	225 (55.7)	141 (67.8)	180 (46.2)		
		Never	40 (9.9)	10 (4.8)	26 (6.7)		
		At the request of the court	80 (19.8)	37 (17.8)	95 (24.4)		
6	Obligation to provide the patient with a copy of the records of hospital/ambulatory treatment by the medical facility	Yes	289 (71.5)	156 (75.0)	264 (67.7)	51.14	0.0001 ***
		No	30 (7.4)	18 (8.7)	53 (13.6)		
		I have no opinion	42 (10.4)	34 (16.4)	29 (7.4)		
		I don't know	43 (10.6)	0 (0.0)	44 (11.3)		

Table 1. Cont.

No.	Patients' Rights	Answer Scale	Responses-Number (%)			Chi-Squared Test (χ^2)	p
			Poland $n = 404$	Spain $n = 208$	Slovakia $n = 390$		
7	Discharge of a patient from a hospital upon the patient's own request	Yes	321 (79.5)	101 (48.6)	296 (75.9)	86.00	0.0001 ***
		No	10 (2.5)	3 (1.4)	20 (5.1)		
		Only if their life is not in danger	47 (11.6)	73 (35.1)	56 (14.4)		
		I don't know	26 (6.4)	31 (14.9)	18 (4.6)		
8	Withdrawal of the patient's objection to organ and tissue donation	Yes	243 (60.2)	150 (72.1)	221 (56.7)	15.17	0.004 **
		No	52 (12.9)	22 (10.6)	54 (13.9)		
		I don't know	109 (27.0)	36 (17.3)	115 (29.5)		

Explanations: * $p < 0.05$; ** $p < 0.01$; *** $p < 0.001$.

In the following analyses, an attempt was made to find a subjective assessment by the nursing students concerning the extent to which patients' rights were respected in healthcare facilities in Poland, Spain and Slovakia. The distribution of the results was significantly different ($\chi^2 = 75.26$; $p < 0.0001$). It was found that 72.1% of nursing students from Spain, 51.2% from Poland and 38.5% of students from Slovakia rated the respect of patients' rights as good (Figure 1). On the other hand, one in five students from the Slovak group (20.8%) also indicated a disadvantageous situation for the patient, indicating that the level of respect for patients' rights was rather low or definitely low (Figure 1).

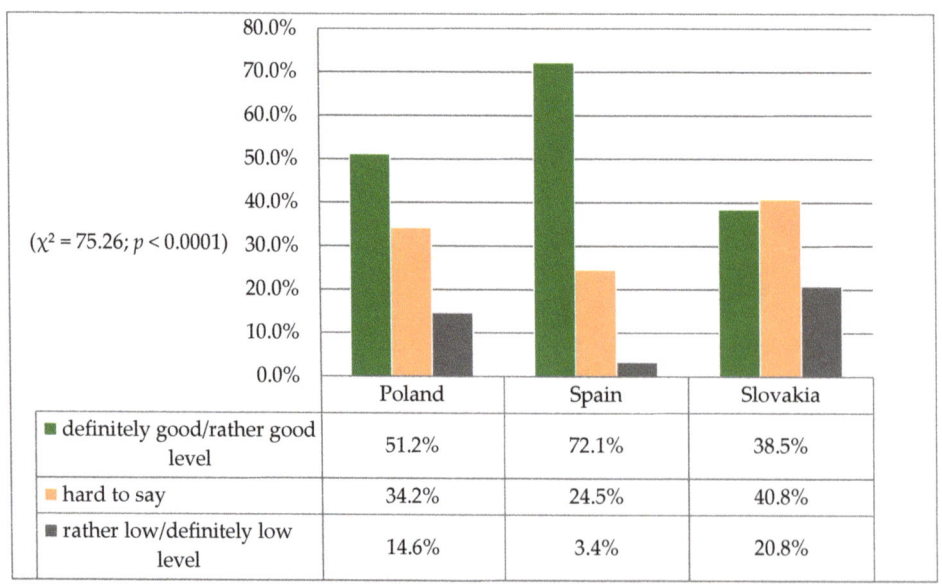

Figure 1. Observance of patients' rights as perceived by nursing students.

3.2. Differences in Nursing Students' Knowledge of Selected Patients' Rights in Personalized Healthcare

Further analyses involved investigating students' knowledge of a patients' rights in personalized healthcare to deposit valuable items to a hospital depository during inpatient treatment in a healthcare facility. The analysis demonstrated statistically significant differences ($\chi^2 = 121.64$; $p < 0.0001$). It was found that the vast majority of Slovak students

(91.3%; $n = 356$) positively responded to the question of whether a patient in healthcare facilities has the right to use a depository for the period of hospitalization. One of the most important patients' rights in personalized healthcare concerns the confidentiality of patient-related information. The data obtained show that 86.5% ($n = 867$) of nursing students confirm that the patient has the right to data protection and confidentiality concerning the information on the patient by the medical staff. This means that all information about the patient's health condition, the diagnostic, therapeutic, rehabilitation and nursing activities carried out and any other information obtained in connection with the exercise of the medical profession must not be disclosed to any unauthorized persons and should be treated as confidential. The data in Table 1 allow us to conclude that there is a statistically significant variation in the results among students across countries ($\chi^2 = 66.13$; $p < 0.0001$) in terms of knowledge of the patients' right to the confidentiality of information. A higher percentage of students from Slovakia (91.3%; $n = 356$) than students from Spain (79.3%; $n = 165$) indicated their knowledge of this right. In certain situations, medical practitioners are obliged to disclose information covered by professional secrecy. It was found that more than half of the nursing students (54.5%; $n = 546$) felt that medical staff could be exempted from professional confidentiality if the information covered could contribute to a risk to the health and life of others. The analysis of opinions concerning the issuance of copies of inpatient/ambulatory treatment records by the medical facility to the patient demonstrated statistically significant differences ($\chi^2 = 51.14$; $p < 0.0001$). It was found (Table 1) that 75% of the students ($n = 156$) from Spain confirmed that a medical facility is obliged to provide the patient with the records of inpatient or outpatient treatment, while a slightly lower percentage of students from Poland (71.5%; $n = 289$) and Slovakia (67.7%; $n = 264$) were of the same opinion. The situation was slightly different as regards knowledge declared by the students of the patient's right to be discharged from a hospital at their own request. The data presented show significant variation in responses among students ($\chi^2 = 86.00$; $p < 0.0001$). The vast majority of respondents from Poland (79.5%; $n = 321$) and Slovakia (75.9%; $n = 296$) stated that a patient has the right to be discharged from hospital on their own request. In contrast, a significant proportion (35.1%; $n = 73$) of Spanish students stated that a patient can only be discharged upon their own request from a hospital if their life is not in danger. Patients' rights also include the right to withdraw their objection to the donation of organs and tissues. Data analysis (Table 1) showed significant differences among nursing students ($\chi^2 = 15.17$; $p < 0.004$); the vast majority of students (72.1%; $n = 150$) from Spain confirmed the patient's right to withdraw their objection to organ and tissue donation, while 29.5% ($n = 115$) of students from Slovakia, 27.0% ($n = 109$) from Poland and 17.3% ($n = 36$) from Spain stated that they had no knowledge of this issue.

In the course of the study, students were asked to make a subjective assessment of their level of knowledge in the field of patients' rights, using a rating scale from 2 to 5. In a statistical analysis, significant differences in the level of knowledge (F = 67.43; $p < 0.0001$) were observed between students from Poland, Spain and Slovakia. The highest mean values were obtained by students from Spain (3.54 ± 0.92), while significantly lower scores were found for students from Poland (3.00 ± 0.73) and Slovakia (Table 2).

Table 2. Variation in students' self-assessed knowledge of patients' rights.

Variables	Country of Origin			ANOVA (F)	p Value
	Poland $n = 404$ (40.3%)	Spain $n = 208$ (20.8%)	Slovakia $n = 390$ (38.9%)		
	M ± SD, Me, Min.–Max., 95% CI	M ± SD, Me, Min.–Max., 95% CI	M ± SD, Me, Min.–Max., 95% CI		
Self-assessment of students' knowledge of patients' rights (rating scale 2–5)	3.00 ± 0.73, 3.00, 2.00–5.00, 2.93 ± 3.07	3.54 ± 0.92, 4.00, 2.00–5.00, 3.42 ± 3.67	2.79 ± 0.69, 3.00, 2.00–5.00, 2.72 ± 2.86	F = 67.43	0.0001 ***

Explanations: * $p < 0.05$; ** $p < 0.01$; *** $p < 0.001$. n, subgroup size; M, arithmetic mean; SD, standard deviation; Me, median; Min., minimum; Max, maximum; 95% CI, confidence interval.

After establishing low, average and high scores, special attention was paid to the proportion of the surveyed students who rated their competence in the area of patients' rights as low. As it turned out, as many as 35.9% of students from Slovakia, 26.5% from Poland and 14.9% from Spain were quite critical and indicated in the self-assessment a low level of knowledge of patients' rights (Figure 2).

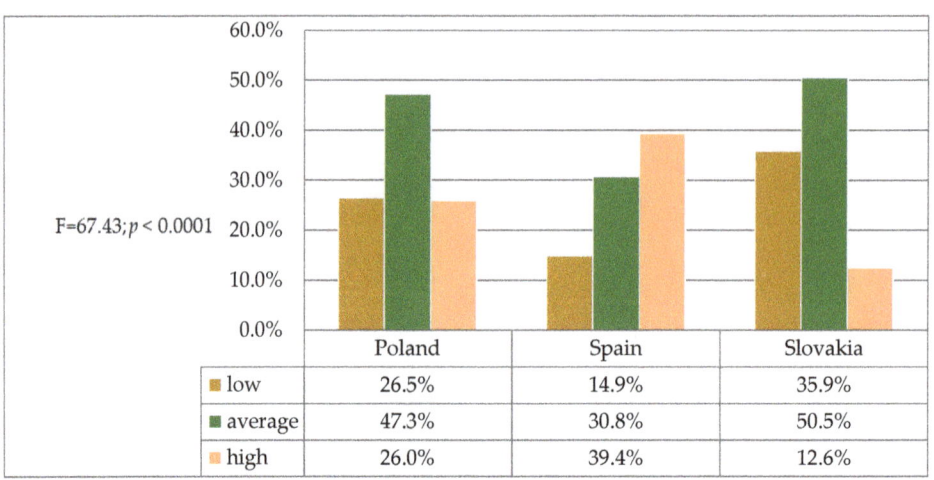

Figure 2. Self-assessment of the level of the students' knowledge of patients' rights—distribution of answers.

Subsequent analyses reported statistically significant differences (F = 3.44; $p < 0.03$) in self-reported knowledge of patients' rights among the age groups of Slovak students. It was proven that students aged 23 years and older received significantly higher mean values in the assessment (3.0 ± 0.68) than students in the ≤20 years age group (2.7 ± 0.67). This is probably linked to the implementation of educational content on the topic of patients' rights in classes in subsequent years. However, no statistically significant differences in self-assessed knowledge were found among Polish and Spanish students (F = 0.11; $p < 0.89$ vs. F = 0.18; $p < 0.83$) in the respective age groups. Analyses demonstrated that, in the Spanish group, the year of study significantly determined the level of students' knowledge of patients' rights (F = 14.68; $p < 0.0001$). Second-year students received higher mean values in the self-assessment (3.8 ± 0.85) than first-year students. Taking into account the year of study in the analyses, no significant differences in self-assessed knowledge of patients' rights were found among students from Poland (F = 0.16; $p < 0.85$) and Slovakia (F = 0.81; $p < 0.44$).

3.3. Assessing the Importance of the Patient's Right to Dignity in Personalized Healthcare

In further analyses, an attempt was made to rank, in the opinion of nursing students, the importance of the patient's right to respect their dignity, since the care of people in health and illness should always be based on respect for their dignity, subjectivity and ensuring intimacy when health services are provided by medical personnel. The right to respect for dignity also includes the right to die in peace. When asked what rank on a 2–5 rating scale the students would give to the patients' right to dignity, significantly different results (F = 133.56; $p < 0.0001$) were obtained, depending on the surveyed students' country of origin (Table 3).

Table 3. Patients' right to dignity—comparison of rankings.

Variables	Country of Origin			ANOVA (F)	p Value
	Poland n = 404 (40.3%)	Spain n = 208 (20.8%)	Slovakia n = 390 (38.9%)		
	M ± SD, Me, Min.–Max., 95% CI	M ± SD, Me, Min.–Max., 95% CI	M ± SD, Me, Min.–Max., 95% CI		
Ranking on a 2 to 5 scale given to the patient's right to dignity by the respondents	3.43 ± 0.77, 4.00, 2.00–4.00, 3.35–3.50	4.37 ± 0.92, 5.00, 2.00–5.00, 4.24–4.49	3.27 ± 0.79, 3.00, 2.00–4.00, 3.19–3.35	F = 133.56	0.0001 ***

Explanations: * $p < 0.05$; ** $p < 0.01$; *** $p < 0.001$. n, subgroup size; M, arithmetic mean; SD, standard deviation; Me, median; Min., minimum; Max., maximum; 95% CI—confidence interval.

The analyses showed that Spanish students obtained significantly higher mean values (4.37 ± 0.92) in the ranking of the patient's right to dignity than students from the other two countries. Subsequent analyses explored the influence of selected sociodemographic characteristics such as age and year of study within the country on the ratings indicated by students regarding the patient's right to dignity. The analysis found no statistically significant differences in the rank given to the patient's right to dignity across age groups in any of the analyzed countries. However, in Spain, the year of study was found to significantly (F = 3.72; $p < 0.03$) influence the level of students' ranking of the patient's right to dignity. Spanish first-year students gave a significantly higher ranking to the patient's right to dignity (4.6 ± 0.73) than third-year students (4.1 ± 1.08; $p < 0.02$). In contrast, there were no statistically significant differences in the ranking given to the patient's right in students from different years of study in Poland and Slovakia. Therefore, it may be concluded that the results of the studies conducted in Poland, Spain and Slovakia confirm the differences in the knowledge of patients' rights among nursing students, but they require further scientific consideration.

4. Discussion

We attempted to determine the role and importance of patients' rights in personalized healthcare from the perspective of nursing students in Poland, Spain and Slovakia. It was recognized that the individualized nature of medical services involves respecting the rights of the patient, which protect the patient's autonomy (freedom) from interference by other parties and provides the basis for claiming the legitimate conditions for the exercise of those rights. According to the procedures applicable in a given healthcare facility, the patient should be informed of their rights, which should be recorded in an understandable and legible manner and available in the patients' areas.

The results of the authors' own research show that only one-third of the respondents were informed about their rights before admission to hospital or during the provision of health services and that the information on patients' rights and the Patients' Ombudsman was posted in a publicly accessible place. The analyses of research results obtained by many other authors quite often reveal an unfavorable situation of the patient concerning their rights in various medical entities operating in the medical services market. For example, a study conducted by Ansari et al. among 500 Iranian patients in inpatient and outpatient care found that 93.5% of them did not receive any information on patients' rights [26]. Moreover, a study conducted by Egyptian researchers on a group of 514 patients hospitalized at the Minia University Hospital found that about 76% of patients did not know about the existence of the patients' rights charter and 98.1% of those surveyed said that the medical team did not inform them of the treatment options available [27]. This means that healthcare providers should place greater emphasis on raising patients' awareness of their rights and involving them in decisions about their treatment choices. Abedi et al. also indicated the need to increase patients' awareness of their rights during the delivery of healthcare services [28]. As stated by Agrawal et al., to take effective educational measures to improve general awareness not only among patients but also among various stakeholders in the healthcare system, it is important to assess the awareness of hospitalized patients of their rights [29]. As shown by the results of a study conducted by Tabassum et al. in two hospitals in Lahore (Pakistan) from the public and the private sectors, most patients (64%) were not aware of their rights. However, the level of awareness of patients' rights was higher in patients receiving medical care in a private hospital than in a public hospital [30]. It is also worth referring to the findings of Mohammadi et al. who, in their study, indicated the need to inform patients about ethical and legal issues related to privacy and confidentiality, before and during admission to hospital [31].

As shown by an analysis of the authors' own study results, significantly more patients in Poland (62.4%) than in Slovakia (37.7%) or Spain (16.5%) were informed about their rights. Other researchers have also attempted to assess existing barriers to compliance with patients' rights on the basis of a meta-analysis. The most important factors cited as obstacles to respecting patients' rights included, among others: excessive workload of nurses, staff shortage, organizational factors and a lack of awareness of the patients' rights charter among patients, nurses, doctors and students [32]. In the current study, the degree of observing patients' rights in healthcare institutions in the opinion of nursing students in Poland, Spain and Slovakia is significantly different. Almost 75% of Spanish students rated the level of observing patients' rights in their country as good. The respect for patients' rights in Polish and Slovak healthcare institutions was rated much lower by the students. Undoubtedly, there is a need to search for subjective and objective factors affecting the level of respecting patients' rights in medical facilities.

Interesting results were also presented by Mousavi et al. who showed that the rights of patients admitted to the Intensive Care Unit are more affected than those of patients admitted to other hospital wards. They pointed to inadequate nurse-to-patient ratios, socio-economic problems, working hours and high workload in a limited time as the main factors affecting the quality of nursing practice in terms of respecting patients' rights, among others [33]. In contrast, Waddington and Mesherry raise the important issue of informed consent for the treatment of people with psychosocial disabilities in Europe [34]. In other studies conducted by Sabzevari et al. among medical staff of the hospitals affiliated with the Mashhad University of Medical Sciences, the highest level of respect for patients' rights was found in the area of respect for patients' privacy and confidentiality, which was assessed as excellent by all respondents (100%). The lowest value of compliance with patients' rights was associated with the presentation of adequate and appropriate information addressed to patients, which was rated excellent by 48.1% respondents [35].

Human dignity and subjectivity require that medical personnel observe the highest standards of ethical conduct and respect the intimacy of the patient. In the authors' own study, Spanish nursing students ranked the patient's right to respect for dignity with the highest mean values, demonstrating the importance of this right in personalized medical care.

Of all the staff caring for patients, it is nurses who spend the most time with the patients, see their behavior and recognize their needs. Thus, the quality of nursing care depends on the knowledge and experience of nurses. As Sheikhtaheri et al. proved in their study on a group of Iranian nurses, the mean score of nurses' knowledge of patients' rights was acceptable, while more experienced and educated nurses showed more knowledge about patients' rights. However, compliance with patients' rights by the nurses involved in the study was questionable [36]. In the current study, the level of nursing students' knowledge of patients' rights significantly varied. The highest average values were obtained by students from Spain, while the most critical in self-evaluation were those from Slovakia.

An attempt to determine the extent to which doctors and nurses in Oman were aware of the importance of patients' rights and their observance was undertaken by Al-Saadi et al. Their research showed that overall awareness of the importance of patients' rights among medical staff was high (91.5%), although compliance with these rights in practice was much lower (63.8%) [37].

Nurses often take on the role of the patient's spokesperson, yet daily nursing practice also includes certain shortcomings with regard to respecting patients' rights [38]. During their studies, nursing students acquire knowledge, clinical skills and social competences in order to fulfill their duties towards patients and their families with due diligence in their professional work.

Aydin Er et al. presented the results of a study involving 238 nursing students from the West Black Sea Universities in Turkey in which the majority of the nursing students held desirable attitudes toward patient information, truth-telling and protection of patients' privacy and medical records. The authors proposed that ethics education, covering both patient's rights and the obligations of nurses to defend these rights, be introduced to the study curriculum [39]. Based on a review of the literature on the topic, genuine contacts of nursing students with patients during clinical classes are of key importance in the development of the skills necessary for students working with patients. The concept of learning from patients has emerged recently, thus transferring the emphasis of learning from professionals as the example to follow to relations created between the student and the patient [40]. This development is particularly important in the domain of social competences, where nursing students should always see to the patient's welfare, respect patient's dignity and autonomy, display understanding for ideological and cultural differences and respond with empathy in contacts with patients and their families [20].

As indicated by Kim, in order for future nurses to be well prepared for their professional roles, it is desirable to revise the curriculum in the nursing program to strengthen interpersonal care behaviors, biomedical ethics and students' sensitivity to human rights [41]. Moreover, mentors involved in clinical nursing education are expected to provide the optimal educational environment for achieving and demonstrating the desired level of competence in conjunction with professional ethics and patients' rights [42]. Finally, it should be added that modern nursing entails an ethical responsibility to respect and protect patients' rights. The presented results of the authors' own research reflect a certain fragment of reality and provide a contribution to further scientific investigations.

5. Limitations and Implications for Professional Practice

The results of this study help to outline implications for professional practice. Firstly, they point to a need to analyze study programs in conjunction with assessing the effectiveness of clinical teaching in the nursing program, with particular emphasis on the courses that involve learning outcomes related to professional ethics and patients' rights. Secondly, there is a need to disseminate the information on patients' rights among the population in a given country. Thirdly, medical practitioners, as part of their postgraduate training, should deepen their knowledge, improve their professional skills and develop their social skills throughout their careers. This will ensure a sufficiently high level of medical care for the patient, which will translate into therapeutic safety and patient satisfaction with the medical services provided. The presented study is the first one of this type conducted on the international scale in selected European countries, i.e., Poland, Spain and Slovakia, but it has its limitations, such as the size of the surveyed group, and needs to be replicated with a larger number of respondents.

6. Conclusions

1. The degree to which patients' rights are respected in healthcare facilities in Poland, Spain and Slovakia in the subjective assessment of nursing students is significantly different and is not always favorable for the patient.
2. A variation in the level of nursing students' knowledge of selected patients' rights in personalized healthcare was observed, requiring in-depth educational activities at the university level in respective countries.

3. The degree of knowledge of patients' rights among nursing students is not uniform and includes the right to information on the patient's health, the confidentiality of patient-related information and medical records, to withdraw their objection to organ and tissue donation, to pastoral care and to deposit valuable items.
4. The right to respect dignity, which also includes the right to die in peace and dignity in personalized medical care, was rated the highest by Spanish first-year students.

Author Contributions: Conceptualization, E.K. and A.B.; methodology, E.K., M.J. and E.G.; software, E.K.; validation, E.K., H.K. and M.M.; formal analysis, E.K.; investigation, E.K.; resources, E.K. and A.K.; data curation, E.K.; writing—original draft preparation, E.K.; writing—review and editing, E.K. and E.G.; visualization, E.K.; supervision, E.K. and A.A.; project administration, E.K. and A.K.; funding acquisition, E.K. All authors have read and agreed to the published version of the manuscript.

Funding: This work was a part of a research project, financed by the University of Warmia and Mazury in Olsztyn (No 63-610-001), Poland.

Institutional Review Board Statement: The study was conducted according to the guidelines of the Declaration of Helsinki, and approved by the Senate Committee on Ethics of Scientific Research at the Higher School in Olsztyn, Poland. (protocol code No. 4/2020, on 12.03.2020).

Informed Consent Statement: Informed consent was obtained from all subjects involved in the study.

Data Availability Statement: The data presented in this study are available on request from the corresponding author.

Conflicts of Interest: The authors declare no conflict of interest.

References

1. Wium-Andersen, I.K.; Vinberg, M.; Lars Vedel Kessing, L.V.; McIntyre, R.S. Personalized medicine in psychiatry. *Nord. J. Psychiat.* **2017**, *71*, 12–19. [CrossRef] [PubMed]
2. Sigman, M. Introduction: Personalized medicine: What is it and what are the challenges? *Fertil Steril.* **2018**, *109*, 944–945. [CrossRef] [PubMed]
3. Anaya, J.M.; Duarte-Rey, C.; Sarmiento-Monroy, J.C.; Bardey, D.; Castiblanco, J.; Rojas-Villarraga, A. Personalized medicine. Closing the gap between knowledge and clinical practice. *Autoimmun Rev.* **2016**, *15*, 833–842. [CrossRef]
4. Markocka-Mączka, K.; Grabowski, K.; Taboła, R. *Holistyczne Podejście do Pacjenta, Profilaktyka i Edukacja Zdrowotna [Holistic Approach to the Patient, Prevention and Health Education]*; Wyd. Naukowe NeuroCentrum: Lublin, Poland, 2017; pp. 171–176.
5. Jacek, A.; Ożóg, K. Przestrzeganie praw pacjenta przez personel medyczny [Respecting patient's rights by medical staff]. *Hygeia Public Health* **2012**, *47*, 264–271.
6. Olejniczak, M.; Michowska, M.; Basińska, K. Opinie studentów Gdańskiego Uniwersytetu Medycznego na temat przestrzegania praw pacjenta w czasie odbywania zajęć klinicznych [Opinions of Gdańsk Medical University students on respecting patients' rights during their clinical practice]. *Ann. Acad. Med. Gedan.* **2011**, *41*, 79–87.
7. WHO. Patients' Rights. Available online: https://www.who.int/genomics/public/patientrights/en/ (accessed on 26 July 2020).
8. Powszechna Deklaracja Praw Człowieka [Universal Declaration of Human Rights]. Available online: https://www.unesco.pl/fileadmin/user_upload/pdf/Powszechna_Deklaracja_Praw_Czlowieka.pdf (accessed on 26 July 2020).
9. Convention for the Protection of Human Rights and Dignity of the Human Being with regard to the Application of Biology and Medicine: Convention of Human Rights and Biomedicine. Available online: http://conventions.coe.int/Treaty/en/Treaties/Html/164.htm (accessed on 26 July 2020).
10. European Charter of Patients' Rights. Available online: http://www.patienttalk.info/european_charter.pdf (accessed on 26 July 2020).
11. European Charter of Patients' Rights, Rome. 2002. Available online: http://ec.europa.eu/health/ph_overview/co_operation/mobility/docs/health_services_co108_en.pdf (accessed on 26 July 2020).
12. Viberg, N.; Forsberg, B.C.; Borowitz, M.; Molin, R. International comparisons of waiting times in health care—Limitations and prospects. *Health Policy* **2013**, *112*, 53–61. [CrossRef]
13. Dyrektywa Parlamentu Europejskiego i Rady 2011/24/UE z Dnia 9 marca 2011 r. w Sprawie Stosowania Praw Pacjentów w Transgranicznej Opiece Zdrowotnej (Dz. U. UE L z Dnia 4 Kwietnia 2011 r.) [Directive 2011/24 / EU of the European Parliament and of the Council of 9 March 2011 on the Application of Patients' Rights in Cross-Border Healthcare (Journal of Laws UE L of 4 April 2011)]. Available online: http://www.kpk.nfz.gov.pl/images/downloads/dyrektywa.pdf (accessed on 30 July 2020).
14. Quinn, P.; De Hert, P. The Patients' Rights Directive (2011/24/EU)—Providing (some) rights to EU residents seeking healthcare in other Member States. *Comput. Law Secur. Rev.* **2011**, *27*, 497–502. [CrossRef]

15. Azzopardi-Muscat, N.; Baeten, R.; Clemens, T.; Habicht, T.; Keskimäki, I.; Kowalska-Bobko, I.; Sagan, A.; van Ginneken, E. The role of the 2011 patients' rights in cross-border health care directive in shaping seven national health systems: Looking beyond patient mobility. *Health Policy* **2018**, *122*, 279–283. [CrossRef]
16. Heinonen, N.; Tynkkynen, L.-K.; Keskimäki, I. The transposition of the patients' rights directive in finland—Difficulties encountered. *Health Policy* **2019**, *123*, 526–531. [CrossRef]
17. Minvielle, E. Toward Customized Care Comment on "(Re) Making the Procrustean Bed? Standardization and Customization as Competing Logics in Healthcare". *Int. J. Health Policy. Manag.* **2018**, *7*, 272–274. [CrossRef]
18. Elewa, A.H.; ElAlim, E.A.; Etway, E.G. Nursing interns' perception regarding patients' rights and patients' advocacy. *SOJ. Nur. Health Care* **2016**, *2*, 1–6. [CrossRef]
19. Dyrektywa 2005/36/WE Parlamentu Europejskiego i Rady z dnia 7 Września 2005 r w Sprawie Uznawania Kwalifikacji Zawodowych (Dz.U. L 255 z 30.9.2005, s. 22). [Directive 2005/36 / EC of the European Parliament and of the Council of 7 September 2005 on the Recognition of Professional Qualifications (OJ L 255, 30.9.2005, p. 22). Available online: https://eur-lex.europa.eu/legal-content/PL/TXT/PDF/?uri=CELEX:02005L0036-20140117&from=EN (accessed on 31 July 2020).
20. Rozporządzenie Ministra Zdrowia z Dnia 26 Lipca 2019 r. w Sprawie Standardów Kształcenia Przygotowującego Do Wykonywania Zawodu Lekarza, Lekarza Dentysty, Farmaceuty, Pielęgniarki, Położnej, Diagnosty Laboratoryjnego, Fizjoterapeuty i Ratownika Medycznego (Dz. U. z 21.08.2019 r., poz. 1573) [Regulation of the Minister of Health of 26 July 2019 on the Standards of Education Preparing for the Profession of a Doctor, Dentist, Pharmacist, Nurse, Midwife, Laboratory Diagnostician, Physiotherapist and Paramedic] (Journal of Laws of 21 August 2019, Item 1573). Available online: https://isap.sejm.gov.pl/isap.nsf/DocDetails.xsp?id=WDU20190001573 (accessed on 31 July 2020).
21. Poorchangizi, B.; Borhani, F.; Abbaszadeh, A.; Mirzaee, M.; Farokhzadian, J. The importance of professional values from nursing students' perspective. *BMC Nurs.* **2019**, *18*, 26. [CrossRef]
22. Kupcewicz, E.; Grochans, E.; Mikla, M.; Kadučáková, H.; Jóźwik, M. Role of global self-esteem in predicting life satisfaction of nursing students in poland, spain and slovakia. *Int. J. Environ. Res. Public Health* **2020**, *17*, 5392. [CrossRef] [PubMed]
23. Kupcewicz, E.; Grochans, E.; Kadučáková, H.; Mikla, M.; Jóźwik, M. Analysis of the relationship between stress intensity and coping strategy and the quality of life of nursing students in poland, spain and slovakia. *Int. J. Environ. Res. Public Health* **2020**, *17*, 4536. [CrossRef]
24. Szymczak, W. *Podstawy Statystyki Dla Psychologów [Fundamentals of Statistics for Psychologists]*; DIFIN: Warszawa, Poland, 2018.
25. Vandenbroucke, J.P.; von Elm, E.; Altman, D.G.; Gøtzsche, P.C.; Mulrow, C.D.; Pocock, S.J.; Poole, C.; Schlesselman, J.J.; Egger, M.; For the STROBE Initiative. Strengthening the reporting of observational studies in epidemiology (strobe): Explanation and elaboration. *Int. J. Surg.* **2014**, *12*, 1500–1524. [CrossRef] [PubMed]
26. Ansari, S.; Abeid, P.; Namvar, F.; Dorakvand, M.; Rokhafrooz, D. Respect to the bill of patients' rights in the educational hospitals in Ahvaz, Iran. *Middle East J. Sci. Res.* **2013**, *4*, 440–444. [CrossRef]
27. Mohammed, E.S.; Seedhom, A.E.; Ghazawy, E.R. Awareness and practice of patient rights from a patient perspective: An insight from Upper Egypt. *Int. J. Qual Health Care* **2018**, *1*, 145–151. [CrossRef] [PubMed]
28. Abedi, G.; Shojaee, J.; Moosazadeh, M.; Rostami, F.; Nadi, A.; Abedini, E.; Palenik, C.J.; Askarian, M. Awareness and observance of patient rights from the perspective of iranian patients: A systematic review and meta-analysis. *Iran. J. Med. Sci.* **2017**, *42*, 227–234.
29. Agrawal, U.; D'Souza, B.C.; Seetharam, A.M. Awareness of Patients' Rights among Inpatients of a Tertiary Care Teaching Hospital- A Cross-sectional Study. *J. Clin. Diagn. Res.* **2017**, *11*, IC01–IC06 [CrossRef]
30. Tabassum, T.; Ashraf, M.; Thaver, I. Hospitalized patients' awareness of their rights-a cross sectional survey in a public and private tertiary care hospitals of punjab, pakistan. *J. Ayub. Med. Coll. Abbottabad.* **2016**, *28*, 582–586.
31. Mohammadi, M.; Larijani, B.; Emami Razavi, S.H.; Fotouhi, A.; Ghaderi, A.; Madani, S.J.; Shafiee, M.N. Do patients know that physicians should be confidential? study on patients' awareness of privacy and confidentiality. *J. Med. Ethics Hist. Med.* **2018**, *11*, 1.
32. Hadian Jazi, Z.; Dehghan Nayeri, N. Barriers in the performance of patient's rights in iran and appropriate offered solutions review article. *J. Holist. Nurs. Midwifery* **2014**, *24*, 69–79.
33. Mousavi, S.M.; Mohammadi, N.; Ashghali Farahani, M.; Hosseini, A.F. Observing patients' rights and the facilitating and deterrent organizational factors from the viewpoint of nurses working in intensive care units. *J. Client Cent. Nurs. Care* **2017**, *3*, 27–36. [CrossRef]
34. Waddington, L.; Mesherry, B. Exceptions and exclusions: The right to informed consent for medical treatment of people with psychosocial disabilities in Europe. *Eur. J. Health. Law.* **2016**, *23*, 279–304. [CrossRef] [PubMed]
35. Sabzevari, A.; Kiani, M.A.; Saeidi, M.; Jafari, S.A.; Kianifar, H.; Ahanchian, H.; Jarahi, L.; Zakerian, M. Evaluation of patients' rights observance according to patients' rights charter in educational hospitals affiliated to mashhad university of medical sciences: Medical staffs' views. *Electron. Physician.* **2016**, *8*, 3102–3109. [CrossRef]
36. Sheikhtaheri, A.; Jabali, M.S.; Dehaghi, Z.H. Nurses' knowledge and performance of the patients' bill of rights. *Nurs. Ethics* **2016**, *23*, 866–876. [CrossRef]
37. Al-Saadi, A.N.; Slimane, S.B.A.; Al-Shibli, R.A.; Al-Jabri, F.Y. Awareness of the Importance of and Adherence to Patients' Rights Among Physicians and Nurses in Oman: An analytical cross-sectional study across different levels of healthcare. *Sultan. Qaboos Univ. Med. J.* **2019**, *19*, e201–e208. [CrossRef] [PubMed]

38. Water, T.; Ford, K.; Spence, D.; Rasmussen, S. Patient advocacy by nurses—Past, present and future. *Contemp. Nurse* **2016**, *56*, 696–709. [CrossRef]
39. Aydin Er, R.; Ersoy, N.; Celik, S. The nursing students' views about the patient's rights at the west black sea universities in turkey. *Nurs. Midwifery Stud.* **2014**, *3*, e19136. [CrossRef] [PubMed]
40. Suikkala, A.; Koskinen, S.; Leino-Kilpi, H. Patients' involvement in nursing students' clinical education: A scoping review. *Int J. Nurs. Stud.* **2018**, *84*, 40–51. [CrossRef]
41. Kim, S.-Y. The Relationship between Human Rights Sensitivity, Interpersonal Caring Behavior, and Biomedical Ethics in Nursing Students Who Have Experienced Clinical Practice. *J. Korea Acad. Industr. Coop. Soc.* **2020**, *21*, 410–418. [CrossRef]
42. Clavagnier, I. Patients' rights. *Rev. Infirm.* **2017**, *66*, 47–48. [CrossRef] [PubMed]

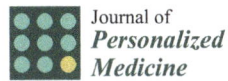

Article

Maternal Psychological and Biological Factors Associated to Gestational Complications

David Ramiro-Cortijo [1,2,†], Maria de la Calle [3,†], Vanesa Benitez [4], Andrea Gila-Diaz [2,5], Bernardo Moreno-Jiménez [6], Silvia M. Arribas [2,*] and Eva Garrosa [6,*]

1. Department of Medicine, Beth Israel Deaconess Medical Center, Harvard Medical School, 330 Brookline Avenue, Boston, MA 02215, USA; dramiro@bidmc.harvard.edu
2. Department of Physiology, Faculty of Medicine, Universidad Autónoma de Madrid, C/Arzobispo Morcillo 2, 28029 Madrid, Spain; andrea.gila@uam.es
3. Obstetric and Gynecology Service, Hospital Universitario La Paz, Universidad Autónoma de Madrid, Paseo de la Castellana 261, 28046 Madrid, Spain; maria.delacalle@uam.es
4. Department of Agricultural and Food Chemistry, Faculty of Science, Universidad Autónoma de Madrid, C/Francisco Tomas y Valiente 7, 28049 Madrid, Spain; vanesa.benitez@uam.es
5. Pharmacology and Physiology PhD Program, Doctoral School, Universidad Autónoma de Madrid, C/Francisco Tomas y Valiente 2, 28049 Madrid, Spain
6. Department of Biological and Health Psychology, Faculty of Psychology, Universidad Autonoma de Madrid, C/Ivan Pavlov 6, 28049 Madrid, Spain; bernardo.moreno@uam.es
* Correspondence: silvia.arribas@uam.es (S.M.A.); eva.garrosa@uam.es (E.G.)
† These authors have equal contribution.

Citation: Ramiro-Cortijo, D.; de la Calle, M.; Benitez, V.; Gila-Diaz, A.; Moreno-Jiménez, B.; Arribas, S.M.; Garrosa, E. Maternal Psychological and Biological Factors Associated to Gestational Complications. *J. Pers. Med.* **2021**, *11*, 183. https://doi.org/10.3390/jpm11030183

Academic Editors: Riitta Suhonen, Minna Stolt and David Edvardsson

Received: 17 January 2021
Accepted: 2 March 2021
Published: 5 March 2021

Publisher's Note: MDPI stays neutral with regard to jurisdictional claims in published maps and institutional affiliations.

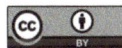

Copyright: © 2021 by the authors. Licensee MDPI, Basel, Switzerland. This article is an open access article distributed under the terms and conditions of the Creative Commons Attribution (CC BY) license (https://creativecommons.org/licenses/by/4.0/).

Abstract: Early detection of gestational complications is a priority in obstetrics. In our social context, this is linked to maternity age. Most studies are focused on biological factors. However, pregnancy is also influenced by social and psychological factors, which have not been deeply explored. We aimed to identify biopsychosocial risk and protective factors associated with the development of maternal and fetal complications. We enrolled 182 healthy pregnant women, and plasma melatonin and cortisol levels were measured in the first trimester by chemiluminescent immunoassays. At different time points along gestation, women answered several questionnaires (positive and negative affect schedule, hospital anxiety and depression scale, pregnancy concerns scale, life orientation test, resilience scale, life satisfaction scale and life–work conflicts scale). They were followed up until delivery and categorized as normal pregnancy, maternal or fetal complications. Maternal complications were associated with low melatonin (OR = 0.99 [0.98; 1.00]; p-value = 0.08) and life satisfaction (OR = 0.64 [0.41; 0.93]; p-value = 0.03) and fetal complications were associated with high cortisol (OR = 1.06 [1.02; 1.13]; p-value = 0.04), anxiety (OR = 2.21 [1.10; 4.55]; p-value = 0.03) and life–work conflicts (OR = 1.92 [1.04; 3.75]; p-value = 0.05). We conclude that psychological factors influence pregnancy outcomes in association with melatonin and cortisol alterations. High maternal melatonin and life satisfaction levels could be potential protective factors against the development of maternal complications during pregnancy. Low anxiety and cortisol levels and reduced work–life conflicts could prevent fetal complications.

Keywords: anxiety; life satisfaction; life–work concerns; melatonin; cortisol; biopsychosocial model; obstetric complications

1. Introduction

Maternity is highly influenced by social factors, including education, economic or racial aspects. In industrialized societies, a key social determinant is the delay of maternity age [1], related to the gradual access of the women to higher education, employment and pregnancy control. The use of assisted reproduction techniques (ART) has made possible maternity beyond biological limits [2]. Pregnancy at an age over the optimum childbearing age has biological consequences, including higher rate of pregnancy complications and infertility. In addition, the use of ART increases the rates of multiple pregnancies [3], which are also a risk factor for complications, including preterm delivery (labor before 37 weeks of gestation) and fetal growth restriction (FGR) [4].

Almost 17% of pregnant women experience some type of pregnancy complication, which affects maternal and infant's health [5]. Detecting women at risk as early as possible is a priority in obstetrics. Despite intensive research, there are still unknown causes that increase the risk of pregnancy complications. The majority of studies have focused on biological factors, some of which have been identified. However, pregnancy is influenced not only by biological determinants, but also by other factors. The biopsychosocial approach is ingrained in the "general systems theory", which states that a system is characterized by the complex interactions of its components [6]. In the obstetric field, there is a psychological and social domain that should be incorporated into clinical practice to improve healthcare. Therefore, insight into pregnancy complications should be approached from a biopsychosocial point of view.

The psychological sphere likely exerts an important influence on pregnancy. Getting pregnant at an advanced age, the need of ART and a multiple pregnancy represent important stress factors which may negatively influence pregnancy outcome. There is evidence that individuals under high stress take poorer care of themselves and are more likely to engage in health-impairing behaviors, which may affect maternofetal health [7,8]. The importance of psychological factors on maternal health also is evidenced by the fact that antenatal optimism is the most protective factor against maternal postnatal adverse outcomes, e.g., depression or other mood disorders [9]. Maternal psychological factors may also influence long-term offspring health. For example, psychological stress in pregnancy, specifically in early stages, has been associated with higher risk of mental disorders in the offspring [10]. Life concerns, anxiety or problems in concealing work and personal life exert an influence on the biological environment of pregnant mothers and could be the link between psychological responses and negative influences on maternofetal health.

The interaction between psychological and biological factors and their impact on pregnancy outcomes have not been sufficiently explored [8]. Melatonin and cortisol are important hormones in gestation and can be potential biological factors implicated in this relationship. Melatonin is synthesized by the pineal gland with a peak at night [11], and during pregnancy it is also produced by the placenta [12]. Melatonin is a key hormone for pregnancy maintenance due to its pleiotropic roles [13], including its remarkable effects as an antioxidant [14]. We have evidence that, in the first trimester of pregnancy, a poor antioxidant status is linked with the development of pregnancy complications, and melatonin is an important contributor protecting against oxidative damage [3]. Our data indicate that maternal plasma melatonin is lower in women with preterm birth [15]. Daytime melatonin levels have been demonstrated to be influenced by anxiety and depression [16], perhaps due to the reduction in the number of sleep hours, which are directly proportional to melatonin circulating levels [17]. Therefore, it is possible that the dysregulation of this hormone under stressful conditions will influence pregnancy outcome.

Cortisol is another important hormone that may influence pregnancy outcome. Cortisol is synthesized by the hypothalamus–pituitary–adrenal axis and has cell catabolic and immune system suppression effects [18]. Cortisol secretion is closely linked to stress conditions, and it has been related to maternal mood, showing associations with psychological stress [19] and anxiety [20]. The maternal psychological stress and the associated increase in cortisol levels have been linked with adverse neonatal outcomes [21]. In this sense, we have evidence from twin pregnancies that the levels of maternal cortisol in early pregnancy are negatively associated with birth weight [15].

We hypothesize that social and psychological spheres exert an impact on obstetric outcome, influencing biological factors. We aimed to identify biopsychosocial risk and protective factors associated with the development of maternal and fetal complications in our social context, characterized by an advanced maternity age. We also explored the relationship between psychological variables and melatonin and cortisol, key hormones implicated in pregnancy and stress.

2. Materials and Methods

2.1. Cohort Selection

This is a retrospective, non-interventional and observational study from the Hospital Universitario La Paz (HULP, Madrid, Spain). Pregnant women were enrolled at 8 weeks of gestation at Obstetrics and Gynecology service. Women were first informed about the study proposal, and those who accepted anonymously and voluntarily to participate in the study signed a consent. The exclusion criterion was women who had previous diseases (hypertension, obesity, diabetes mellitus, inflammatory or immune deficiency diseases or record of previous pregnancy complications). The inclusion criterion was good comprehension of the Spanish language. Finally, 182 healthy pregnant women were enrolled. The study flow-chart is shown in Figure 1.

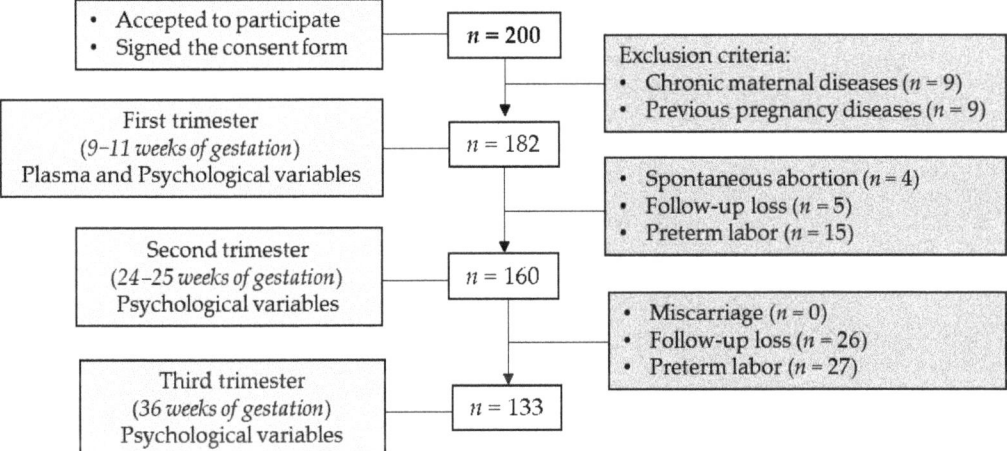

Figure 1. Flow-chart of study participants. Exclusion criteria: chronic maternal disease (i.e., hypertension, obesity, diabetes mellitus, inflammatory or immune deficiency diseases previous pregnancy) and diagnoses of obstetrical complications before. Sample size (n) is shown between brackets.

This study was performed in accordance with the Declaration of Helsinki regarding studies in human subjects and it was approved by HULP and Universidad Autónoma de Madrid Ethical Committees (PI-1490 and CEMU/2013-10, respectively).

2.2. Maternal and Neonatal Data Collection and Group Classification

Maternal and neonatal data were collected from the medical record. Maternal data collected were maternal age (years), civil status (single/married), educational level (undergraduate/university degree), employment situation (working/unemployment, of herself and, in the case of having a partner, also of the partner), family core-economic income (euros/month), smoking habits (yes/no) and alcohol intake during pregnancy (yes/no), gestational age (weeks of gestation), twin gestation (binary variable) and assisted reproduction techniques (ART, binary variable). In addition, obstetric adverse outcomes (diagnosed by the obstetrician staff based on hospital guidelines) were also recorded and included: *hyperemesis gravidarum* (defined as more than 3 episodes of vomiting/day, weight loss of 5% and ketones in the urine), pregnancy-induced hypertension (defined as blood pressure $\geq$ 140/110 mmHg without preeclampsia alterations before 20 weeks of gestation), gestational diabetes mellitus (defined as blood glucose levels > 140 mg/dL in the glucose tolerance test), preeclampsia (defined as pregnancy-induced hypertension and protein in the urine), pregnancy anemia (defined as hemoglobin < 11 g/dL in the first trimester or < 10.5 g/dL in the second or third trimester) and intrahepatic cholestasis of pregnancy (defined as pruritus and alterations in the blood/liver function tests including serum bile acids levels). Women who developed any of these complications during pregnancy were included in the "maternal complications" group.

Neonatal data recorded were infant sex and the following fetal adverse clinical outcome: any alterations in the physiologic systems reported by echography during pregnancy follow-up, FGR (defined as intrauterine growth below the third percentile or below the tenth percentile with hemodynamic alterations by Doppler echography; binary variable) and preterm labor (defined as gestational age low than 37 weeks; binary variable). Pregnancies with any of these fetal outcomes were included in the "fetal complications" group.

2.3. Maternal Plasma Variables in the First Trimester

At 9–11 weeks of gestation, blood samples were extracted from 8:00 to 9:00 am, by venipuncture in Vacutainer® lithium heparin gel tubes for plasma separation (Becton Dickinson comp., Madrid; Spain), following the protocols established by the medical staff. Plasma was obtained by centrifugation ($2100 \times g$, 15 min at 4 °C), within a maximum of 2 h after extraction and stored at -80 °C to assay melatonin and cortisol.

To determine melatonin levels, plasma was evaporated to dryness with an evaporator centrifuge (Speed Vac SC 200; Savant; Hyannis, MA, USA). The residues were dissolved in distilled water and melatonin levels were determined by a competitive enzyme immunoassay kit (Melatonin ELISA; IBL International, Hamburg; Germany) according to the manufacturer's instructions. The kit is characterized by an analytical sensitivity of 1.6 pg/mL and high analytical specificity (low cross-reactivity). Melatonin was expressed as pg/mL. This method was extensively described in Aguilera et al. [22].

To assess plasma cortisol, a competitive immunoassay using direct chemiluminescent technology was used, being analyzed with an Advia Centaur instrument (Siemens Healthineers, Madrid; Spain). Cortisol was expressed as µg/dL.

2.4. Maternal Psychological Variables during Pregnancy

Women answered psychological applications in each trimester of pregnancy at Weeks 9–11 (first trimester), 24–25 (second trimester) and 36 (third trimester), during a programmed visit to the hospital. Missing data referred to women with miscarriage, preterm delivery or follow-up loss, coinciding with the visit of pregnant women to the hospital. Psychological applications are described below:

Positive and Negative Affect Schedule [23], Spanish version [24]. This standardized application scores the positive and negative affectivity using 20 items with a Likert answer of 5 points ranging from "nothing" (1) to "extremely" (5). Some of the positive items were "active" or "strong" and some of the negative items were "restless" or "distressed".

Hospital Anxiety and Depression Scale [25], Spanish version [26]. This standardized application scores the anxiety using a questionnaire with seven items with a Likert answer of 4 points ranging from "no anxiety" (0) to "high anxiety" (3).

Pregnancy concerns scale. It is an ad-hoc scale, which was elaborated according to the recommended phases for the creation of psychological scales [27] and was previously used by our research group [28]. This scale evaluates personal concerns about gestation worries. It is a scale with 10 items with a Likert answer of 4 points ranging from "none" (0) to "many" (3). Some items were "the health of my newborn" or "the effect of the drugs on the fetus".

Life Orientation Test [29], Spanish version [30]. This application scores personal optimism. We used a short scale of five items with a Likert answer of 5 points ranging from "completely agree" (1, low optimism) to "completely disagree" (5, high optimism). Some examples of the items are "I am always optimistic about my future" and "I usually think the things are not going right".

Resilience scale [31], Spanish version [32]. This application scores the ability to cope with daily difficulties/problems. We used a short scale of six items with a Likert answer of 7 points ranging from "completely disagree" (1, low resiliency) to "completely agree" (7, high resiliency). Some items in the scale were "In any situation, I can be efficient" and "When I believe in myself, I can go through difficult times".

Life Satisfaction scale [33], Spanish pregnancy version [34]. This application scores subjective satisfaction with your own life. The scale has five items with a Likert answer of 5 points ranging from "completely disagree" (1, low life satisfaction) to "completely agree" (7, high life satisfaction). Some items in the scale were "In general, my real life is close to my ideal life" or "If I were born again, I don't think I'd change anything in my life".

Life–work conflicts scale. It is an ad-hoc scale, which was elaborated according to the phases for the construction of psychological scales [27] and was previously used by our research group [28]. This application scores the association between work and family life difficulties. It is a scale with six items with a Likert answer of 4 points ranging from "never" (0, minimum conflicts) to "always" (3, maximum conflicts). Some items were "I am irritable at home because my work is exhausting" and "I have to cancel plans with my partner/family/friends due to work commitments".

The points of data collection and reliability of psychological applications are summarized in Table 1.

Table 1. Timing for data collection and reliability of the psychological application.

	Cronbach's α	1T	2T	3T
Maternal and neonatal data	-	X	X	X
Maternal plasma variables	-	X		
Maternal psychological variables				
Negative affect	0.80	X	X	X
Positive affect	0.73	X	X	X
Anxiety	0.84	X	X	X
Pregnancy concerns	0.82	X	X	X
Optimism	0.66	X		X
Resilience	0.66	X		X
Life satisfaction	0.87		X	X
Life–work conflicts	0.88		X	

First trimester (1T), second trimester (2T) and third trimester (3T) of pregnancy. Cronbach's α was used to assess the reliability of psychological applications in this study.

2.5. Statistical Analysis

Statistical analysis was performed using R software (version 3.6.0, R Core Team, 2018, Vienna; Austria) within R Studio interface, using MASS, pscl, oddsratio, ggplot2, ggpubr and cowplot packages. Continuous variables were expressed as median and interquartile range (IQR) and qualitative variables as relative frequency. The univariate analysis for the maternal characteristics, plasma and psychological variables were compared using the Mann–Whitney test. The correlation between hormonal levels and psychological factors was analyzed by the rho-Spearmen test. The association between quantitative variables was assessed by the Chi-squared test. Those variables that showed a p-value < 0.10 in the univariate analysis were considered as modulatory variables in the regression models. This criterion was proved as the most parsimonious analysis in the models [35].

Regression models were created through stepwise procedures to estimate the major contribution of maternal/neonatal characteristics, maternal plasma and psychological variables to maternal and fetal complications. We conducted a stepwise analysis of potential confounders in five sequential categories: (1) maternal characteristics: maternal age, gestational age, twin gestation, ART, infant sex, FGR and preterm labor; (2) maternal plasma variables at first trimester: melatonin and cortisol; (3) psychological variables at first trimester; (4) psychological variables at second trimester; and (5) psychological variables at third trimester. The regression models show adjusted odds ratios (OR) with 95% of confidence interval (CI) and determination coefficients (R^2). In the regression models, the collinearity variables were discharged. The p-value < 0.05 was considered significant. In addition, p-value < 0.10 was reported as a quasi-significant trend.

3. Results

The prevalence of maternal complications in the cohort was 46.2% (84/182) and the prevalence of fetal complications was 25.0% (45/182). There was no statistical association between maternal and fetal complications (χ^2 = 0.759; p-value = 0.38).

3.1. Maternal Characteristics and Development of Obstetric Complications

Overall, 67.5% (123/182) of the women in the study had graduate degree, being the rest undergraduate degree. There were no women with less than an undergraduate education. Overall, 67.0% (122/182) had a partner; and the partner was employed for 95.1% (116/122). Overall, 86.2% (157/182) of the women were employed during the study period. Regarding the economic level of the family core, 74.1% (135/182) of the cohort earned more than 2000 euros/month.

We did not find statistical differences in any of the socioeconomic parameters analyzed (civil status, educational level, economic status and alcohol or tobacco consumption) between women with and without maternal complications. No differences were found in relation to either infant sex or maternal age. The group of women with maternal complications showed a significantly lower gestational age and higher use of ART, twin pregnancies and preterm labor, compared to women without maternal complications (Table 2).

Table 2. Maternal characteristics according to maternal and fetal complications.

	Maternal Complications			Fetal Complications		
	No (n = 98)	Yes (n = 84)	p-Value	No (n = 125)	Yes (n = 45)	p-Value
Maternal age (years)	35.0 (6.0)	35.0 (7.0)	0.51	34.0 (6.0)	35.0 (5.0)	0.039
Civil status						
Single	26.6% (21)	26.7% (24)	0.40	28.3% (33)	27.5% (11)	0.87
Married	73.4% (58)	71.1% (64)		71.8% (84)	72.5% (29)	
Educational level						
Undergraduate	21.0% (17)	34.5% (32)	0.49	27.3% (33)	29.2% (12)	0.77
Graduate	77.7% (63)	64.5% (60)		71.1% (86)	70.7% (29)	
Employment situation						
Working	93.8% (76)	87.1% (81)	0.16	91.7% (111)	85.4% (35)	0.25
Unemployment	6.2% (5)	9.7% (9)		5.7% (7)	14.6% (6)	
Smoking habits	14.8% (12)	17.2% (16)	0.61	14.0% (17)	19.5% (8)	0.35
Alcohol intake	42.0% (34)	39.1% (36)	0.70	38.3% (46)	48.8% (20)	0.24
Gestational age (weeks)	38.0 (3.0)	37.5 (2.0)	0.006	38.0 (2.4)	35.8 (2.5)	0.001
Twin pregnancies	38.1% (37)	67.5% (56)	0.001	41.9% (52)	80.0% (36)	0.001
ART	25.5% (25)	49.4% (41)	0.001	28.0% (35)	60.0% (27)	0.001
Male [1]	52.3% (46)	60.8% (48)	0.27	57.6% (68)	51.3% (20)	0.49
Male [2]	41.9% (13)	52.9% (27)	0.33	54.2% (26)	42.9% (12)	0.34
Preterm labor	17% (16)	32.9% (26)	0.015	0% (0)	52.4% (22)	0.001
Fetal growth restriction	4.3% (4)	12.2% (9)	0.060	0% (0)	33.3% (15)	0.001

Data show median and interquartile range (IQR) in quantitative variables and relative frequency (n) in qualitative variables. [1] Sex in single and first newborn in twin pregnancies. [2] Sex of the second newborn in twin pregnancies. Assisted reproduction techniques (ART). The p-value was obtained by Mann–Whitney U and Chi-squared tests, for quantitative or qualitative variables, respectively.

Regarding differences between women who developed or not fetal complications, no statistical differences were found in socioeconomic parameters or infant sex. However, women with fetal complications had significantly higher age, use of ART, twin pregnancies, preterm labor and FGR, compared to women without fetal complications (Table 2).

In our cohort, ART and twin pregnancy were significantly associated (χ^2 = 79.512; p-value = 0.001), as well as preterm labor and FGR (χ^2 = 4.391; p-value = 0.036). Based on these collinearities, the variables twin pregnancy and preterm labor were included in the logistic regression models.

3.2. Maternal Plasma Variables in the First Trimester

In pregnancies without any obstetric adverse outcome, plasma melatonin levels were 16.0 (27.3) pg/mL. Melatonin levels tended to be lower in women who developed a maternal complication compared to those who did not develop a maternal complication, it but did not reach statistical significance (*p*-value = 0.09; Figure 2A). Melatonin levels were not significantly different between women with and without fetal complications (Figure 2B).

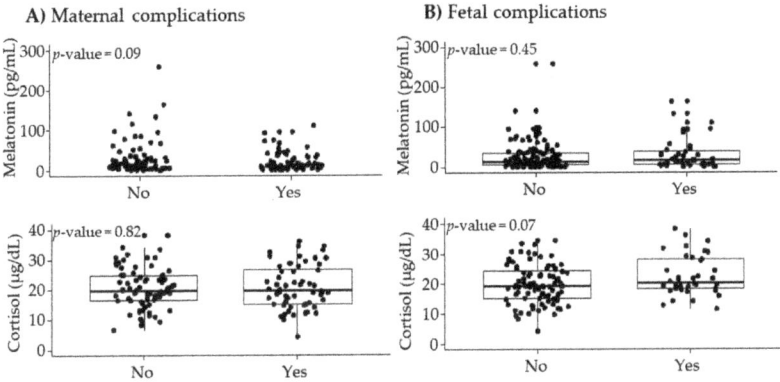

Figure 2. Maternal plasma melatonin and cortisol levels according to maternal (**A**) and fetal (**B**) complications. Data show median and interquartile range (IQR). The *p*-value was obtained by Mann–Whitney U test.

In pregnancies without any obstetric adverse outcomes, plasma cortisol levels were 19.2 (8.7) μg/dL. Cortisol levels did not show statistical differences between women with and without maternal complications (Figure 2A). Cortisol tended to be higher in the group who developed fetal complications but did not reach statistical significance (*p*-value = 0.07) (Figure 2B).

3.3. Psychological Variables during Pregnancy

Psychological variables were reported according to the gestational trimester. Table 3 shows the scores of the study groups and mothers without any obstetric adverse outcome (maternal or fetal complications).

Regarding maternal complications, in the first trimester, we did not detect statistical differences between groups in any of the parameters evaluated. In the second trimester, women who developed maternal complications showed significantly lower scores in life satisfaction compared to those without maternal complications. In the third trimester, the group of maternal complications scored statistically lower in both life satisfaction and resilience than women without maternal complications (Table 3).

Regarding the group of fetal complications, in the first trimester, women with fetal complications showed a significantly higher score in anxiety compared to women without fetal complications. In the second and third trimesters, no statistical differences in the psychological variables were detected between mothers with and without fetal complications (Table 3).

Table 3. Psychological variables according to maternal (n = 84) and fetal (n = 45) complications.

	First Trimester							Second Trimester							Third Trimester					
	Ref.	Maternal Complic.			Fetal Complic.			Ref.	Maternal Complic.			Fetal Complic.			Ref.	Maternal Complic.			Fetal Complic.	
		No	Yes	p-Value	No	Yes	p-Value		No	Yes	p-Value	No	Yes	p-Value		No	Yes	p-Value	No	Yes	p-Value
Negative affect	1.7 (0.7)	1.8 (0.8)	2.0 (1.0)	0.16	1.8 (0.8)	2.1 (0.7)	0.13	1.7 (0.8)	1.8 (0.8)	2.0 (0.7)	0.054	1.8 (0.9)	2.0 (0.8)	0.12	1.9 (1.1)	1.9 (1.1)	2.1 (1.0)	0.15	2.0 (0.9)	2.1 (1.1)	0.49
Positive affect	3.4 (0.7)	3.4 (0.7)	3.3 (0.8)	0.76	3.3 (0.8)	3.3 (0.9)	0.63	3.5 (0.8)	3.4 (0.8)	3.4 (0.8)	0.80	3.4 (0.7)	3.2 (0.7)	0.056	3.6 (0.7)	3.5 (0.7)	3.5 (0.8)	0.36	3.5 (0.8)	3.5 (0.7)	0.81
Anxiety	0.9 (0.6)	0.9 (0.7)	0.9 (0.7)	0.90	0.9 (0.6)	1.1 (0.7)	0.041	1.0 (0.9)	1.0 (0.9)	1.0 (0.9)	0.62	1.0 (0.7)	1.1 (1.1)	0.18	0.9 (0.7)	1.0 (0.7)	1.1 (1.0)	0.14	1.0 (0.9)	1.1 (1.0)	0.36
Pregnancy concerns	1.6 (0.1)	1.6 (0.7)	1.7 (0.7)	0.96	1.7 (0.8)	1.6 (0.7)	0.52	1.8 (0.1)	1.8 (0.9)	1.8 (0.8)	0.68	1.7 (0.8)	1.9 (0.8)	0.78	1.9 (0.1)	1.9 (0.7)	1.8 (0.8)	0.063	1.9 (0.8)	1.8 (0.8)	0.83
Optimism	3.4 (0.9)	3.4 (1.4)	3.2 (1.2)	0.28	3.2 (1.2)	3.6 (1.4)	0.28	-	-	-	-	-	-	-	3.4 (0.9)	3.4 (0.9)	3.2 (1.0)	0.49	3.2 (0.8)	3.5 (1.0)	0.17
Resilience	6.0 (0.1)	6.2 (0.7)	6.0 (1.0)	0.20	6.0 (0.8)	6.2 (0.7)	0.35	-	-	-	-	-	-	-	3.0 (0.1)	6.0 (0.9)	5.3 (1.8)	0.001	5.7 (1.2)	5.7 (1.5)	0.47
Life satisfaction	-	-	-	-	-	-	-	5.8 (0.9)	5.8 (0.9)	5.5 (1.0)	0.015	5.8 (1.1)	5.6 (1.2)	0.59	5.8 (0.8)	5.8 (1.0)	5.4 (1.2)	0.010	5.8 (1.0)	5.6 (1.8)	0.61
Life–work conflicts	-	-	-	-	-	-	-	0.8 (0.1)	0.8 (1.0)	1.0 (1.3)	0.70	0.8 (1.2)	1.2 (1.2)	0.061	-	-	-	-	-	-	-

Data show median and interquartile range (IQR). Reference data (Ref.) show the psychological score in our cohort in pregnancies without any obstetric adverse outcomes (n = 72). Complications (complic.). The p-value was obtained by Mann–Whitney U test.

In the cohort (n = 182), we found in the first trimester a significant and positive correlation between resilience and melatonin levels (rho = 0.18; p-value = 0.021). Although without significant differences, in the second trimester, we found a negative correlation among negative affect (rho = -0.15; p-value = 0.09), pregnancy concerns (rho = -0.15; p-value = 0.07) and melatonin levels. Furthermore, in pregnant women with maternal and fetal complications, we found in the second trimester a significant and positive correlation between positive affect and melatonin levels (rho = 0.55; p-value = 0.033). However, we did not find a statistical correlation between cortisol levels and any of the psychological scores.

Since a high proportion of women in the study had pregnancies derived from ART (n = 66), we also analyzed differences in psychological variables according to use of ART. In the first trimester, ART had significantly higher scores of negative affect (ART = 2.1 (1.0); non-ART = 1.7 (0.8), p-value = 0.026) and anxiety (ART = 1.1 (0.6); non-ART = 0.7 (0.4), p-value = 0.006). In the third trimester, ART also had significantly higher scores of negative affect (ART = 2.3 (1.1); non-ART = 2.0 (1.0), p-value = 0.010) and anxiety (ART = 1.3 (0.8), non-ART = 1.0 (0.7), p-value = 0.007). Furthermore, ART had significantly lower scores of positive affect (ART = 3.4 (0.7); non-ART = 3.5 (0.8), p-value = 0.033) and life satisfaction (ART = 5.4 (1.6); non-ART = 5.8 (1.0), p-value = 0.017).

3.4. Logistic Regression Models Associated with Maternal and Fetal Complications

The models showed that maternal complications were associated with preterm labor, indicating that maternal complications are a risk factor for prematurity. Data also evidence that melatonin levels in the first trimester and the psychological variable "life satisfaction" in the third trimester were negatively associated with maternal complications and, therefore, could be considered protective factors (Figure 3A).

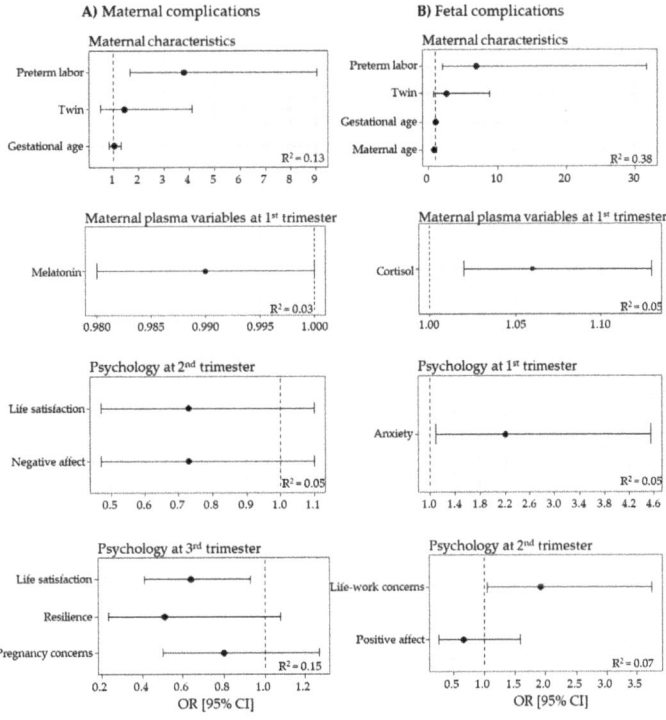

Figure 3. Logistic regression models, obtained by stepwise procedures, for maternal (**A**) and fetal (**B**) complications. Data show odds ratio (OR) [95% confidence interval (CI)] and determination coefficients (R^2).

In the models of fetal complications, preterm labor was a risk factor associated with fetal complications. Other risk factors for fetal complications were maternal cor-tisol levels and anxiety in the first trimester, and life–work concerns in the second tri-mester (Figure 3B).

4. Discussion

The objective of this study was to identify biopsychosocial risk and protective factors associated with the development of adverse obstetric outcomes. Our data show that maternal psychological features exert an influence on pregnancy outcomes; in particular, high scores in life satisfaction could be a protective factor to prevent maternal complications, while anxiety and life–work conflicts may be risk factors of fetal complications. The present study also points out the relationship between maternal melatonin and cortisol levels in early pregnancy and obstetric outcomes. We explored the association between maternal psychological parameters and these plasma hormones. Although we did not find a significant correlation with cortisol, we found some associations between psychological variables and melatonin. Melatonin levels were positively associated with resilience in the first trimester and with positive affect in the second trimester, while a negative association was found with pregnancy concerns. In summary, our data reveal the relationship between social, psychological and biological spheres, which can exert an influence on pregnancy outcomes. Our data point out the need to study pregnancy from a more global biopsychosocial approach.

Pregnancy complications are increasing in our society due to several factors and represent an important health problem. Thus far, they have been studied mainly from a clinical point of view. The incorporation of the psychological and social domain into clinical practice may help to understand their origin and to improve healthcare. The relevance of considering multiple spheres to predict the clinical outcomes has been demonstrated in perinatology [36]. In this work, we considered this global approach, analyzing the social, psychological and biological spheres. These different aspects are discussed below.

Social factors. Regarding the social sphere, poverty and racial disparities have usually been explored as key determinants of health. In the studied population, these factors do not seem to play an important influence on the obstetric and neonatal outcome, since the population studied is of middle-high socioeconomic level. A relevant characteristic in our population was the age, which was above the optimum for maternity. This fact reflects a key aspect in high-income countries: the delay in the maternity age. In our social context, there has been a gradual access of the women to higher education and employment, as well as in pregnancy control [37]. These sociocultural determinants may be some of the factors implicated in the continuing rise in the age of childbearing observed from the second half of the twentieth century [38]. High-income countries enacted comprehensive maternity legislation providing women with rights, such as a period of employment protection for childbirth [39]. Legislation can help solving the problem of work–family conflicts; however, delayed maternity age and its impact on women's health remains a problem. In fact, in our population, we found that maternity age was associated with adverse fetal outcomes.

The association between advanced maternity age and adverse outcome may have biological grounds. On the one hand, it is linked to infertility. ART has made possible maternity beyond biological limits. However, the main consequence is an increased rate of twin pregnancies, which are a risk factor for obstetric complications, particularly preterm labor [38,40]. This was confirmed in the present study, evidencing that twin pregnancies were nearly seven times more likely to develop a complication compared to singletons. It is important to note that obstetric adverse outcomes are not a direct effect of ART, but rather of the fact that the use of ART is associated with twin pregnancies. In fact, it has been found that the rate of obstetric complications in twin pregnancies derived from ART is not higher than in spontaneous twin pregnancies, even at 45 years old [41]. In addition, an important aspect to explore would be the relationship of particular ART techniques and obstetrical outcomes, which we did not collect it.

In addition to the biological influence on pregnancy outcome, psychological factors were considered. Getting pregnant at an advanced age, the process of repetitive ART cycles and a multiple pregnancy represent important stress factors for the mother, which may exert negative influences. Therefore, the psychological sphere should be considered.

Psychological factors. Psychological stress during pregnancy affects the maternal–fetal binomial health and is known to have effects on pregnancy hypertension, fetal programming and gestational timing [42]. According to the literature, pregnancy is a period of significant life change for a woman and her partner, and it can be perceived as a stressful situation. Research has found that negative life events were associated with an increased risk of fetal complications and emotional distress in the mother [43]. Our data support that pregnant women with high negative affect scores are associated with maternal and fetal complications. In the same line, other studies have found that psychological optimism, pessimism or anxiety are associated with birth outcomes [44]. Our data show that maternal anxiety in the first trimester is a risk factor for later development of fetal complications.

Pregnancy represents a challenge, and, for many women, it may be a stressful period, particularly if there are insufficient psychosocial resources or additional stressors. One of them is the use of ART, which implies a high level of uncertainty. We therefore explored the possible influence on psychological factors and pregnancy outcomes. As expected, we found higher scores of negative affect and anxiety and lower positive affect and life satisfaction in pregnancies derived from ART. If the response to a stressor is inadequate, it may lead to a negative influence on health. Our data show that ART-derive pregnancies were at higher risk of maternal and fetal complications. This has been proposed to be directly linked to advanced maternity age and the association with twin pregnancies; however, our data reveal high levels of anxiety, which may also contribute to the worse outcome and could be taken into consideration.

According to the Commission on the Social Determinants of Health from the World Health Organization [45], a stressful workplace is considered one of the most important psychological stressors, while stable family core and social behaviors are key positive aspects for mental health [46]. Our data support that pregnant women with maternal and fetal complications scored low in life satisfaction and high in life–work concerns. Today, health professionals should be aware of the influence of psychological processes and social behavior disadvantage on disease; in fact, sociodemographic disadvantages are also postulated as independent risk factors for adverse pregnancy outcomes [47].

It is important to note that the psychological scores in the second and third trimesters may be biased because pregnancy problems have already been diagnosed and maternal behaviors could be affected.

Biological factors. Pregnancy is a period of biological changes, which interacts with the psychological sphere. A stressful job, the problems associated with the pressure of getting pregnant at an advanced age, the use of ART and twin pregnancies are important psychological factors which may influence the biological domain [43]. Even though the biological milieu has been thoroughly studied in relation to obstetric complications, the relationship between psychological and biological spheres has not been fully addressed before. In our study, we assessed two key hormones, melatonin and cortisol, since they are relevant in pregnancy and have been previously shown to be affected by psychological conditions.

Melatonin has been associated with the psychological alterations, and it has been proposed that low levels of this hormone may underlie the pathophysiology of depression and other mood disorders, which are also relatively frequent the context of pregnancy. In addition, this hormone is relevant in the maintenance of a normal pregnancy. Therefore, we hypothesized that melatonin could be a keystone between psychological processes and pregnancy disorders. Our data show a negative correlation between melatonin levels and pregnancy concerns. In addition, we demonstrated that women with maternal complications tended to have lower melatonin levels. This association may be related to poorer antioxidant defenses, since oxidative stress is a key mechanism in pregnancy complications [48] and the role of melatonin as protective hormone in pregnancy is related to its powerful antioxidant actions [14]. In fact, previous data of our group demonstrate that low plasma melatonin was associated with low levels of antioxidants and development of maternal complications [3] and with preterm delivery in twin gestation [15]. We suggest that low melatonin can contribute to a poor antioxidant balance in early pregnancy and participate in pregnancy complications later on. Melatonin is a hormone with a circadian rhythm and its highest levels occur during sleep. Therefore, the reasons for low melatonin levels can be directly related to sleep deficiency. Sleep disturbances can be linked to psychological factors. For example, it has been shown that life–work conflicts and pregnancy concerns are key factors influencing sleep [48]. According to our data, pregnancy concerns tended to be increased in women with maternal complications. Therefore, it is possible that the association between low melatonin and poor pregnancy outcome could be partially related to a reduction of the number of sleep hours. Additionally, the effects of job-related stressors on work–family conflict are most often viewed from the perspective of conservation of resources theory [49]. According to the theory, individuals have a finite amount of time, attention and energy, and, therefore, higher time commitment or demand from one role puts pressure on other roles [50,51]. We analyzed the possible relationship between melatonin and resilience in the first trimester and found a positive association. We propose that melatonin can be a hormone affected by psychological variables, being associated with positive and negative mood in pregnancy. This hypothesis needs to be studied further since the present work had some limitations, such as assessing melatonin at daytime and at a single and point. It would be desirable to analyze also night levels along pregnancy, together with evaluation of sleep quality and psychological variables.

Cortisol is a hormone with multiple physiological roles and well known to be secreted in stressful situations. In pregnancy, maternal cortisol passage to the fetus is limited by the placental barrier 11β-dehydrogenase enzyme (11β-HSD-2), which transforms cortisol into cortisone, an inactive glucocorticoid [52,53]. It has been demonstrated that 11β-HSD-2 is inhibited as a consequence of maternal psychological stress, affecting fetal growth [54,55]. There is also evidence that pregnant women who had anxiety showed a reduction of uterine blood flow [56] which is related to FGR. These studies are in accordance with our data showing high anxiety scores in women who developed fetal complications together with a trend towards high levels of cortisol in the first trimester. Our data add evidence to the link between maternal stress during early pregnancy and adverse maternal-fetal outcome, through alterations in the hormonal milieu. However, although we analyzed the possible association between cortisol levels and the psychological variables, such as anxiety, we did not find any potential relationship. Our study had some limitations regarding cortisol measurements, which could account for this. Firstly, the assessment at a single time point in the morning; evaluation of the hormone at different time points would have been more informative, allowing analyzing other parameters such as the diurnal cortisol slope and cumulative cortisol output across the day. It is also possible that venipuncture could have caused additional stress and cortisol release; this effect has been mainly observed in children related to fear of pain and is likely minimized in our population of adults with a programmed intervention. Cortisol measurements in saliva could avoid this possible problem.

Strengths and Limitations

The main strength of this study was the longitudinal approach in the psychological variables. This condition adds power to the design compared to cross-sectional studies, by virtue of observing the temporal order of events. The second strength of the study was the exploration of multiple spheres in the pregnancy context. The new methodological approaches to research in human biomedicine must consider the biological, psychological and social points of view. Thirdly, the logistic regression models with the stepwise method allow estimating the contribution of biological, psychological and social areas sequentially.

Regarding limitations, the first is the assessment of the biochemical variables only at a one-time point since cortisol and melatonin exhibit circadian rhythms. This was due to ethical limitations, which restricted the blood collection only in the morning and in the first trimester, coincident with a routine analysis. Although blood samples were extracted in the same conditions and the levels were determinate under the same protocols for all women, this aspect needs to be taken into account in future studies. The second limitation is the sample size, which is smaller in the third trimester than in the first one, related to prematurity, stillbirths or loss to follow-up, resulting in fewer women completing the psychological applications at the end of pregnancy. It would also be desirable to have a more heterogeneous population reflecting other social environments, since the present sample is homogeneous in terms of age, education and income. Thirdly, the analysis of the biological markers at different time points along gestation, and the inclusion of other molecules such as inflammatory mediators, oxidative stress markers or placental and vascular growth factors, known to be related to pregnancy disorders would help to complete the relationship between biological and psychological variables and their role in pregnancy outcomes.

In addition, it would be necessary to carry out new studies to check whether the results are maintained in other cohorts with another methodologies (i.e., Monte Carlo simulation analysis). However, the key element is to start from a theoretical model that justifies the analyses performed, not only focus on the method [57]. Gaining knowledge on factors from these three spheres would help building up the biopsychosocial model of pregnancy, which would aid maternal counseling to improve pregnancy outcomes.

5. Conclusions

In this work, using logistic regression models, we detected a relationship between some maternal psychological and biological factors (melatonin and cortisol) and the development of complications.

To help preventing maternal complications, high melatonin levels at the beginning of gestation and life satisfaction in mid-pregnancy could be protective factors. Our results also suggest that low anxiety and cortisol levels at the beginning of pregnancy and reducing problems of work–life conciliation could help prevent fetal complications. Considering these data, it may be interesting to promote health public guidelines to support resources, which will improve life satisfaction and life–work conciliation during pregnancy. In addition, to know the social-reality of each pregnant women, intervening from primary care to specialized clinical psychology would help humanize pregnancy. These policies contribute to the decline in the rate of adverse obstetric outcomes with a direct impact on the healthcare cost, particularly in societies with advanced maternity age.

Author Contributions: Conceptualization, B.M.-J., S.M.A. and E.G.; methodology, B.M.-J. and E.G.; software, D.R.-C. and E.G.; validation, B.M.-J., S.M.A. and E.G.; formal analysis, D.R.-C. and E.G.; investigation, D.R.-C., M.d.l.C., V.B. and A.G.-D.; data curation, D.R.-C. and A.G.-D.; writing—original draft preparation, D.R.-C., M.d.l.C., V.B. and A.G.-D.; writing—review and editing, B.M.-J., S.M.A. and E.G.; and supervision, S.M.A. and E.G. All authors have read and agreed to the published version of the manuscript.

Funding: This research received no external funding.

Institutional Review Board Statement: The study was conducted according to the guidelines of the Declaration of Helsinki, and approved by the Human Research Ethical Committee of Hospital Universitario La Paz and Institutional Review Board of Universidad Autónoma de Madrid (protocol code PI-1490 and CEMU/2013-10, respectively; October 2013).

Informed Consent Statement: Informed consent was obtained from all subjects involved in the study.

Data Availability Statement: The raw datasets used for this study contained health personal information and the Ethical Committee requirements has forbidden the data transfer. However, a particular report could be sent to the corresponding authors by email.

Acknowledgments: The authors would to thank all study pregnant and nursing research staff.

Conflicts of Interest: The authors declare no conflict of interest.

References

1. Varea, C.; Teran, J.M.; Bernis, C.; Bogin, B. The impact of delayed maternity on foetal growth in Spain: An assessment by population attributable fraction. *Women Birth* **2018**, *31*, e190–e196. [CrossRef]
2. Nicoloro-SantaBarbara, J.M.; Lobel, M.; Bocca, S.; Stelling, J.R.; Pastore, L.M. Psychological and emotional concomitants of infertility diagnosis in women with diminished ovarian reserve or anatomical cause of infertility. *Fertil. Steril.* **2017**, *108*, 161–167. [CrossRef] [PubMed]
3. Ramiro-Cortijo, D.; Herrera, T.; Rodriguez-Rodriguez, P.; Lopez De Pablo, A.L.; De La Calle, M.; Lopez-Gimenez, M.R.; Mora-Urda, A.I.; Gutierrez-Arzapalo, P.Y.; Gomez-Rioja, R.; Aguilera, Y.; et al. Maternal plasma antioxidant status in the first trimester of pregnancy and development of obstetric complications. *Placenta* **2016**, *47*, 37–45. [CrossRef]
4. Cheong-See, F.; Schuit, E.; Arroyo-Manzano, D.; Khalil, A.; Barrett, J.; Joseph, K.S.; Asztalos, E.; Hack, K.; Lewi, L.; Lim, A.; et al. Prospective risk of stillbirth and neonatal complications in twin pregnancies: Systematic review and meta-analysis. *BMJ* **2016**, *354*, i4353. [CrossRef]
5. APA. Pregnancy Statistics. Available online: https://americanpregnancy.org/ (accessed on 20 March 2019).
6. Edozien, L.C. Beyond biology: The biopsychosocial model and its application in obstetrics and gynaecology. *BJOG* **2015**, *122*, 900–903. [CrossRef]
7. Ng, D.M.; Jeffery, R.W. Relationships between perceived stress and health behaviors in a sample of working adults. *Health Psychol.* **2003**, *22*, 638–642. [CrossRef] [PubMed]
8. Nicoloro-SantaBarbara, J.; Busso, C.; Moyer, A.; Lobel, M. Just relax and you'll get pregnant? Meta-analysis examining women's emotional distress and the outcome of assisted reproductive technology. *Soc. Sci. Med.* **2018**, *213*, 54–62. [CrossRef]
9. Robakis, T.K.; Williams, K.E.; Crowe, S.; Kenna, H.; Gannon, J.; Rasgon, N.L. Optimistic outlook regarding maternity protects against depressive symptoms postpartum. *Arch Womens Ment. Health* **2015**, *18*, 197–208. [CrossRef]
10. Hermes, M.; Antonow-Schlorke, I.; Hollstein, D.; Kuehnel, S.; Rakers, F.; Frauendorf, V.; Dreiling, M.; Rupprecht, S.; Schubert, H.; Witte, O.W.; et al. Maternal psychosocial stress during early gestation impairs fetal structural brain development in sheep. *Stress* **2020**, *23*, 233–242. [CrossRef]
11. Claustrat, B.; Brun, J.; Chazot, G. The basic physiology and pathophysiology of melatonin. *Sleep Med. Rev.* **2005**, *9*, 11–24. [CrossRef] [PubMed]
12. Soliman, A.; Lacasse, A.A.; Lanoix, D.; Sagrillo-Fagundes, L.; Boulard, V.; Vaillancourt, C. Placental melatonin system is present throughout pregnancy and regulates villous trophoblast differentiation. *J. Pineal Res.* **2015**, *59*, 38–46. [CrossRef]
13. Gomes, P.R.L.; Motta-Teixeira, L.C.; Gallo, C.C.; Carmo Buonfiglio, D.D.; Camargo, L.S.; Quintela, T.; Reiter, R.J.; Amaral, F.G.D.; Cipolla-Neto, J. Maternal pineal melatonin in gestation and lactation physiology, and in fetal development and programming. *Gen. Comp. Endocrinol.* **2020**, *300*, 113633. [CrossRef]
14. Reiter, R.J.; Tamura, H.; Tan, D.X.; Xu, X.Y. Melatonin and the circadian system: Contributions to successful female reproduction. *Fertil. Steril.* **2014**, *102*, 321–328. [CrossRef]
15. Ramiro-Cortijo, D.; Calle, M.; Rodriguez-Rodriguez, P.; Pablo, A.L.L.; Lopez-Gimenez, M.R.; Aguilera, Y.; Martin-Cabrejas, M.A.; Gonzalez, M.D.C.; Arribas, S.M. Maternal Antioxidant Status in Early Pregnancy and Development of Fetal Complications in Twin Pregnancies: A Pilot Study. *Antioxidants (Basel)* **2020**, *9*, 269. [CrossRef]
16. Sundberg, I.; Rasmusson, A.J.; Ramklint, M.; Just, D.; Ekselius, L.; Cunningham, J.L. Daytime melatonin levels in saliva are associated with inflammatory markers and anxiety disorders. *Psychoneuroendocrinology* **2020**, *112*, 104514. [CrossRef]
17. Abbott, S.M. Non-24-hour Sleep-Wake Rhythm Disorder. *Neurol. Clin.* **2019**, *37*, 545–552. [CrossRef]
18. Quax, R.A.; Manenschijn, L.; Koper, J.W.; Hazes, J.M.; Lamberts, S.W.; van Rossum, E.F.; Feelders, R.A. Glucocorticoid sensitivity in health and disease. *Nat. Rev. Endocrinol.* **2013**, *9*, 670–686. [CrossRef]
19. Shelton, M.M.; Schminkey, D.L.; Groer, M.W. Relationships among prenatal depression, plasma cortisol, and inflammatory cytokines. *Biol. Res. Nurs.* **2015**, *17*, 295–302. [CrossRef]
20. Sarkar, P.; Bergman, K.; O.'Connor, T.G.; Glover, V. Maternal antenatal anxiety and amniotic fluid cortisol and testosterone: Possible implications for foetal programming. *J. Neuroendocr.* **2008**, *20*, 489–496. [CrossRef]
21. Bleker, L.S.; Roseboom, T.J.; Vrijkotte, T.G.; Reynolds, R.M.; de Rooij, S.R. Determinants of cortisol during pregnancy—The ABCD cohort. *Psychoneuroendocrinology* **2017**, *83*, 172–181. [CrossRef]
22. Aguilera, Y.; Rebollo-Hernanz, M.; Herrera, T.; Cayuelas, L.T.; Rodriguez-Rodriguez, P.; de Pablo, A.L.; Arribas, S.M.; Martin-Cabrejas, M.A. Intake of bean sprouts influences melatonin and antioxidant capacity biomarker levels in rats. *Food Funct.* **2016**, *7*, 1438–1445. [CrossRef]
23. Watson, D.; Clark, L.A.; Tellegen, A. Development and validation of brief measures of positive and negative affect: The PANAS scales. *J. Pers. Soc. Psychol.* **1988**, *54*, 1063–1070. [CrossRef]
24. Moriondo, M.; Palma, P.; Medrano, L.A.; Murillo, P. Adaptación de la Escala de Afectividad Positiva y Negativa (PANAS) a la población de Adultos de la ciudad de Córdoba. *Univ. Psychol.* **2012**, *11*, 187–196. [CrossRef]
25. Zigmond, A.S.; Snaith, R.P. The hospital anxiety and depression scale. *Acta Psychiatr. Scand.* **1983**, *67*, 361–370. [CrossRef]
26. Lopez-Roig, S.; Terol, C.M.; Pastor, M.A. Ansiedad y depresión. Validación de la Escala HAD en pacientes oncológicos. *Rev. Psicol. Salud.* **2000**, *12*, 127–155.
27. Fernández, J.M.; Pedrero, E.F. Diez pasos para la construcción de un test. *Psicothema* **2019**, *31*, 7–16.

28. Ramiro-Cortijo, D.; de la Calle, M.; Gila-Diaz, A.; Moreno-Jimenez, B.; Martin-Cabrejas, M.A.; Arribas, S.M.; Garrosa, E. Maternal Resources, Pregnancy Concerns, and Biological Factors Associated to Birth Weight and Psychological Health. *J. Clin. Med.* **2021**, *10*, 695. [CrossRef] [PubMed]
29. Scheier, M.F.; Carver, C.S.; Bridges, M.W. Distinguishing optimism from neuroticism (and trait anxiety, self-mastery, and self-esteem): A reevaluation of the Life Orientation Test. *J. Pers. Soc. Psychol.* **1994**, *67*, 1063–1078. [CrossRef] [PubMed]
30. Ferrando, P.J.; Chico, E.; Tous, J.M. Propiedades psicométricas del test de optimismo Life Orientation Test. *Psicothema* **2002**, *14*, 673–680.
31. Wagnild, G.M.; Young, H.M. Development and psychometric evaluation of the Resilience Scale. *J. Nurs. Meas.* **1993**, *1*, 165–178.
32. Rodriguez, M.; Pereyra, M.G.; Gil, E.; Jofre, M.; De Bortoli, M.; Labiano, L.M. Propiedades psicométricas de la escala de resiliencia versión argentina. *Rev. Evaluar.* **2009**, *9*, 72–82.
33. Diener, E.; Emmons, R.A.; Larsen, R.J.; Griffin, S. The Satisfaction with Life Scale. *J. Pers. Assess.* **1985**, *49*, 71–75. [CrossRef]
34. Cabañero Martínez, M.J.; Richart Martínez, M.R.; Cabrero García, J.; Orts Cortés, M.I.; Reig Ferrer, A.; Tosal Herrero, B. Fiabilidad y validez de la Escala de Satisfacción con la Vida de Diener en una muestra de mujeres embarazadas y puérperas. *Psicothema* **2004**, *16*, 448–455.
35. Konnikova, Y.; Zaman, M.M.; Makda, M.; D'Onofrio, D.; Freedman, S.D.; Martin, C.R. Late Enteral Feedings Are Associated with Intestinal Inflammation and Adverse Neonatal Outcomes. *PLoS ONE* **2015**, *10*, e0132924. [CrossRef] [PubMed]
36. Jackson, W.M.; O'Shea, T.M.; Allred, E.N.; Laughon, M.M.; Gower, W.A.; Leviton, A. Risk factors for chronic lung disease and asthma differ among children born extremely preterm. *Pediatr. Pulmonol.* **2018**, *53*, 1533–1540. [CrossRef]
37. Ramiro-Cortijo, D.; Rodríguez-Rodríguez, P.; Lopez De Pablo, Á.L.; López-Giménez, M.R.; González, M.C.; Arribas, S.M. Fetal undernutrition and oxidative stress: Influence of sex and gender. In *Handbook of Famine, Starvation and Nutrient Deprivation: From Biology to Policy*; Preedy, V.R., Patel, V.B., Eds.; Springer International Publishing: Springer Nature Switzerland AG: London, UK, 2019; pp. 1–19.
38. Avnon, T.; Haham, A.; Many, A. Twin pregnancy in women above the age of 45 years: Maternal and neonatal outcomes. *J. Perinat. Med.* **2017**, *45*, 787–791. [CrossRef]
39. Berkman, L.F.; Soh, Y. Social Determinants of Health at Older Ages: The Long Arm of Early and Middle Adulthood. *Perspect. Biol. Med.* **2017**, *60*, 595–606. [CrossRef]
40. Okun, N.; Sierra, S.; Genetics, C.; Special, C. Pregnancy outcomes after assisted human reproduction. *J. Obstet. Gynaecol. Can.* **2014**, *36*, 64–83. [CrossRef]
41. Jauniaux, E.; Ben-Ami, I.; Maymon, R. Do assisted-reproduction twin pregnancies require additional antenatal care? *Reprod. Biomed. Online* **2013**, *26*, 107–119. [CrossRef]
42. Glover, V. Maternal depression, anxiety and stress during pregnancy and child outcome; what needs to be done. *Best Pract. Res. Clin. Obstet. Gynaecol.* **2014**, *28*, 25–35. [CrossRef]
43. Tani, F.; Castagna, V. Maternal social support, quality of birth experience, and post-partum depression in primiparous women. *J. Matern. Fetal. Neonatal. Med.* **2017**, *30*, 689–692. [CrossRef]
44. Preis, H.; Chen, R.; Eisner, M.; Pardo, J.; Peled, Y.; Wiznitzer, A.; Benyamini, Y. Testing a biopsychosocial model of the basic birth beliefs. *Birth* **2018**, *45*, 79–87. [CrossRef]
45. Sheiham, A. Closing the gap in a generation: Health equity through action on the social determinants of health. A report of the WHO Commission on Social Determinants of Health (CSDH) 2008. *Community Dent. Health* **2009**, *26*, 2–3.
46. Rowe, H. Biopsychosocial obstetrics and gynaecology—A perspective from Australia. *J. Psychosom. Obstet. Gynaecol.* **2016**, *37*, 1–5. [CrossRef]
47. Lindquist, A.; Noor, N.; Sullivan, E.; Knight, M. The impact of socioeconomic position on severe maternal morbidity outcomes among women in Australia: A national case-control study. *BJOG* **2015**, *122*, 1601–1609. [CrossRef] [PubMed]
48. Ahmad, I.M.; Zimmerman, M.C.; Moore, T.A. Oxidative stress in early pregnancy and the risk of preeclampsia. *Pregnancy Hypertens* **2019**, *18*, 99–102. [CrossRef]
49. Hobfoll, S.E. Conservation of Resources Theory: Its Implication for Stress, Health, and Resilience. In *The Oxford Handbook of Stress, Health, and Coping*; Folkman, S., Ed.; Oxford University Press: New York, NY, USA, 2011; pp. 1–38.
50. Edwards, J.R.; Rothbard, N.P. Work and family stress and well-being: An integrative model of person-environment fit within and between the work and family domains. *Organ. Behav. Hum. Decis. Process.* **2004**, *77*, 85–129. [CrossRef]
51. Ten Brummelhuis, L.L.; Bakker, A.B. A resource perspective on the work-home interface: The work-home resources model. *Am. Psychol.* **2012**, *67*, 545–556. [CrossRef]
52. Mastorakos, G.; Ilias, I. Maternal and fetal hypothalamic-pituitary-adrenal axes during pregnancy and postpartum. *Ann. N. Y. Acad. Sci.* **2003**, *997*, 136–149. [CrossRef]
53. Merlot, E.; Couret, D.; Otten, W. Prenatal stress, fetal imprinting and immunity. *Brain Behav. Immun.* **2008**, *22*, 42–51. [CrossRef]
54. Brunton, P.J. Effects of maternal exposure to social stress during pregnancy: Consequences for mother and offspring. *Reproduction* **2013**, *146*, R175–R189. [CrossRef]
55. Monk, C. Stress and mood disorders during pregnancy: Implications for child development. *Psychiatr. Q.* **2001**, *72*, 347–357. [CrossRef]

56. Littleton, H.L.; Bye, K.; Buck, K.; Amacker, A. Psychosocial stress during pregnancy and perinatal outcomes: A meta-analytic review. *J. Psychosom Obstet. Gynaecol.* **2010**, *31*, 219–228. [CrossRef]
57. Collins, C.S.; Stockton, C.M. The Central Role of Theory in Qualitative Research. *Int. J. Qual. Methods* **2018**, *17*, 1–10. [CrossRef]

MDPI
St. Alban-Anlage 66
4052 Basel
Switzerland
Tel. +41 61 683 77 34
Fax +41 61 302 89 18
www.mdpi.com

Journal of Personalized Medicine Editorial Office
E-mail: jpm@mdpi.com
www.mdpi.com/journal/jpm

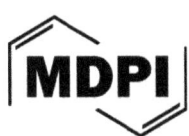

www.ingramcontent.com/pod-product-compliance
Lightning Source LLC
LaVergne TN
LVHW070500100526
838202LV00014B/1763